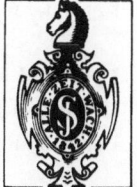

Clinical Practice in Urology
Series Editor: Geoffrey D. Chisholm

Adenocarcinoma of the Prostate

Edited by

Andrew W. Bruce and John Trachtenberg

With 37 Figures

Springer-Verlag
London Berlin Heidelberg New York
Paris Tokyo

Andrew W. Bruce, FRCS, FRCS(C)
Professor and Chairman, Division of Urology, University of
Toronto, Suite 14–205, The Eaton Wing, Toronto General Hospital,
200 Elizabeth Street, Toronto, Ontario, Canada M5G 2C4

John Trachtenberg, MD, FRCS(C)
Associate Professor, Division of Urology, University of Toronto,
Toronto General Hospital, Suite 14–209, The Eaton Wing,
200 Elizabeth Street, Toronto, Ontario, Canada M5G 9Z9; and
Career Scientist, Ministry of Health, Province of Ontario

Series Editor

Geoffrey D. Chisholm, ChM, FRCS, FRCSEd
Professor of Surgery, University of Edinburgh; and Consultant
Urological Surgeon, Western General Hospital, Edinburgh, Scotland

ISBN-13: 978-1-4471-1400-0   e-ISBN-13: 978-1-4471-1398-0
DOI: 10.1007/978-1-4471-1398-0

British Library Cataloguing in Publication Data
Adenocarcinoma of the prostate.—(Clinical practice in urology series). 1. Prostate
gland—Cancer   I. Bruce, A. W.   II. Trachtenberg, J.   III. Series   616.99′463
RC280.P7

Library of Congress Cataloging-in-Publication Data
Adenocarcinoma of the prostate.
(Clinical practice in urology)
Includes bibliographies and index.
1. Prostate gland—Cancer. 2. Adenocarcinoma. I. Bruce, A.W. (Andrew W.),
1925–   . II. Trachtenberg, J. (John), 1949–   .   III. Series. [DNLM:
1. Adenocarcinoma. 2. Prostatic Neoplasms. WJ 752 A232]   RC280.P7A34
1987   616.99′463   87–9506

© Springer-Verlag Berlin Heidelberg 1987
Softcover reprint of the hardcover 1st edition 1987

The use of registered names, trademarks etc. in this publication does not imply, even
in the absence of a specific statement, that such names are exempt from the relevant
laws and regulations and therefore free for general use.

Product Liability: The publisher can give no guarantee for information about drug
dosage and application thereof contained in this book. In every individual case the
respective user must check its accuracy by consulting other pharmaceutical literature.

Filmset by Wilmaset, Birkenhead, Merseyside
Printed by Henry Ling, The Dorset Press, Dorchester

Series Editor's Foreword

Carcinoma of the prostate increasingly dominates the attention of urologists for both scientific and clinical reasons. The search for an explanation and the prediction of the variable behaviour of the malignant prostatic cell continues unabated. The search for more precise tumour staging and more effective treatment is equally vigorous. Editors Andrew Bruce and John Trachtenberg have assembled acknowledged leaders in prostate cancer to present those areas of direct interest to the clinician. There are a number of other topics that might have been considered but most of these, such as experimental tumour models or biochemical factors affecting cell growth, still lack immediate application for the clinician.

Carcinoma of the prostate continues to have its highest incidence in the western world, and the difference in comparison with the incidence in the Far East appears to be real and not masked by diagnostic or other factors. A number of other epidemiological aspects need careful analysis: Is the incidence increasing? Is the survival improving? Is the prognosis worse in the younger patient? Epidemiological data are easily misused and misinterpreted so that a precise analysis of the known facts makes an important opening chapter to this book.

The comprehensive review of the main methods for grading prostatic cancer provides more evidence that there is, as yet, no wholly reliable method for determining the malignant potential of the cell. It is also evident that the measurement of hormone receptors, either cytosolic or nuclear, is not yet sufficiently precise for predicting tumour response. Nevertheless, the two chapters on this topic illustrate the importance of recent studies and how they have added to our understanding of morphology and function of the malignant cell.

The steady progress in more precise tumour staging is described in chapters on tumour markers and imaging and these provide up to date assessments of the methods available. The chapter on staging indicates the importance of using tried and trusted and available methods for a system to be internationally useful. The chapter on the diagnosis and significance of pelvic lymph node metastases addresses a series of important questions and gives the clinician clear answers.

Doctors Bruce and Trachtenberg have planned the chapters on management so that acknowledged leaders can present their evidence in support of their views. The controversial management of localised cancer faces the central fact that the selection of patient and of treatment must take account of a wide range of factors in order to obtain the best results in terms of cancer control and quality of life. The present status of interstitial radiotherapy and the case for external beam radiotherapy for certain tumours are given by leaders in these fields but the reader can be assured that there is more than sufficient evidence on the advantages and disadvantages of these methods to draw independent conclusions.

Recent years have witnessed a surge in developments in hormonal control and chemotherapy but the one absolute fact that can be established from these recent reports is the need for properly conducted clinical trials before any new drug or combination can be proclaimed as a breakthrough. It is therefore most appropriate that this book concludes with a chapter on clinical trials in prostatic cancer: perhaps it should have been the opening chapter, for here are spelled out the traps for the unwary in their endeavours to conquer this frustrating cancer.

Edinburgh, June 1987   Geoffrey D. Chisholm

Preface

Prostatic cancer is the most common urologic malignancy, yet it remains one of the great enigmas for the treating physician. That this disease can appear so benign in many, while so devastatingly malignant in others, is one of the mysteries of clinical medicine. The past three decades have witnessed major advances in the basic understanding of carcinogenesis, as well as exciting advances in the diagnostic and therapeutic modalities for dealing with many cancers. While much information about prostatic cancer has been gleaned in this period, it is only too frustrating to have to admit that survival of patients with this disease has not changed substantially. Thus it is not difficult to understand the prevailing undercurrent of controversy that exists in regard to the diagnosis and treatment of this neoplasm. In this book, a group of authorities in the field provide us with their experience and special expertise. The aim of the text is to highlight the areas of difficulty and for the participants to present their personal approach to each problem area.

The book is divided into two sections. The first deals with recent important advances in basic science as it relates to prostatic cancer. A fundamental view of the immense scope of this problem is presented in the introductory chapter, which explores the epidemiology of the disease. Histologic grading methods used are discussed and the variables associated with the different methods are presented. The clinical methods of staging this neoplasm are reviewed and updated, and special emphasis is given to the new advances available in imaging technology. Other chapters address the factors that should improve our ability to detect those patients at high risk of developing the disease and those patients who are likely to be treatment failures. The second section of the book deals with the specific problems of treating the patient in each stage of the disease: from small volume localized disease to disseminated hormone-resistant patterns. The authors have attempted to summarize the present controversies within their own areas of interest, to explain and support their approach to the problem, and finally to predict what research developments are likely to have an impact on disease detection and management in the future. Integration of these therapeutic concepts may yield a more favorable prognosis for our patients.

Finally, we wish to express to all our contributors our most grateful thanks for their support and patience.

Toronto   Andrew W. Bruce
March 1987   John Trachtenberg

Contents

Contributors

Malcolm Bagshaw, MD
Professor and Chairman, Department of Therapeutic Radiology,
Stanford University Medical Center, Stanford, California 94305,
USA

Peter N. Bretan, MD
Department of Urology, School of Medicine, University of California
San Francisco, San Francisco, California 94143, USA

Francisco Bretas, MD
Scott Department of Urology, Baylor College of Medicine, Houston,
Texas, USA

Andrew W. Bruce, FRCS, FRCS(C)
Professor and Chairman, Division of Urology, University of Tor-
onto, Suite 14–205, The Eaton Wing, Toronto General Hospital, 200
Elizabeth Street, Toronto M5G 2C4, Ontario, Canada

William J. Catalona, MD
Professor and Chairman, Division of Urologic Surgery, Washington
University School of Medicine, St Louis, Missouri, USA

B. K. Choe, MD
University of Illinois, Clinical Sciences Bldg. 518J, Dept. of Surgery,
P.O. Box 6998, Chicago, Illinois 60680, USA

John G. Connolly, MD
Professor, Division of Urology, University of Toronto Women's
College Hospital, 76 Grenville Street, Toronto, Ontario, Canada,
M5S 1B2

James I. Harty, FRCSI, FACS
Division of Urology, Department of Surgery, University of Louisville
School of Medicine, Louisville, Kentucky 40292, USA

Robert P. Huben, MD
Chief, Department of Urology, Roswell Park Memorial Institute,
Buffalo, New York, USA

Betty G. Mobbs, MD
Associate Professor, Department of Surgery, Room 7336, Medical
Sciences Building, University of Toronto, Toronto, Ontario, Canada
M5S 1B2

F. K. Mostofi, MD
Chairman, Department of Genitourinary Pathology, Armed Forces
Institute of Pathology, Washington DC 20306, USA

Gerald P. Murphy, MD
Chairman and Co-ordinator Urologic Co-operation Oncology Group,
Professor of Urology, Department of Urology, State University of
New York at Buffalo, 139 Parker Hall, Buffalo, New York 14214,
USA

Carl A. Olsson, MD
Professor and Chairman, Department of Urology, College of
Physicians and Surgeons of Columbia University, Director J. Bentley
Squier Urological Clinic, Presbyterian Hospital in the City of New
York, Columbia Presbyterian Medical Center, 622 West 168th Street,
New York, New York 10032, USA

Peter T. Scardino, MD
Professor of Urology, The Scott Department of Urology, Baylor
College of Medicine, Suite 1003, 6560 Fannin Street, Houston, Texas
77030, USA

Howard I. Scher, MD
Associate Attending Physician, Solid Tumor Service, Department of
Medicine, Memorial Sloan- Kettering Cancer Center, 1275 York
Avenue, New York, New York 10021, USA

Pramod C. Sogani, MD, FRCS(C)
Associate Attending Surgeon, Solid Tumor Service, Department of
Medicine, Memorial Sloan-Kettering Cancer Center, 1275 York
Avenue, New York, New York 10021, USA

John Trachtenberg, MD, FRCS(C)
Associate Professor, Division of Urology, University of Toronto,
Toronto General Hospital, Suite 14–209, The Eaton Wing, 200 Elizabeth
Street, Toronto, Ontario, Canada M5G 9Z9

Willet F. Whitmore Jr., MD
Attending Surgeon and Professor of Surgery, Cornell Medical
Center, Memorial Sloan-Kettering Cancer Center, 1275 York
Avenue, New York, New York 10021, USA

Richard D. Williams, MD
Professor and Chairman, Department of Urology, University of
Iowa, Iowa City, Iowa, 52245, USA

J. M. G. Wilson, FRCP
Millhill House, 77 Millhill, Musselburgh, Midlothian EH21 7RP,
Scotland, UK (Formerly at the Scottish Health Service, Common
Services Agency, Information Service Division)

Alan Yagoda, MD
Attending Physician, Acting Chief, Solid Tumor Service, Depart-
ment of Medicine, Memorial Sloan- Kettering Cancer Center, 1275
York Avenue, New York, New York 10021, USA

Chapter 1

Epidemiology

J.M.G. Wilson

Introduction

Despite being one of the most common cancers among Western males, the etiology of carcinoma of the prostate remains elusive. Epidemiologic studies provide intriguing clues but the combination that will release the lock and reveal the mystery has yet to be found. To a greater or lesser extent, age, race, geography, sexual activity, hormone levels, diet, trace metals, and virus infections may all play a part in establishing the risk of developing prostatic cancer. But it is in the nature of epidemiologic studies that, while demonstrating associations, they stop short of providing the vital links between cause and effect; for this, biologic studies are necessary. This chapter attempts to summarize the present state of epidemiologic knowledge, to bring together some of the world data on survival, and to analyze published work on clinical and pathologic survival studies. Excellent extended reviews of the epidemiology by Owen (1976), Mandel and Schuman (1980), Alderson (1981), Greenwald (1982), and Mettlin (1983) have been published elsewhere. However, before discussing these and other questions it may be helpful to consider aspects of data collection and interpretation that are fundamental to understanding the epidemiologic picture: first, the problems of large-scale data collection by many different centers, and the comparability of their data; and second, the nature of epidemiologic information itself, where the relationship between prevalence, incidence, mortality, and survival merits interpretation.

Quality of Data

The primary data for mortality at the national level are obtained through death certification (World Health Organization 1977), and for morbidity by means of cancer registration schemes, either regional or national (e.g., Waterhouse et al. 1982, p. 17). There are large differences in the recorded levels of these rates both between and within countries, as well as between different ethnic and social groups within countries. To what extent are these differences real and how much, or little, may be attributable to differing practices in registering cancers and certifying deaths? Completeness of registration depends in the first place upon the general effectiveness and efficiency of the medical services and the accessibility, both geographic and economic, of these services to the population, as well as on the completeness of the population census, and secondly upon the efficiency and width of coverage of the cancer registration organization. More detailed clinical factors are also important: the diagnostic skill of the clinician, the precise diagnostic rubric used, and the efficiency of the clinical team in registering cases all affect the quality and quantity of the cancer registry. In the same way, variations in practice in the certification of deaths can produce unreal variations in mortality data: in addition to factors concerning registration, the statement on the death certificate of the underlying cause of death is crucial; variations from the rules set out by the World Health Organization (WHO) in the ninth edition of the International Classification of Diseases (World Health Organization 1977) can lead to apparent, but unreal, differences in mortality rates between or within countries.

There are therefore pitfalls in making comparisons without proper attention to the source and accuracy of the data. Fortunately it is possible to carry out cross-checks and in this way to identify reliable centers producing comparable statistics. The WHO International Agency for Research on Cancer (Waterhouse et al. 1982, p. 671) acknowledges the problem of completeness and accuracy in cancer registration, and provides ways of estimating this by examining (a) the proportion of cases that have been diagnosed histologically, and (b) the proportion that have been registered as a result of death certification, as well as the ratio, for each site, of deaths to cases registered in the same period. Comparison of registration with death certification makes possible an updating of cases that may not have been registered and also serves as a check on the efficiency of registration. If the proportion of cases registered as a result of death certification is high, the probability is that the recorded incidence is below the real one. Not all cancers are fatal, and if a large number are only being detected because of death certification, it is likely that an unknown proportion of nonfatal cases are escaping registration.

Interpretation of Data

The relationship between the incidence and prevalence of a disease, its mortality, and the length of survival of patients forms a time-related complex. The number of cases of cancer in a population, the prevalence, is the resultant of

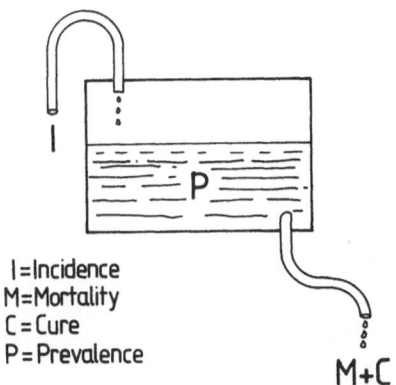

I = Incidence
M = Mortality
C = Cure
P = Prevalence

Fig. 1.1. Relationship of incidence (*I*), mortality (*M*), cure (*C*), and prevalence (*P*).

the incidence and mortality, and the length of survival. To appreciate this dynamic relationship more clearly it may be helpful to consider it in the form of a simple model: the filling and emptying of a tank of water (Fig. 1.1). The water enters the tank at a certain rate—the incidence—and empties at another (or the same) rate, representing the mortality and rate of cure. The level of water in the tank will rise until equilibrium is reached between the input and output rates, this level representing the prevalence of the condition in the population. The prevalence will, of course, change in response to alterations in incidence and mortality. Where we are considering the long-term prognosis of a particular disease, one further outcome is important: death due to causes other than the disease in question. In the water tank analogy the average duration of a disease would be represented by the average time the molecules of water remain in the tank. This mean duration can be determined by the relationship:

$$\frac{\text{prevalence}}{\text{incidence}} = \text{duration}$$

For a chronic disease like cancer, the cases occurring in 1 year suffer a falling off in survival over subsequent years according to the sum of the interactions between the aggressiveness of the disease, the stage at which the disease was diagnosed, and the varying resistance of the patients according to age and other factors. As a new batch of cases occurs each year, so there is left a steadily diminishing band of survivors from the previous and earlier years. The sum of all these survivors, from the newly incident cases to the few cases still not regarded as cured after say 10–15 years, constitutes the prevalence. In a similar way cases removed by death, in decreasing numbers in any particular cohort as the number at risk diminishes, add up to the annual mortality. The average duration of the disease is indicated, as we have seen, by dividing the prevalence by the incidence, expressed either by the numbers of cases or by rates. Table 1.1, using as an example data extrapolated from the Scottish cancer registration statistics, brings these relationships together for annual registrations of carcinoma of the prostate at ages 45 and over. The table shows the average number newly incident each year, and the number surviving in the next and subsequent years up to a total of 15 years (the available data extend only over a 10-year period, but for

Table 1.1. Carcinoma of the prostate: example of a 15-year life table[a] showing numbers, aged 45 and over, surviving each year (with derived prevalence, incidence, mean duration, and annual mortality)

Year	0–1	1–2	2–3	3–4	4–5	5–6	6–7	7–8	8–9	9–10	10–11	11–12	12–13	13–14	14–15	All years	No. deaths
0	560																
0–1	365	560															195
1–2	285	365	560														77
2–3	230	285	365	560													46
3–4	192	230	285	365	560												28
4–5	167	192	230	285	365	560											16
5–6	149	167	192	230	285	365	560										10
6–7	135	149	167	192	230	285	365	560									6
7–8	120	135	149	167	192	230	285	365	560								5
8–9	113	120	135	149	167	192	230	285	365	560							2
9–10	107	113	120	135	149	167	192	230	285	365	560						1
10–11	101	107	113	120	135	149	167	192	230	285	365	560					1
11–12	95	101	107	113	120	135	149	167	192	230	285	365	560				1
12–13	90	95	101	107	113	120	135	149	167	192	230	285	365	560			1
13–14	84	90	95	101	107	113	120	135	149	167	192	230	285	365	560		1
14–15	78	84	90	95	101	107	113	120	135	149	167	192	230	285	365	2311	
																	391

Number

		Crude rate/100 000 males, aged 45 and over, Scotland
Annual incidence (I)	= 560 p.a.	22.3
Prevalence (P)	= 2311	91.7
Mean duration (D)	= P/I = 2311/560 = 4.1 years	
Annual mortality	= 391	15.6
Case fatality	= 391/2311 = 16.9% p.a.	

[a] Data extrapolated from Scottish cancer registrations, 1966–1976.

the purpose of arriving at an approximate number of prevalent cases they have been extrapolated to 15 years).

The usual measure of the progress against cancer is the proportion of patients surviving from year to year. The first column of Table 1.1 shows the number of patients with carcinoma of the prostate at ages 45 and over surviving year by year. The survival rate at 5 years is 167 out of 560, i.e., 29.8%. This is the actual, observed, proportion surviving; but a large proportion of these patients, particularly the oldest ones, will in fact have died from other causes, and it is therefore usual to correct the observed proportion by allowing for other causes of death, using the expected survival rate for the whole population at risk. In this example the expected survival rate for males of all ages over 45 at 5 years is 62.7%. Thus the so-called 5-year relative survival rate (RSR5), that which would have occurred from the cancer alone if other causes of death had not been operating, is $29.8/62.7 \times 100 = 47.5\%$.

Longitudinal survival data are not always available. An index of the lethality of a cancer is given by the ratio of the incidence to the mortality: the larger the ratio, the better the survival. For male lung cancer in Scotland in 1981 the ratio of incidence to death was 1.1:1; for cancer of the prostate it was 1.9:1 (Scottish Health Service Common Services Agency, Information Services Division 1984). These ratios relate to RSR5s (1971–73) of 11% and 44% respectively. The ratio of incidence to death correlates to a highly significant degree with the RSR5 over a range of 13 cancers.

We can now consider the frequency and mortality of cancer of the prostate, both its between-country and within-country incidence, and its place in comparison with other cancers.

Incidence

World Incidence

It may first be useful to set the condition in its world perspective. This in turn yields further epidemiologic information. Table 1.2, showing both age-standardized world and cumulative incidence rates (Waterhouse et al. 1982), is arranged in descending order of incidence for 69 countries, areas, or population groups, divided into those with high, medium, or low rates. In the top group are, broadly, the Western developed countries. Within the United States the highest incidence by far is among blacks. In the middle band are a number of European countries; the lower rates for the United Kingdom compared with North America are notable. In the lowest range are a number of Far Eastern countries, Japan in particular having a remarkably low rate, of the order of only one-tenth that of the United States and Canada. Some of these differences may be explained by artifacts such as those mentioned above; but it is highly unlikely that the extremes between peoples such as the Japanese, North Americans, and Europeans are not due to real differences in the cancer attack rate. That said, it is probable that the aggressive diagnostic methods used more widely in countries with highly developed medical services play some part in accounting for high incidence rates: an increase in the diagnosis of nonclinical cancers can inflate the incidence considerably.

Table 1.2. Carcinoma of the prostate: age-standardized[a] and cumulative incidence rates[b], by country

Country and registration area	World rate 30.0–100.0	Cumulative rate, age range 0–74	Country and registration area	World rate 15.0–29.9	Cumulative rate, age range 0–74	Country and registration area	World rate 0–14.9	Cumulative rate, age range 0–74
1 USA, Alameda, Black	100.2	12.0	25 Jamaica, Kingston	28.6	3.6	49 Poland, Warsaw City	14.6	1.7
2 USA, Bay Area, Black	92.2	11.8	26 Germany, F.R., Hamburg	28.5	3.2	50 Hungary, Vas	13.3	1.6
3 USA, LA, Black	79.1	9.7	27 Australia, NSW	28.4	3.0	51 Poland, Cieszyn	13.2	1.8
4 Hawaii, White	59.7	6.8	28 Finland	27.2	2.9	52 USA, Bay Area, Japanese	12.7	1.4
5 USA, LA, Spanish	47.7	4.6	29 USA, LA, Chinese	26.6	2.9	53 Poland, Cracow	11.0	1.1
6 USA, Bay Area, White	47.4	5.4	30 Hawaii, Chinese	25.8	2.3	54 Japan, Nagasaki	10.2	1.1
7 Canada, Saskatchewan	46.2	5.3	31 France, Doubs	25.7	3.0	55 Hungary, Szabolcs	10.1	1.2
8 USA, Alameda, White	44.5	5.1	32 Denmark	23.6	2.6	56 Rumania, Cluj	9.7	1.1
9 Sweden	44.4	4.8	33 UK, Scotland, N.E.	23.4	2.4	57 Czechoslovakia	8.1	1.0
10 USA, LA, White	44.3	5.3	34 UK, Scotland, S.E.	23.0	2.4	58 Singapore, Malayan	7.2	0.5
11 USA, Connecticut	42.7	4.6	35 France, Bas Rhin	23.0	2.7	59 India, Bombay	6.8	0.5
12 Hawaii, Hawaiian	42.5	3.9	36 Italy, Varese	22.8	2.2	60 Singapore, Indian	6.7	0.8
13 USA, New York State	39.9	4.4	37 Brazil, Sao Paolo	22.2	2.5	61 Poland, Katowice	6.6	0.8
14 New Zealand, Maori	39.8	3.3	38 USA, LA, Japanese	21.5	2.1	62 India, Poona	6.2	0.6
15 Canada, Br. Columbia	39.8	4.5	39 Spain, Zaragoza	20.7	1.6	63 Hong Kong	5.1	0.6
16 Australia, South	39.6	4.4	40 UK, Oxford	20.7	2.3	64 Japan, Miyagi	4.9	0.5
17 Switzerland, Vaud	39.0	3.7	41 UK, South Thames	20.1	2.0	65 Israel, Non-Jews	4.9	0.5
18 Norway	38.9	4.4	42 Cuba	19.9	2.3	66 Singapore, Chinese	4.8	0.5
19 Switzerland, Geneva	36.3	3.9	43 USA, Bay Area, Chinese	18.6	1.5	67 Japan, Fukuoka	4.1	0.4
20 Hawaii, Japanese	35.9	3.2	44 UK, Birmingham	18.6	2.0	68 Japan, Osaka	3.4	0.3
21 Canada, Ontario	34.1	3.5	45 Germany, GDR	18.1	2.3	69 China, Shanghai	0.8	0.1
22 Germany, F.R., Saar	32.9	3.7	46 Spain, Navarra	17.6	1.6			
23 New Zealand, Non-Maori	30.7	3.1	47 Yugoslavia, Slovenia	15.8	1.7			
24 Hawaii, Filipino	30.5	3.7	48 Israel, All Jews	15.5	1.7			

[a]Rate per 100 000 males, standardized to standard world population.
[b]Rate percent. Source: Waterhouse et al. 1982.

Within-Country Incidence

Having examined the variations in incidence between different national and regional cancer registries throughout the world, we may now focus on a typical country where there is a moderately high incidence of cancer of the prostate, and consider the latter's importance in relation to other cancers and, indeed, in the context of all causes of physical illness and death. In Scotland in 1982 (Scottish Health Service Common Services Agency, Information Services Division 1984) cancer of the prostate accounted for 1 in 14 (7.2%) of all male hospital admissions for cancer; these in turn were responsible for 1 in 11 hospital admissions of males for all causes other than psychiatric illnesses. Of all male cancer deaths, 1 in 16 (6.4%) are attributable to cancer of the prostate, while total cancer deaths together account for more than one-fifth (23%) of all male deaths in Scotland. Thus 1 in 65 (1.5%) of all male deaths is certified as due to carcinoma of the prostate, a crude mortality of 18.9 per 100 000 male population. Not only is it, as Table 1.3 shows, one of the most frequent of the cancers, but over the past 15 years it has been advancing its position both in Scotland (where it is now the third most common cancer) and in other countries. This move up the league table is explained by a relative decrease in carcinoma of the stomach, as well as an increase in the registrations of cancer of the prostate over and above the increase in registrations for all cancers.

Table 1.3 also shows the much greater frequency of prostatic carcinoma in the United States, where its proportion of all the cancers is twice that in Scotland. This is the same difference seen in Table 1.2 in the form of age-standardized and cumulative rates.

Table 1.3. Frequency of nine cancers compared with all cancers, Scotland 1963–66, 1977–80; United States, white males, 1969–71

Malignant neoplasms	ICD-8 No.	Scotland						USA		
		1963–1966			1977–1980			1969–1971		
		No.	%	Rank order	No.	%	Rank order	No.	%	Rank order
Lung	162	8 881	29.1	1	13 047	29.7	1	17 020	21.0	1
Skin	172	3 281	10.7	2	4 574	10.4	2	–	–	(3)[a]
Stomach	151	2 886	9.4	3	2 874	6.5	5	3 299	4.1	7
Prostate	185	2 112	6.9	4	3 377	7.8	3	12 796	15.8	2
Colon	153	2 067	6.8	5	2 893	6.6	4	7 753	9.6	4
Rectum	154	1 544	5.1	6	1 844	4.2	7	4 175	5.2	6
Bladder	188	1 379	4.5	7	2 690	6.1	6	5 478	6.8	5
Pancreas	157	988	3.2	8	1 237	2.8	8	2 845	3.5	8
Esophagus	150	601	2.0	9	1 089	2.5	9	1 103	1.4	9
Other cancers		6 829	22.3		10 288	23.4		54 469	32.8	
All cancers		30 568	100.0		43 917	100.0		81 006	100.0	

Sources: 1. Scottish Cancer Registration Scheme
Cancer Registration Statistics, 1963–77 and 1971–80 Scottish Health Service Common Services Agency, Information Services Division, Edinburgh, 1981, 1984
2. Third National Cancer Survey: Incidence Data
National Cancer Institute Monograph 41, US Department of Health, Education and Welfare, 1975

[a]Skin cancers not listed separately; from the percentage of "other cancers" the probability is that skin cancers were proportionately fewer than those of the prostate.

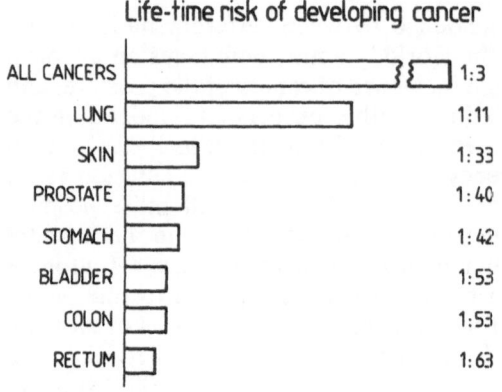

MALES
Life-time risk of developing cancer

ALL CANCERS	1:3
LUNG	1:11
SKIN	1:33
PROSTATE	1:40
STOMACH	1:42
BLADDER	1:53
COLON	1:53
RECTUM	1:63

Fig. 1.2. Lifetime risk of cancers in males [source: Cancer Statistics: incidence, survival and mortality; series SMPS 43 (HMSO 1981); Crown copyright 1981; reproduced with the permission of the Controller of Her Majesty's Stationery Office].

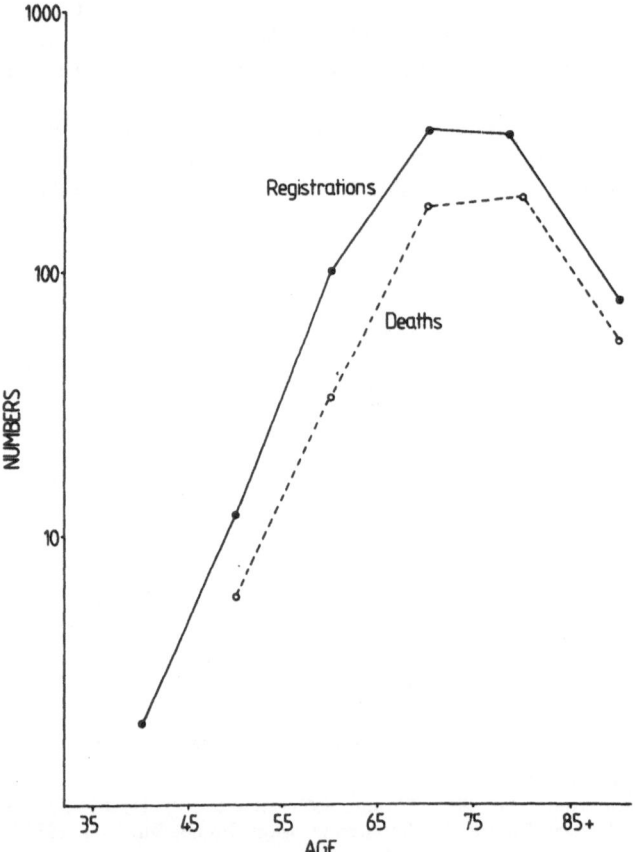

Fig. 1.3. Carcinoma of the prostate: number of registrations and deaths, by age, Scotland 1981 (sources: Scottish Cancer Registration Scheme, Scottish Health Service Common Services Agency, Information Services Division, unpublished series 1981; Registrar General Scotland, Annual Report 1981, HMSO, Edinburgh 1982)

Another way of expressing the relative frequency of a disease is by comparing the lifetime risk of its development with that of other conditions. This can be estimated by calculating the cumulative incidence, as shown in Table 1.2. Figure 1.2 shows that in England and Wales there is a 1 in 40 probability of carcinoma of the prostate developing during a male's lifetime, compared with a 1 in 11 probability of lung cancer, a 1 in 53 probability of cancer of the bladder, and a 1 in 3 probability of any cancer.

Age Incidence and Mortality

The importance of a disease to a community depends, of course, not only upon its frequency but also upon its effect on life expectancy and quality of life. These in turn depend upon a number of factors, including (a) the age at which the disease begins, (b) the degree to which it threatens life, i.e., the force of

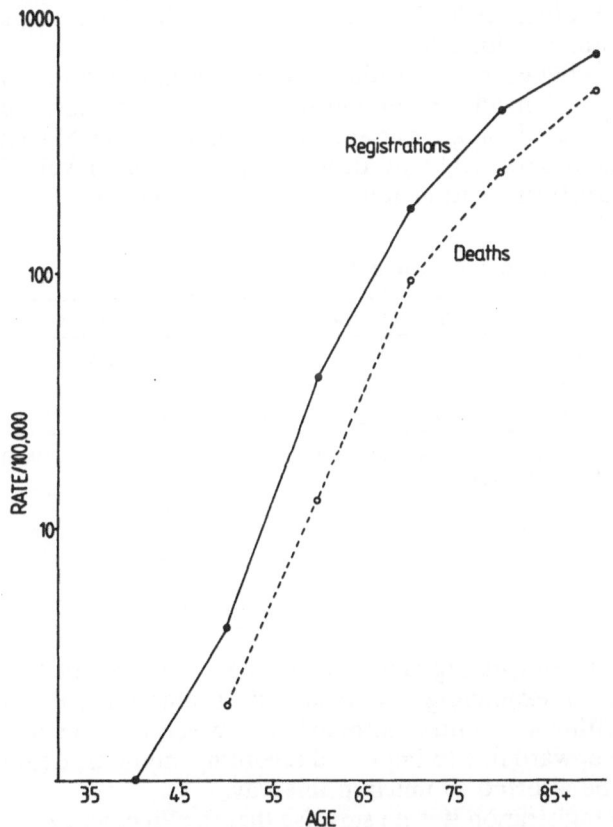

Fig. 1.4. Carcinoma of the prostate: incidence and death rate per 100 000 male population, by age, Scotland 1981 (sources: Scottish Cancer Registration Scheme, Scottish Health Service Common Services Agency, Information Services Division, unpublished series 1981; Registrar General Scotland, Annual Report 1981, HMSO, Edinburgh 1982)

mortality, measurable as the ratio of incidence to mortality, and (c) the length of survival.

Since carcinoma of the prostate occurs mainly in older men, its incidence increasing with age, it may be argued that its importance to the health of the whole community is not so great as that of a disease of similar incidence occurring in younger men, such as cancer of the bladder: 10% of bladder cancers occur in men under the age of 55, and 34% in men under 65, compared with less than 2% and 16% of cases of prostatic carcinoma respectively. However, a man reaching the age of 55 in Scotland or England and Wales has an average life expectancy of a further 17 years; and it is during this period that he is at increasing risk of developing cancer of the prostate. Figures 1.3 and 1.4 show the numbers and rates by age for registrations and deaths in Scotland in 1981. The highest number of cases occurs at ages 65–74, while the incidence climbs steeply as age advances. The form of these curves is similar to that for other cancer registries, with, of course, differences in the levels of the age-specific rates: In the 1969–71 US Third National Cancer Survey (Cutler and Young 1975), for example, the incidence rates for white males were at a considerably higher level in each age group; thus at ages 75–84 the incidence reached 656–837 per 100 000 males, compared with the Scottish 1970 rate of 350 (the United States age grouping is for 5 years, the Scottish for 10).

In Figs. 1.3 and 1.4 the gap between registrations and deaths at the different ages, indicating the relation of incidence to mortality, is one measure of lethality. We can see that the gap is smaller at ages 45–54 than at ages 55–64; after that the gap narrows progressively as deaths approach the level of registrations. The ratio of registrations to deaths is shown in Table 1.4.

Table 1.4.   Carcinoma of the prostate: registrations and deaths, Scotland, 1981

	45–54	55–64	65–74	75–84	85+	All ages
Registrations	12	103	353	339	81	890
Deaths	6	34	184	197	58	479
Ratio of registrations to deaths	2.0	3.0	1.9	1.7	1.4	1.9

Source: Scottish Health Service Common Services Agency, Information Services Division (1984) Scottish Health Statistics 1983. HMSO, Edinburgh

Time Trends in Incidence and Mortality

In spite of the difficulties in interpreting time trend data, owing to factors already discussed, it is worth examining the recorded secular changes in incidence and mortality. Within a country, although the baseline of cancer registrations may be moving upward due to improved recording methods, death certification is less likely to be affected so much in this way.

Because of this improving registration it is no surprise that the "incidence" of cancer of the prostate in Scotland rose between 1963–1967 and 1976–1980 by an average of 56%. This compares with a rise in registration rates over the same period of 40% for all cancers in males. The largest increases were at ages 55–64 (from 27 to 42 per 100 000) and ages over 85 (from 449 to 703 per 100 000).

Allowing for increasingly complete registration of cases, some of this rise in rates is probably attributable to changing and more efficient diagnostic practice, both in the clinical and the pathologic fields. To what extent, if any, there has been an actual increase in cancer incidence can only be guessed at.

It seems likely, however, that the real incidence of cancer of the prostate is fairly stable in Scotland, as also in England and Wales. Mortality data support this view: apart from some increase in mortality at ages 75 and over between 1950–1952 and 1960–1962, rates have remained relatively constant in all age groups from the 1930s up to 1983 (Registrar General, Scotland 1984). These rates approximate closely to those of England and Wales (Office of Population Censuses and Surveys/Cancer Research Campaign 1981; Office of Population Censuses and Surveys 1980, 1982, 1983a, b, 1984).

Survival

The primary relationship between incidence, mortality, survival, and prevalence has already been discussed. An increase in incidence will lead to increasing prevalence unless the end process of mortality, cure, or spontaneous remission also increases, or the duration of the disease is in some way shortened, e.g., by increased virulence. In fact the mean duration of a cancer is a statistic in which the dynamics of the disease are buried. A fuller picture is given by the life-table presentation of Table 1.1, where the number or proportion of a cohort surviving year by year is obtained by following the various exits from the pool of prevalence from death, cure, or loss of contact due to migration or other causes. As explained above, however, the so-called cumulative observed survival rate (the proportion of new patients surviving year by year) offers an unrealistically gloomy picture of the actual prognosis of cancer of the prostate; a truer idea of survival is provided by the relative survival rate (RSR), which is usually derived from the observed rate, as described above.

For purposes of illustration, and for deriving an approximate prevalence, Table 1.1 followed survival for a period of 15 years on the assumption that by then all the original patients either would have died or could be regarded as cured. Often, this is an unrealistically long time for the accurate follow-up of registrations; as time passes cases are lost to follow-up due to changes of address, migration, and possibly misleading death certification. This can be seen from the fact that applying the expected to the observed survival rates leads to an apparent increase in the RSR in the later years of follow-up. For practical purposes, therefore, survival rates up to 5 years are the most useful indices.

In the example of cumulative survival illustrated in Table 1.1, the extrapolation from 10 up to 15 years may also be giving an untrue picture in another way, since incidence and mortality have been assumed to remain constant. In reality, with changing clinical practice this is unlikely to be true, especially since it is probable that cases without symptoms are being increasingly diagnosed through, for example, transurethral resections for supposedly benign prostatic hyperplasia and more complete morbid histologic examinations. The incidence will thus apparently increase since registrations include not only living patients notified by hospitals but also those who die when there is any mention of cancer on the death certificate, regardless of whether this was the underlying cause of death. Mortality data, on the other hand, are compiled from the certifications on which the underlying cause of death is given as cancer. From this it follows that survival will appear to be lengthened and prevalence increased.

Apart from revealing a larger number of nonclinical or early clinical cases, aggressive diagnosis will also lead to earlier diagnosis. Through this the total time from diagnosis to death will be automatically extended, and thus survival time apparently improved although it may not in fact be affected. Of course, as a result of early clinical intervention, survival may well in reality be improved; an apparent and a real increase in the survival rate may thus go hand in hand. For these reasons the survival rate and the incidence–mortality ratio may both show a rise even though there has in fact been little or no change in the underlying natural history of the condition or the effectiveness of treatment. Thus secular changes in survival data, as a measure perhaps of the effectiveness of treatment, need to be treated with reserve. By the same token comparisons of survival rates between countries, or between different regions within some countries, have to be seen in this light. As we shall see, the recorded RSR5s in the United States for prostatic cancer at all ages are considerably higher than those in the United Kingdom; but the reasons for the different rates are undoubtedly complex and close examination of clinical details would be needed for their complete elucidation. This limitation does not, however, invalidate the survival rate as a means of interpreting contemporary differences within countries, such as survival at different ages. These points are illustrated in Fig. 1.5, where it can be

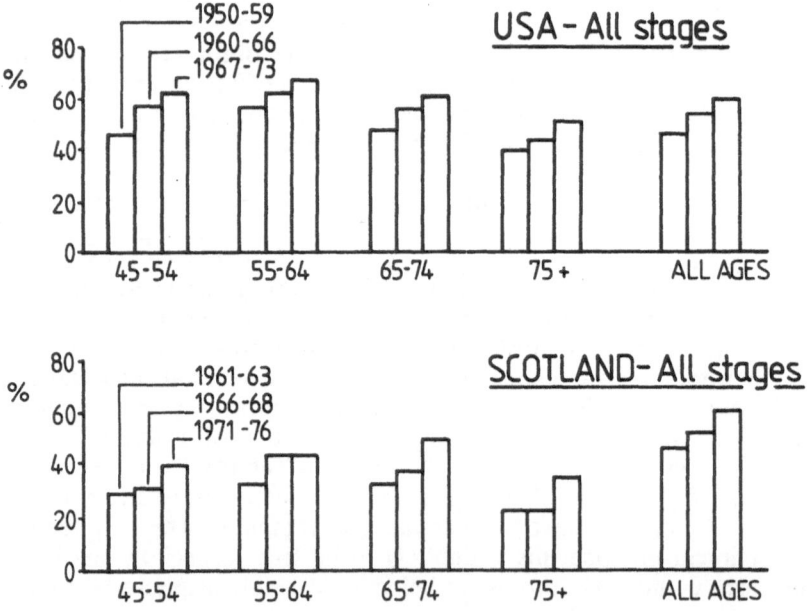

Fig. 1.5. Carcinoma of the prostate: 5-year relative survival rates, by age, all stages, by years of registration, in Scotland and parts of the United States (whites) (sources: Scottish Cancer Registration Scheme, Cancer registration and survival statistics, Scotland 1963–1977. Scottish Health Service Common Services Agency, Information Services Division, 1981; Axtell et al. 1976).

seen that in the United States and Scotland the recorded survival rates increased progressively over three periods. The recorded United States levels were consistently higher than the Scottish, and the relative levels of the survival rates at different ages were maintained.

The belief that apparent improvement in survival is at least in part due to an inflated incidence of relatively benign cases as a result of improved diagnosis is supported by evidence on two counts: first, the knowledge that there is a large pool of nonclinical carcinoma of the prostate awaiting diagnosis, a pool which is fed increasingly as age rises; and second, the finding that the overall proportion of latent tumors has been increasing. On the first count, there are numerous studies (Mandel and Schuman 1980) showing an increasing amount of latent carcinoma of the prostate as age increases. Breslow and his colleagues (1977), in a worldwide autopsy study of the frequency of latent carcinoma, found an average prevalence of 20% in men over the age of 44, ranging from 10% at the lower ages to 40% at age 80 and over. This trend was similar in five of the seven countries studied, but was not found in Israel or Singapore. The authors observed that the prevalence of latent carcinoma at autopsy followed closely the age-standardized incidence and mortality rates for all seven countries (Sweden, the Federal Republic of Germany, Jamaica, Israel, Hong Kong, Singapore, and Uganda), and they concluded that the behavior of latent cancer of the prostate is similar to that of clinical carcinoma in its geographic and age distribution. Rosenberg's New York series of 500 consecutive autopsies (1965) gave similar findings, the proportion of latent to fatal cases increasing with age. On the second point, an increase in the proportion of latent cases for all ages combined has been reported from the California Tumor Registry (Enstrom and Austin 1977): for the years 1942–1954 the proportion of latent (not in situ) cases to all cases registered was 41%; by 1955–1969 this proportion had risen to 63%.

Survival by Age

Although survival as a measure of prognosis possesses the drawbacks discussed above, it can be used, as we have seen, as a valid instrument for comparing contemporary differences in survival, such as survival at different ages. There are two main approaches to prognosis; each has its own advantages and shortcomings, but each complements the other. Most studies aimed at throwing light on the question of whether the outlook for prostatic cancer is poorer in younger than older men have been based on clinical and/or pathologic follow-up. The other chief approach is through the analysis of large-scale data on survival collected by national or regional cancer registries. The first kind of study has the advantage that it can eliminate some of the problems due to changing diagnostic practice by differentiating between preclinical and clinical stages and between histologic gradings, thus enabling like to be compared with like. On the other hand, clinical and pathologic studies tend to suffer from the disadvantage of relatively small numbers, with the ensuing difficulty of drawing statistically valid conclusions. The large-scale data collected and analyzed by cancer registries, while avoiding the pitfall of small numbers, suffer from the countervailing drawback that detail is lacking for ensuring that like is being compared with like.

Table 1.5.   Cancer of the prostate, Scotland: 5-year survival rate, by age, 1966–1976

Age	Number of registrations	Observed survival (%)	Expected survival (%)	Relative survival (%)	Standard error
45–54	116	37.5	94.3	39.7	5.2
55–64	912	40.7	85.8	47.5	2.1
65–74	2512	35.4	69.6	50.8	1.5
75–84	2103	20.8	48.1	43.2	2.1
All ages, 45–84	5643	31.0	68.0	45.6	1.0

Source: Scottish Cancer Registration Scheme, Scottish Health Service Common Services Agency, Information Services Division, unpublished series

In an attempt to combine the advantages, and as far as possible eliminate the disadvantages of these two methods of study, Wilson et al. (1984) analyzed both the available cancer registry data and the published clinical and pathologic studies for evidence on survival at different ages in cancer of the prostate.

Cancer Registration Data

Survival in Scotland

Table 1.5 shows the age-specific 5-year survival rates for the aggregated registrations of the years 1966–1976. The RSR5 is lower, though not significantly, at ages 45–54 than at all higher ages. In Fig. 1.6 we can see from the year by year age-specific rates that survival at ages 45–54 is at first better than at older ages, but that after 2 years survival deteriorates more rapidly than in the older groups. A possible reason might be a greater initial natural resistance in younger men, which later breaks down suddenly under the spreading assault of malignancy.

International Comparisons

In Fig. 1.7 the Scottish rates are compared with similar age-specific survival rates for England and Wales (Office of Population Censuses and Surveys 1982) and a group of cancer registries in the United States (Axtell et al. 1976). In both England and Wales and the United States, as in Scotland, survival at ages 45–54 is poorer than in the age group 55–64; thereafter survival again deteriorates. Survival in Finland shows the same pattern (Hakulinen et al. 1981). The clinical stage at which the disease is diagnosed appears to be a key to differences in survival at different ages. The reason for the worse survival in younger men appears to be the resultant of slightly better survival in localized disease being outweighed by a much poorer survival for nonlocalized cancer in this youngest age group, as can be seen in Fig. 1.8, which shows survival by broad clinical stage in Finland and the United States. Corriere et al. (1970), in their follow-up series, found a considerably higher proportion of cancers in clinical stages C and D in men aged under 55 than in men aged 55–64 (70% vs 43%). It can also be

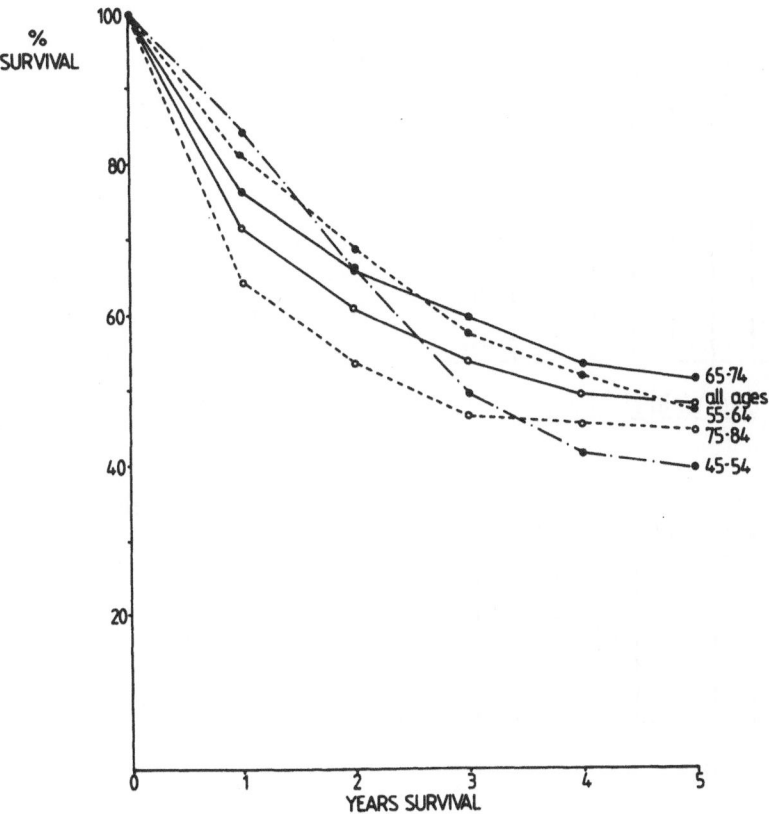

Fig. 1.6. Carcinoma of the prostate: 1966–1976 registrations, Scotland; relative survival rate by year, 1–5 years, by age, all stages (source: Scottish Cancer Registration Scheme, Scottish Health Service Common Services Agency, Information Services Division, unpublished series)

calculated from the Finnish registration data that there is a higher proportion of nonlocalized cancer at ages 45–64 than in the age group 65–74 (Wilson et al. 1984).

Clinical and Pathologic Studies

A number of papers dealing with age and prognosis were studied in an endeavor to determine the extent to which the evidence of the cancer registration data was supported or refuted. Apart from relatively small numbers, bias in the selection of case series posed a problem. Types of selection can be demonstrated from the following examples:

1. Autopsy cases only (Rosenberg 1965)
2. Particular treatment groups, such as patients who have undergone radical surgery (Turner and Belt 1957; Belt and Schroeder 1972)

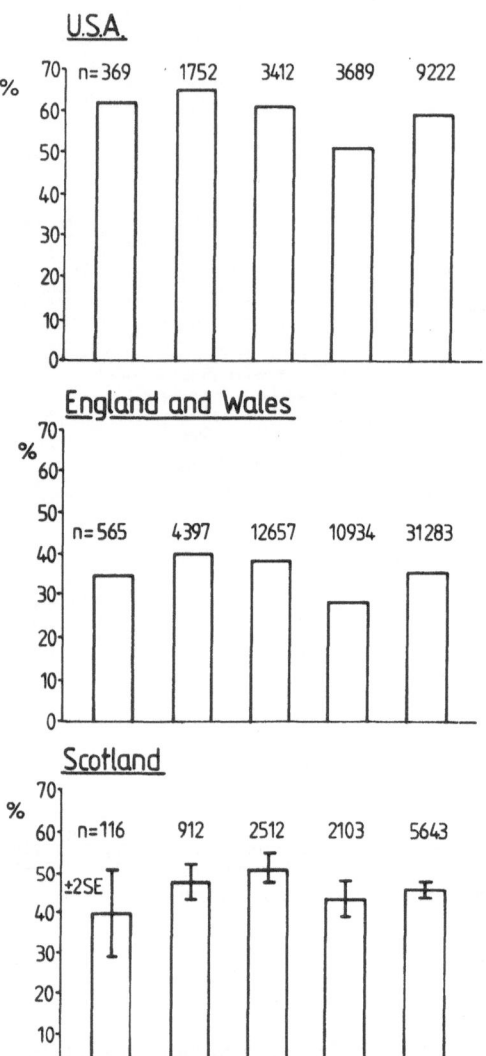

Fig. 1.7. Carcinoma of the prostate: 5-year relative survival rate by age, all stages. *Top*: Parts of United States (whites), registrations 1966–1973 (Source: Axtell et al. 1976). *Middle*: England and Wales, registrations 1971–1975 (source: Office of Population Censuses and Surveys 1982). *Bottom*: Scotland, registrations 1966–1976 (source: Scottish Cancer Registration Scheme, Scottish Health Service Common Services Agency, Information Services Division, unpublished series)

3. Comparison of groups of patients from different hospitals with differing admission and discharge policies (Silber and McGavran 1971)
4. Inclusion of groups of patients especially liable to either early or late diagnosis, such as members of the armed forces on the one hand (Byar and Mostofi 1969) and the "medically indigent" on the other (Cook and Watson 1968)

In addition to the problems presented by these biases, some studies fail to make allowance for the expected population survival rate, a statistic that is in any case problematic when applied to a selected population.

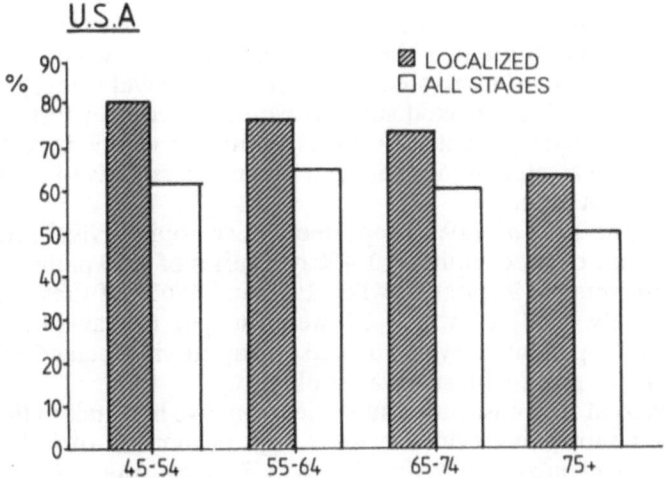

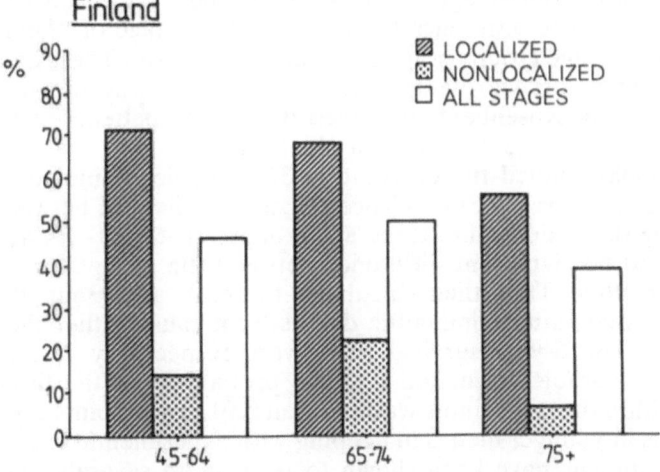

Fig. 1.8. Carcinoma of the prostate: 5-year relative survival rate, by age and clinical stage, parts of the United States (whites) 1967–1973, Finland 1967–1974 (sources: USA—Axtell et al. 1976; Finland—Hakulinen et al. 1981).

Bearing in mind these biases, the principal published studies can be briefly summarized as follows:

Franks (1956), in an autopsy study of 53 men with prostatic cancer, found that a considerably higher proportion of the younger men had gross metastases as compared with the older. However, his numbers of younger subjects were small: at ages 50–59 there were only four cases, but all had advanced metastatic disease.

The study by *Turner and Belt* (1957) suffered from the limitations that it was confined to men who had undergone perineal resection and that it dealt with survival from the date of operation only. The 5-year survival rate, which was uncorrected for general mortality, showed steadily improving survival from ages 46–50 up to 61–65 (correction for expected survival would, of course, further improve the survival of the older patients). Another limitation of this report, however, was that the numbers cited in the table and the numbers derived from the distribution curve did not agree.

The autopsy study by *Tjaden et al.* (1965) reported a very poor survival rate among 56 men under the age of 50, comprising 1.4% of a series of 4009 patients' records at Iowa State University Hospital between 1938 and 1963. Of these 56 cases, 38 had been rapidly fatal, of which 37 were judged to have been inoperable. Only 13% of the patients survived 5 years, mean survival being 22.7 months. No comparison was given with survival at older ages.

Rosenberg's study (1965) of 500 consecutive autopsies from five hospitals in the New York area provides supporting evidence for a high proportion of lethal cancers in younger men. He estimated that, for all ages, 37% of cancers had been "fatal," i.e., directly responsible for death, while 57% he classified as "latent," considering these to have no discernible effect on life expectancy. A small proportion, 6%, were classed as "serious," with metastases or local spread which did not, however, lead to death. Rosenberg found a considerable difference in the proportion of "fatal" cases at different ages: 57% at ages 51– 60, 37% at ages 61–75, and 27% at ages 76–80. The difference between the percentage of "fatal" cases in the 51–60 and 61–75 age groups is significant at the 5% level. These data suggest, therefore, that in patients who die the tumor is more frequently the cause of death in the younger man. Rosenberg concluded that young patients suffer from a more "virulent" form of the disease than older men.

Cook and Watson (1968) studied the outcome in 367 "medically indigent" patients admitted to the Ellis Fischel State Cancer Hospital, Missouri between 1939 and 1961. Dividing the patients into three age groups, 51–60, 61–70, and 71–80, the authors found no significant difference between the groups for six clinical comparability factors. They then calculated for each age group the proportion surviving by year, after eliminating deaths from causes other than cancer of the prostate. The 5-year survival rates were respectively 23.2%, 27.9%, and 33.6%. The authors calculated that the probability of the three survival curves being within the same limits was less than 0.01. They pointed out that the worse prognosis in younger men is in keeping with experimental cancer findings, where young animals have been shown to react more severely than older ones to transplanted tumors, such as Rous sarcoma.

Byar and Mostofi (1969), as a result of their study of 51 patients under the age of 50, concluded that these younger men enjoyed a better survival rate for prostatic cancer than a group of 210 patients over the age of 50 (mean age 69), selected from the Veterans Administration Cooperative Urological Research Group study. For cancer deaths only, the 5-year survival rates were 86% and 63% respectively. However, as the authors say, and as Johnson and his colleagues have pointed out (1972), 38% of the younger group were men on active duty in military service whose tumors were discovered through routine physical examination. Byar and Mostofi also showed that survival was better in their younger group by histologic grade of tumor. Survival by clinical stage by age was not reported.

Corriere et al. (1970), in a review of all clinical records of patients attending the Hospital of the University of Pennsylvania between 1955 and 1964 with a diagnosis of cancer of the prostate confirmed by pathology, reported a rise in survival of patients with the disease as age increases. At ages 35–59, 60% of patients were dead at 5 years after diagnosis, compared with 57% at ages 60–74 81% at ages 75–95. However, in the two older groups, as would be expected, a higher proportion, 26% and 61% respectively, had died of causes other than cancer, compared with 12% in the youngest group. Of deaths at 5 years directly attributed to cancer of the prostate, 48% occurred at ages 35–59, compared with 32% at ages 60–74 and 21% at ages 75–95. However, as noted, deaths from all causes at 5 years in this oldest age group was very high, with only 19% surviving. If the normally expected survival rates for this population could be applied to the observed 5-year survival rates, it is likely that the corrected survival rate would be of the order of 40%–45% for the youngest group, 50%–60% for the intermediate group, and 30%–40% for the oldest group: an order of magnitude in keeping with the cancer registry survival rates reported above.

Corriere and his colleagues also reported the clinical stage by age at diagnosis of 492 patients. An important finding, which matched that deduced from the Finnish and United States registration data, was that there is a higher proportion of more advanced cases (clinical stages C and D) in younger patients than in older ones. At ages 45–54, 13 of 19 patients were at stages C and D at diagnosis, compared with 55 of 128 patients aged 55–64. This difference is just statistically significant.

Silber and McGavran (1971) analyzed the records of 65 men under the age of 56 who had been patients at Barnes Hospital, St. Louis, between 1950 and 1968, diagnosed as suffering from cancer of the prostate. Their median age was 53, and they were compared with 78 matched cases of median age 73 from the Ellis Fischel State Cancer Hospital, Missouri. In patients with localized disease the observed survival rate at 5 years for the younger group of 28 men was 77%, compared with 21% for the 38 older men from the cancer hospital. Allowing for differences in general mortality, the corrected survival rates are 83% and 30% respectively, a highly significant difference. In patients with fixed prostatic and/ or metastatic disease the observed 5-year survival rates were 24% for the 37 younger patients and 21% for the 78 older men. Silber and McGavran concluded that "these data provide no support for the impression that younger men with cancer of the prostate have a less favorable survival than do older men." However, when the survival rates for fixed and/or metastatic disease are corrected for general mortality at the younger and older ages, the RSR5s are 26% for the under–56 age group and 30% for the group of median age 73. This difference, although not statistically significant, is nevertheless in line with the trend of poor survival in younger men with nonlocalized disease demonstrated by the cancer registration data reviewed above.

Belt and Schroeder (1972) of the University of California Medical Center in Los Angeles analyzed the data for 464 patients seen between 1920 and 1970. All patients had undergone radical prostatectomy. They reported an observed 5-year survival rate of 66% for the 19 patients under the age of 50, compared with 81% for men aged 51–60, and 71% for those aged 61–70. These survival rates, corrected for general mortality, become 70%, 88%, and 86% respectively: differences that are not statistically significant. Of the 19 patients under the age of 50, 9 had died of cancer of the prostate with fixed metastatic disease; this was a very significantly larger proportion than the 21 of 122 patients aged 51–60 (47.3% vs 17.2% respectively). This study of surgical patients therefore strongly suggests a poorer prognosis in the younger patient.

Johnson et al. (1972) studied 26 cases of prostatic carcinoma in men under the age of 50 (mean age 46.2 years), and compared the outcome with that in 599 patients over 50 (mean age 66.5), all of whom had been diagnosed and treated at the M.D. Anderson Hospital, Texas. All 26 patients had presented clinically, and cases diagnosed through incidental postmortem or surgical findings were excluded. Of the 26 patients under the age of 50, 16 (62%) were found to have widespread metastatic disease (stage D), and 8 (31%) had tumors extending into the extracapsular structures (stage C). This compared with 34% stage D and 20% stage C disease in the 599 patients over the age of 50. The difference in the proportion of stage D cases is highly significant statistically. The RSR5 for all stages for men aged less than 50, as calculated by the authors, was 14%, compared with 43% for the 599 patients over 50 years. Survival by clinical stage was also much worse for the younger men: 15% compared with 42% for local spread cases (stage C), and nil survival compared with 22% for widely disseminated cancers. All these differences were statistically significant. There were only two cases of localized disease (stage B) diagnosed among the 26 men under 50. The authors concluded that the main reason for their findings of such a poor outcome in younger men was late diagnosis due to failure to consider the possibility of prostatic cancer at this age. But they also concluded that cancers in younger men have a greater force of malignancy (Rosenberg's "virulence"), as evidenced by the much poorer survival even at the same clinical stage of the disease, when compared with older men.

The findings of *Hanash et al.* (1972), based on the follow-up of 200 consecutive histologically confirmed cases of cancer of the prostate at the Mayo Clinic, support those of Rosenberg and of Johnson and his co-authors. Hanash et al. reported an RSR5 of 20% for men aged 50–59, compared with 40% at ages 60–69. This difference, though not significant, matches the trend demonstrated elsewhere of worse survival in the younger man. These authors also found much poorer survival in patients with widely disseminated disease, but they did not publish survival data on clinical stage by age.

Harrison (1983) has recently reported on two groups of patients: 46 men under the age of 60 and 193 aged 65–74 attending respectively the General Infirmary, Leeds, and St. James University Hospital, Leeds, between the years 1969 and 1977. The two groups were well matched clinically, there being no significant difference between them for a set of five main symptoms and signs, and the proportion undergoing prostatectomy and biopsy was similar. There was no significant difference between the groups in terms of presence of metastatic disease, the figures being 30% in the under-60s and 28% in those aged 65–74. The RSR5 was slightly, though not significantly, poorer for the younger men: 41% vs 47%. For patients with metastases and for those with histologically well-differentiated tumors, survival appeared to be poorer in the younger group, though not significantly so. There was little difference in survival between the two groups of men with poorly differentiated tumors. Confidence limits for all the survival data presented are wide owing to the small numbers of cases in the subgroups, and it is possible only to conclude, as does the author, that the evidence presented shows no significant difference in survival between the older and younger men, although there is a suspicion of better survival, particularly after 5 years, for the older patients. Harrison concludes that the presence of metastases and the degree of tumor differentiation exert a similar influence in both younger and older patients. However, the survival curves for patients with metastases show that all the younger men are dead by 5 years whereas some 16 (8%–9%) of the older men have survived for 10 years. Again, this difference does not reach a level of significance, but is in the same direction as other evidence and may perhaps be considered as giving some support to the view that younger men suffer from more aggressive malignancy, as postulated by Rosenberg, Cook and Watson, and Johnson et al., or, as these last authors believe, are diagnosed at a later stage of their illness.

Of the 12 studies, the authors of three (Byar and Mostofi 1969; Silber and McGavran 1971; Harrison 1983) consider that their evidence fails to support the hypothesis of a worse prognosis in younger men. However, there appear to be qualifications to this conclusion in all three studies. In that of Byar and Mostofi there is the question of the inclusion of 38% of cases detected by routine examination in the younger group of men on active military service, which would lead to apparently longer survival. In the study by Silber and McGavran the 5-year survival rate for cases with fixed or metastatic cancer, when corrected for normal life expectancy, is slightly worse for the younger men. This is in keeping with the information from cancer registration where data on the stage of disease are available: that the poorer outlook for all stages in the youngest age group is the resultant of a very bad prognosis in nonlocalized disease and a better outlook for the localized cancers. Harrison, in his study, correctly concludes, owing to the small number of cases, that his data show no significant difference in survival between the younger and older men. However, his RSR5 is slightly lower in the younger age group, and the survival curve for patients with metastases is again rather poorer for the younger men.

Thus none of these studies provides unassailable evidence against there being a worse survival rate in younger men, while most give support to this hypothesis and to the explanation that this is at least in part due to the very bad survival in cases of nonlocalized disease.

Etiology

Relationship to Benign Prostatic Hyperplasia

There is a high degree of correlation between international mortality rates for carcinoma of the prostate and benign prostatic hyperplasia (Wynder et al. 1967)—and, of course, between age at incidence for the two conditions, suggesting a possible relationship between them. However, correlation does not necessarily imply causal connection; it can be related to other factors such as systematic differences in certification practice between countries, or the action of some common etiologic element, genetic, sexual, or environmental for example. There are also direct reasons why this association is unlikely to be one of cause and effect: Breslow et al. (1977) have demonstrated that the prevalence of latent carcinoma of the prostate in men aged 75 and over reaches an average of 30%–40%, and in some countries over 50%. Benign prostatic hyperplasia is also a frequent condition in elderly men, and it is thus likely that the two conditions will be found together by chance, especially since the presenting symptoms tend to be the same.

Carcinoma of the prostate and benign prostatic hyperplasia occur in the same part of the prostate only infrequently; benign prostatic hyperplasia involves the inner zone, which is embryologically different from the outer zone in which most cancers arise (Franks 1974)—97% as recorded by Byar and Mostofi (1972). In the study by Breslow et al. the prevalence of small latent carcinomas was 27% in the outer zone, compared with 6% in the inner.

Clinical follow-up investigations into an association have yielded conflicting results. Armenian et al. (1974) found a 3.7 times increase in the death rate from cancer of the prostate in patients discharged from hospital with a diagnosis of benign prostatic hyperplasia, compared with matched controls. In contrast, Greenwald et al. (1974) reported a similar incidence (approximately 3%) when following up patients who had undergone subtotal prostatectomy for benign prostatic hyperplasia and matched controls who had been operated on for some other condition. Both studies had design drawbacks which it would be hard to avoid. In the first, the greater possibility that patients discharged with the diagnosis of benign prostatic hyperplasia might in fact already have cancer cannot be excluded. In the second, although most cancers occur in the outer zone of the gland, subtotal prostatectomy might well diminish the likelihood of developing cancer. The conclusions of Armenian and his colleagues have in particular been questioned by Franks (1974), Williams and Blackard (1974), and Byar (1975).

Geographic and Ethnic Differences

The large differences in incidence of cancer of the prostate between countries, shown in Table 1.2, are reflected in age-standardized mortality rates (Segi et al. 1981). These range, for example, from 21.5 per 100 000 population in Sweden to 2.3 in Japan. The United States and Canada rates fall in between, at 14–15, while Scotland and England and Wales have death rates of between 10 and 12. In the United States, blacks have a far higher incidence than whites, about twice as high. These differences have been much studied (for a review see Mandel and Schuman 1980) but reasons are hard to find. The evidence of migration provides some clues. The study of migrants of one ethnic origin living in another country can help differentiate between environmental and genetic factors. If migrants verge toward the incidence and mortality rates of the host country, this provides evidence for an environmental influence. If, on the other hand, the incidence remains similar to that of the country of origin, a genetic factor is favored. Migration to Hawaii provides an example: Table 1.2 shows that native Hawaiians have an incidence of 42.5 per 100 000; the incidence in Hawaiian whites is 59.7, while that for Hawaiian Japanese is 35.9 and that for Hawaiian Chinese 25.8. Thus the whites have the same or a slightly higher rate in Hawaii than in the United States, while the Japanese and Chinese rates approach that of the Hawaiians themselves and are one order of magnitude higher than in the home country. Similarly, Japanese, Chinese, and Spanish immigrants to

California have higher incidence rates than in their countries of origin. Lilienfeld et al. (1972) have shown that migrants to the United States from 13 European countries and Canada experience higher mortality rates than those of their countries of origin, with the exception of Finland and Sweden. Such evidence, where incidence rates fall between those of migrants' countries of origin and that of their country of adoption, supports the influence of environment.

A genetic factor might be favored by family studies which show more than expected numbers of deaths from prostatic cancer within families (Woolf 1960; Steele et al. 1971; Krain 1974; Schuman et al. 1977). A difficulty is that families may be subject to the same or similar environmental factors, and that this may be the reason for the aggregation rather than a genetic connection.

Dietary and Other Factors

In the further search for pointers to the etiology of cancer of the prostate, a large number of factors other than the above-mentioned have also been examined: dietary, social, hormonal, and infective—unfortunately so far without conclusive results. This evidence has been comprehensively reviewed by a number of authors (Mandel and Schuman 1980; Alderson 1981; Greenwald 1982; Mettlin 1983) and is summarized in Table 1.6. Unfortunately the experimental problems in demonstrating causality from these many associations have so far not been overcome. It is likely that there is no single cause; several factors may need to operate together, for example genetic, environmental, and dietary elements. Ashley (1965), in his study of autopsy material, postulated that a series of three

Table 1.6. Carcinoma of the prostate: etiologic factors

Variable	Factor	Effect
Genetic	Ethnic	Rates low in Japanese, Chinese
	Familial	Aggregation in families
Environmental	Geographic	Migrants verge toward rate of country of adoption
	Urban/rural	Rates higher in built and industrial environment
	Pollution	Positive association with atmospheric pollution but not with smoking tobacco
	Occupation	Rates higher in rubber industry and cadmium exposure
Social	Marital status	Rates higher in men ever-married, widowed, divorced, with children
	Sexual	Rates higher in men with more pre- and extramarital partners, more sexual drive, more frequent coitus, history of sexually transmitted disease
	Socioeconomic	Indeterminate; reports vary
	Religion	Lower rates in Seventh Day Adventists and active Mormons (apart from in Utah)
Hormonal	Androgens	Some evidence of higher levels
	Estrogens	Protection in cirrhosis of liver
Diet	Fat	Positive association with high fat, beef, milk products, and eggs
		Negative association with green and yellow vegetables (Japan)
		Vitamin A intake may be a factor
Infection	Viral	Possible relationship with herpes simplex and cytomegalovirus

"hits" or "events" affecting the prostatic tissue are needed for the development of a latent carcinoma, while an additional four or five "hits" are required for the induction of full malignant potential.

One variable of perhaps particular interest is that of diet. Various authors have demonstrated a strong positive correlation between carcinoma of the prostate and dietary fat (Howell 1974) and milk products, animal protein, eggs, fats, and oils (Lea 1967; Armstrong and Doll 1975; Blair and Fraumeni 1978). Dietary fat is also positively associated with both breast cancer and cancer of the colon and rectum (Wynder et al. 1971; Berg 1975). By contrast, in Japan Hirayama (1979) has demonstrated, in a prospective study of 95% of the census populations of 29 health center districts, that the age-standardized death rate from carcinoma of the prostate is inversely related to the intake of green and yellow vegetables. There was a more than twofold difference in mortality between areas with diets high and low in these vegetables—carrots, spinach, pumpkins, lettuce, etc. A causal factor could lie in the fat-soluble vitamin A content of these vegetables, animal experiments having shown vitamin A to have a protective effect against the risk of developing cancer (Greenwald 1982).

Apart from diet, other most likely causes of "hits" are perhaps hormonal levels and their influence on sexual drive and activity, occupational exposure to trace elements such as cadmium, and infections by herpes simplex and cytomegalus viruses.

Early Detection

The pros and cons of early disease detection have been extensively discussed elsewhere (Wilson and Jungner 1968; Nuffield Provincial Hospitals Trust 1968; Cochrane and Holland 1971; Lancet 1974). Among the accepted principles of screening are four main requirements:

1. A recognizable latent, preclinical, or unreported clinical stage
2. A valid and acceptable test
3. An effective treatment
4. Cost-effectiveness

We can consider these criteria in turn, as applied to the early detection of carcinoma of the prostate.

Latent Stage

There is certainly a recognizable latent lesion (Breslow et al. 1977), although the relationship to invasive cancer remains in doubt. Byar (1977) found that patients with focal lesions incidentally diagnosed experience the survival rate expected for the normal age-matched population, and rarely die of their malignancy. Invasive cancers in their early stages may at first give rise to few or no symptoms, and to this extent be latent.

Latent focal lesions can only be diagnosed incidentally since they cause no symptoms and there is at present no test that will identify them, apart from blind biopsy. Early invasive cancers can be diagnosed at the pre- or unreported symptomatic stage if positively looked for, rather than leaving patients to take the initiative and consult their physician. Chisholm (1983) has pointed out that at the time of presentation some 60% of patients have locally advanced tumors, and 50% of all patients have evidence of metastatic disease. At the same time, among 100 new patients, Chisholm found that 70 presented with prostatism and 23 with urinary retention.

Valid and Acceptable Test

The early reporting of symptoms and preventive physical examination constitute one form of test. Whether routine physical examination should be encouraged on this basis is more open to question, since the proportions of false-positives and missed cases are a drawback that needs to be set against the advantages of earlier diagnosis. In the Federal Republic of Germany, where an annual free routine medical examination is offered every year to all men over 45, the proportion of histologically confirmed cancers of the prostate out of more than 15 000 suspicious cases recorded in 1977 was 13.4%, i.e., 87% of the suspected cases proved to be false-positives (Faul 1982). In Faul's own series of 350 patients with a suspicious finding on rectal examination, biopsy confirmed carcinoma of the prostate in only 26%.

The question of acceptability to the public poses a different problem; the prospect of routine rectal examination deters many men. Faul reports that not more than 20% of men eligible for a free check-up take advantage of the offer; the highest rate of participation, 25%, has been between the ages 45 and 52.

Effective Treatment

The effectiveness of early compared with later treatment is difficult to judge. One problem is the lead-time, the apparent longer survival resulting from earlier diagnosis. In addition, early diagnosis does not necessarily mean early-stage disease; Chisholm (1983), in his series of 100 consecutive new patients, found that one-third had evidence of metastatic disease at the time of presentation. Faul states that in the Federal Republic of Germany it is at present not possible to say whether the routine check-up has altered the outcome for carcinoma of the prostate. Gilbertsen (1971) considered that the 75 patients with carcinoma of the prostate detected by the routine screening of 6000 men over the age of 45 experienced better survival rates than would be expected. His standard for comparison was the United States End Results Survey for men of similar age (Axtell et al. 1972). Thus, while it must be good practice to diagnose this, as any other, cancer as early as possible, at present the results do not appear to show clearly whether prognosis is improved.

Cost-effectiveness

A detection rate on screening in the region of 1.5% (Gilbertsen 1971; Faul 1982) must put in question the worth of routine examination, if detection of cancer of the prostate is the only objective. Of course, most screening programs include a number of tests, and the value of one needs to be set in the perspective of the whole package. However, for carcinoma of the prostate it appears that the dividends from early detection are at present not highly apparent; inviting middle-aged and elderly men to undergo screening for this purpose is therefore probably not worth the cost in clinical and community health resources, unless other, more effective, forms of secondary prevention can be offered at the same time. On the other hand, a program of health education aimed at encouraging middle-aged men to report urinary symptoms early, being relatively inexpensive, could be worthwhile. This could be particularly valuable in view of the evidence, discussed above, that younger men fare worse than older patients.

Conclusions

While the recorded incidence of carcinoma of the prostate is on the increase, it seems likely that this increase may be more apparent than real, being due to progressively more efficient diagnostic and pathologic techniques tapping a very large pool of previously undiagnosed disease, as well as to improved registration. This probability is supported by the fact that over the past 30 years there has been little change in mortality.

Registered survival rates, also, have apparently improved. It is difficult to apportion the contribution due to earlier diagnosis compared with that resulting from improvements in treatment. Reviewing the evidence on survival by age, it appears that younger men as a group experience a poorer survival rate than older patients. This may be due to a combination of later diagnosis and greater malignancy. This view is supported by the fact that there is a higher proportion of nonlocalized to localized disease in men in the youngest age group.

Although there are many etiologic factors that may play a part in initiating cancer of the prostate, none has so far been incriminated as causal. It seems probable that the condition is multifactorial. The wide differences in incidence recorded in different ethnic groups, and in the same ethnic groups both within and between countries, perhaps provide some of the most promising clues. The positive relationship between dietary fat on the one hand, and the negative association with green and yellow vegetables and carotene intake on the other, seem tantalizingly close to a causal connection. Further work in this field, as well as on hormonal relationships, may throw a clearer light on the etiology of cancer of the prostate and then, perhaps, on the way to prevent it developing.

References

Alderson MR (1981) Epidemiology. In: Duncan W (ed) Prostate cancer. Springer, Berlin Heidelberg New York, pp 1–19 (Recent results in cancer research, vol 78)

Armenian HK, Lilienfeld AM, Diamond EL, Bross IDJ (1974) Relation between benign prostatic hyperplasia and cancer of the prostate. Lancet II:115–117

Armstrong B, Doll R (1975) Environmental factors and cancer incidence and mortality in different countries, with special reference to dietary practices. Int J Cancer 15:617–631

Ashley DJB (1965) On the incidence of carcinoma of the prostate. J Pathol Bact 90:217–224

Axtell LM, Cutler SJ, Myers MH (1972) (eds) End results in cancer, report No. 4. National Cancer Institute, Bethesda Md [DHEW Publication No. (NIH) 73–272]

Axtell LM, Asire AJ, Myers MH (1976) (eds) Cancer patient survival report No. 5: a report from the cancer surveillance, epidemiology and end results (SEER) program. National Cancer Institute, Bethesda Md [DHEW Publication No. (NIH) 77–992]

Belt E, Schroeder FH (1972) Total perineal prostatectomy for carcinoma of the prostate. J Urol 107:91–96

Berg JW (1975) Can nutrition explain the pattern of international epidemiology of hormone-dependent cancers? Cancer Res 35:3345–3350

Blair A, Fraumeni JF (1978) Geographic patterns of prostate cancer in the United States. J Natl Cancer Inst 61:1379–1384

Breslow N, Chan CW, Dhom G et al. (1977) Latent carcinoma of prostate at autopsy in seven areas. Int J Cancer 20:680–688

Byar DP (1975) Benign prostatic hyperplasia and cancer of the prostate. Lancet I:866

Byar DP (1977) VACURG studies on prostatic cancer and its treatment. In: Tannenbaum M (ed) Urologic pathology: the prostate. Lea & Febiger, New York, pp 241–267

Byar DP, Mostofi FK (1969) Cancer of the prostate in men less than 50 years old: an analysis of 51 cases. J Urol 102:726–733

Byar DP, Mostofi FK (1972) Carcinoma of the prostate: prognostic evaluation of certain pathologic features in 208 radical prostatectomies. Cancer 30:5–13

Chisholm GD (1983) Perspectives and prospects. In: Duncan W (ed) Prostate cancer. Springer, Berlin Heidelberg New York, pp 173–184 (Recent results in cancer research, vol 78)

Cochrane AL, Holland WW (1971) Validation of screening procedures. In: Acheson ED (ed) Epidemiology of non-communicable disease. Br Med Bull 27:3–8

Cook GB, Watson FR (1968) A comparison by age of death rates due to prostate cancer alone. J Urol 100:669–671

Corriere JN, Cornog JL, Murphy JJ (1970) Prognosis in patients with carcinoma of the prostate. Cancer 25:911–918

Cutler SJ, Young JL (1975) Third national cancer survey: incidence data. National Cancer Institute Monograph 41 [DHEW Pub. No. (NIH) 75–787], Table 5

Enstrom JE, Austin DF (1977) Interpreting cancer survival rates. Science 195:847–857

Faul P (1982) Experience with the German annual preventive check-up examination. In: Jacobi GH (ed) International perspectives in urology, vol 3: Prostate cancer. Williams & Wilkins, Baltimore Md, pp 57–68

Franks LM (1956) Latency and progression in tumours: the natural history of prostate cancer. Lancet II:1037–1039

Franks LM (1974) Benign prostatic hyperplasia. Lancet II:293

Gilbertsen VA (1971) Cancer of the prostate gland: results of early diagnosis and therapy undertaken for cure of the disease. JAMA 215:81–84

Greenwald P (1982) Prostate. In: Schottenfeld D, Fraumeni JF (eds) Cancer epidemiology and prevention. WB Saunders, New York, pp 938–946

Greenwald P, Kirmss V, Polan AK, Dick VS (1974) Cancer of the prostate among men with benign prostatic hyperplasia. J Natl Cancer Inst 53:335–340

Hakulinen T, Pukkala E, Hakama M, Lehtonen M, Saxén E, Teppo L (1981) Survival of cancer patients in Finland in 1953–1974. Ann Clin Res 13 [Suppl 31]:59–61

Hanash KA, Utz DC, Cook EN, Taylor WF, Titus JL (1972) Carcinoma of the prostate: a 15-year follow-up. J Urol 107:450–453

Harrison GSM (1983) The prognosis of prostatic cancer in the younger man. Br J Urol 55:315–320

Hirayama T (1979) Epidemiology of prostate cancer with special reference to the role of diet. In: National Cancer Institute Monograph 53: Second Symposium on Epidemiology and Cancer Registries in the Pacific Basin. National Cancer Institute, Bethesda Md, pp 149–155

Howell MA (1974) Factor analysis of international cancer mortality data and per capita food consumption. Br J Cancer 29:323–336

Johnson DE, Lanieri JP, Ayala AG (1972) Prostatic adenocarcinoma occurring in men under 50 years of age. J Surg Oncol 4:207–216

Krain LS (1974) Some epidemiologic variables in prostatic carcinoma in California. Prev Med 3:154–159

Lancet (1974) Screening for disease: a series reprinted from the Lancet. 5 October–21 December

Lea AJ (1967) Neoplasms and environmental factors. Ann R Coll Surg Engl 41:432–437

Lilienfeld AM, Levin ML, Kessler II (1972) Cancer in the United States, APHA monograph. Harvard University Press, Cambridge, Mass

Mandel JS, Schuman LM (1980) Epidemiology of cancer of the prostate. In: Lilienfeld AM (ed) Reviews in cancer epidemiology, vol 1. Elsevier/North Holland, New York, pp 1–83

Mettlin C (1983) Cancer of the prostate and testis. In: Bourke GJ (ed) The epidemiology of cancer. Croom Helm, London; The Charles Press, Philadelphia, pp 245–259

Nuffield Provincial Hospitals Trust (1968) Screening in medical care: reviewing the evidence. Oxford University Press, London

Office of Population Censuses and Surveys/Cancer Research Campaign (1981) Cancer statistics: incidence, survival and mortality in England and Wales. Studies on Medical and Population Subjects No. 43. HMSO, London, pp 79–82

Office of Population Censuses and Surveys (1980, 1982, 1983a, 1983b, 1984) Mortality statistics: cause, England and Wales. Series DH2, Nos 6–10, Table 3. HMSO, London

Office of Population Censuses and Surveys (1982) Cancer statistics: survival. 1971–1975 registrations, England and Wales. HMSO, London, p 29

Owen WL (1976) Cancer of the prostate: a literature review. J Chron Dis 29:89–114

Registrar General, Scotland (1984) Annual report 1983. HMSO, Edinburgh, Table C 1.4

Rosenberg SE (1965) Is carcinoma of the prostate less serious in older men? J Am Geriatr Soc 13:791–798

Schuman LM, Mandel JS, Blackard C, Bauer H, Scarlett J, McHugh R (1977) Epidemiologic study of prostatic cancer: preliminary report. Cancer Treat Rep 61:181–186

Scottish Health Service Common Services Agency, Information Services Division (1984) Scottish health statistics 1983. HMSO, Edinburgh

Segi M, Hattori H, Noye H, Segi R (1981) Age-adjusted death rates for cancer for selected sites (A-classification) in 40 countries in 1976. Segi Institute of Cancer Epidemiology, Nagoya, Japan, Fig 1–14

Silber I, McGavran MH (1971) Adenocarcinoma of the prostate in men less than 56 years old: a study of 65 cases. J Urol 105:283–285

Steele R, Lees REM, Kraus AS, Rao C (1971) Sexual factors in the epidemiology of cancer of the prostate. J Chron Dis 24:29–37

Tjaden HB, Culp DA, Flocks RH (1965) Clinical adenocarcinoma of the prostate in patients under 50 years of age. J Urol 93:618–621

Turner RD, Belt E (1957) A study of 229 consecutive cases of total perineal prostatectomy for cancer of the prostate. J Urol 77:62–77

Waterhouse J, Muir C, Shanmugaratnam K, Powell J (1982) Cancer incidence in five continents, vol 4. IARC Scientific Publications No. 42, International Agency for Research on Cancer, Lyon

Williams RD, Blackard CE (1974) Benign prostatic hyperplasia and cancer of the prostate. Lancet II:1265

Wilson JMG, Jungner G (1968) Principles and practice of screening for disease. World Health Organization: Public Health Papers 34. World Health Organization, Geneva, Switzerland

Wilson JMG, Kemp IW, Stein GJ (1984) Cancer of the prostate: do younger men have a poorer survival rate? Br J Urol 56:391–396

Woolf CM (1960) An investigation of the familial aspects of carcinoma of the prostate. Cancer 13:739–744

World Health Organization (1977) International classification of diseases, 9th edn., vol 1. World Health Organization, Geneva, pp 699–730

Wynder EL, Hyams L, Shigematsu T (1967) Correlations of international cancer death rates. Cancer 20:113–126

Wynder EL, Mabuchi K, Whitmore WF (1971) Epidemiology of cancer of the prostate. Cancer 28:344–360

Chapter 2

Grading of Prostatic Carcinomas— Current Status*

F.K. Mostofi

Introduction

To provide a much needed estimate of growth and malignant potential of tumors, Broders (1925) proposed that tumors be divided into four grades:

Grade I: Three-fourths of the tumor is differentiated, one-fourth is undifferentiated.
Grade II: The proportion of differentiated and undifferentiated components is about equal.
Grade III: Three-fourths of the tumor is undifferentiated, one-fourth of the tumor is differentiated.
Grade IV: The tumor shows no tendency to cell differentiation.

In subsequent years the reproducibility and the reliability of grading tumors have been controversial. Indeed, even today, grading on the same slides may vary from grade 1 to grade 3 or even 4. This is attributable to the fact that differentiation has not been clearly defined—histology vs cytology—so that some have graded the tumor on structural differentiation, others on cellular differentiation, and still others on cellular anaplasia.

---

*The opinions or assertions contained herein are the private views of the author and are not to be construed as official or as reflecting the views of the Department of the Army or the Department of Defense.

The problem is magnified in carcinoma of the prostate (CaP). Almost 40 grading systems have been proposed, each working well for its advocate but found unsatisfactory by others (Mostofi and Price 1973; Mostofi 1976; Böcking 1982). This is attributable to certain peculiarities of CaP. The behavior of many CaPs is unpredictable. Many are slow-growing tumors, and with or without treatment, the patient may live for many years. The tumor itself presents a wide range of growth patterns.

The NPCP Task Force

In 1979 the National Prostatic Cancer Project (NPCP) convened a meeting in Buffalo, New York, to evaluate four of the many existing grading systems: the Mayo, the Gaeta, the Gleason, and the Mostofi systems. Prior to the conference, a separate task force of the NPCP visited each laboratory to evaluate the system. Each task force presented a report at the meeting.

The Mayo System

Four grades were recognized based on seven histologic criteria: acinar structure, individual cell structure, nuclear characteristics, presence of nucleoli, cytoplasmic characteristics, mitotic activity, and degree of invasiveness. Since there were four grades the system was reported by the task force as not providing a greater degree of discrimination than the Gleason system, and did not provide primary and secondary patterns.

The Gaeta System

As the pathologist for the NPCP, Gaeta had devised a classification taking into account both glands and cells:

Grade I: Well defined, medium and large glands separated by scant stroma. The cells are uniform and of normal size; the nucleoli, if present, are inconspicuous.
Grade II: Medium sized and small glands with moderate amount of stroma. The cells demonstrate slight pleomorphism; the nucleoli are prominent.
Grade III: Small acini, frequent loss of glandular organization, cribriform and scirrhous patterns. The cells demonstrate pronounced pleomorphism; the nuclei are often vesticular, with acidophilic nucleoli.
Grade IV: Round expansile masses of tumor cells. No gland formation. The cells are small or large, uniform or pleomorphic with significant mitotic activity.

In practice, Gaeta graded the tumor according to the more malignant element. If the cells were grade IV, that was the tumor grade, irrespective of the categorization of the glands. The Gaeta system was characterized by the task force as being simple, objective, and reproducible.

The Gleason System

In the early 1960s, while studying the slides of CaP of the Veterans Administration Cooperative Urological Research Group (VACURG) Gleason noticed that many CaPs showed more than one histologic pattern. Each of these patterns was assigned a number. In grading a given tumor, he identified the two most prevalent of these patterns, which are designated the primary and secondary patterns. The sum of the two constituted the grade.

Pattern 1: Very well differentiated small, closely packed uniform glands in essentially circumscribed masses.

Pattern 2: Similar to pattern 1 but with moderate variation in size and shape of glands; still essentially circumscribed but more closely arranged.

Pattern 3: Similar to pattern 2, but marked irregularity in size and shape of glands, with tiny glands or individual cells invading stroma away from circumscribed masses or solid cords and masses with easily identifiable glandular differentiation within most of them; may be papillary or cribriform.

Pattern 4: Raggedly infiltrating, fused glandular tumor frequently with pale cells; may resemble hypernephroma.

Pattern 5: Anaplastic carcinoma with minimal glandular differentiation, infiltrating the prostatic stroma diffusely.

In a subsequent report by Mellinger et al. (1967) it was demonstrated that the primary and secondary patterns were both equally important in determining survival but the correlation was better if stage was added to the pattern.

In several reports, Gleason (1966, 1977) and Mellinger and co-workers (Mellinger et al. 1967; Mellinger 1977) claimed good correlation with clinical behavior but the system had not been accepted by any pathologist as judged by lack of publications other than those of Gleason on the Gleason system.

The task force reported that the Gleason system was quite readily learned and easily reproducible.

The Mostofi System

This system took into account two features: the degree of nuclear anaplasia and the pattern of glandular differentiation. Cellular anaplasia was defined as variations from normal based on size, shape, chromatin distribution, and the character of nuclei. Such variation could be slight, moderate, or marked. Since maturation results in formation of glands and ducts, Mostofi confined differentiation to formation of glands. The glands could be large, small, fused, or cribriform. These were considered differentiated tumors while tumors that formed columns, cords, or solid sheets were classified as undifferentiated. Poorly differentiated tumors consisted of those with minimal gland formation.

In preliminary studies reported by Harada et al. (1977) the two parameters, individually, combined together, or combined with clinical staging provided a good prognostic index but the two parameters had not been correlated with each other. In the Mostofi system there seemed to be a critical level of glandular differentiation in relationship to cancer deaths. For example, up to 40% of tumors could consist of cribriform pattern without affecting mortality rates. According to the task force, the system was simple, clearly definable, and reasonably reproducible.

The NPCP Recommendations

The general recommendations of the NPCP workshop were that CaPs be graded, and that for the purpose of analysis of clinical experience, the Gleason system be employed tentatively at least in conjunction with any other system utilized; that nuclear and cytologic characteristics be considered in prospective studies to further the discriminative capabilities of the Gleason system; and that data be accumulated on the correlation between the histologic grade of the tumor, the natural history of the disease, and the response to various forms of treatment. The recommendations were published in *Cancer* (Murphy and Whitmore 1979). The absolute endorsement of the Gleason system by the NPCP was given despite the fact that the only evaluation of the system had been by Gleason (Gleason et al. 1974). There had been no independent evaluation.

Is the Gleason System Readily Learned, as Claimed by the NPCP?

Gleason reported his observations in 1966. Although this was followed by several reports by Gleason and Mellinger, both of the Veterans Administration (Gleason 1966, 1977; Gleason et al. 1974; Mellinger et al. 1967; Mellinger 1977), the system was not readily accepted by pathologists. The only other report in the literature on the system was by Harada et al. (1977). These authors found it necessary to have two tutorials by Gleason before they felt reasonably competent to use the system.

This is not an exceptional situation as many pathologists who have been required to use the system since the NPCP workshop have found it necessary to take a private tutorial from Gleason.

A disturbing feature for pathologists is that the Gleason system is illustrated by diagrammatic sketches rather than by photomicrographs and that it is based entirely on low power view.

Reproducibility of the System

Gleason has personally estimated reproducibility at 80% (Murphy and Whitmore 1979). Harada et al. (1977) reported that after two tutorials from Gleason, their reproducibility was 70%. Reproducibility by the same individual on the same slides on two different examinations was 64% for the primary patterns, and 44% for the secondary patterns. For the sum of the two, agreement was reached in 38% (Harada et al. 1977).

Reliability of the Gleason System

Studies of the Gleason system since its endorsement by the NPCP have given conflicting results, but the number of cases studied has been small and the majority of patients fall into the moderately differentiated group (score of 5–7). The situation is discussed in detail by Grayhack and Assimos (1983). Donohue et al. (1981) reported negative lymph nodes in 24 patients with well differentiated tumors (Gleason 2–4), but histologically positive lymph nodes were present in 50% (6 of 12) of moderately (Gleason 5–7) and poorly differentiated (Gleason 8–10) tumors (4 of 8). Prout et al. (1980) reported absent pelvic lymph node metastases in 12 patients with well differentiated tumors, and Kramer et al. (1981) had 29 such patients (with Gleason 2–4). On the other hand, Fowler and Whitmore (1981) found nodal metastases in 11 of 69 patients with well differentiated carcinoma, and Donohue et al. (1981) had 14 positive nodes among 72 such patients (16%).

For well differentiated B_2 tumors Donohue et al. (1981) reported an incidence of nodal metastasis in 37% while Fowler and Whitmore found nodal involvement in 39%.

Similar discrepancies exist with higher grades and stages. Corriere et al. (1970) reported local spread in 25% of Gleason grade 1 and 28% of Gleason grade 2 tumors (the authors state that they used Gleason's system and it is probably the predominant pattern that they used rather than the sum). They also reported that 62.5% of patients with Gleason grade 4 and 81.8% of patients with Gleason grade 5 had stage C and D tumors, respectively, on admission. On the other hand, Kramer et al. (1980) claimed that 100% of patients with stage A, B and C disease with Gleason grades 9 and 10 tumors and 90% of Gleason grade 8 tumors had positive lymph nodes. But there were only a total of nine patients in the former and 20 patients in the latter group. In contrast, Barzell et al. (1977) reported metastases in 9 of 15 stage B and C patients with Gleason grades 8, 9, and 10 (poorly differentiated) tumors, and Donohue et al. (1981) found metastases in 18 of 37 stage A_2, B_1, and B_2 tumors with Gleason grades 8, 9, and 10.

In 115 patients, Wilson et al. (1983) found lymph node metastases as follows: in the Gleason group 2–4, 2 of 6 stage A_2, 4 of 35 B_1, 0 of 13 B_2, and 2 of 7 C; in Gleason group 5–6, 5 of 8 stage A_2, 4 of 12 B_1, 8 of 12 B_2, and 2 of 4 C; and in Gleason group 7–8 (they considered 4 and 5 as 4), 1 of 2 stage A_2, 2 of 6 B_1, 3 of 6 B_2, and 3 of 4 C.

Cantrell et al. (1981) reported on 117 patients with stage A CaP who had not received any treatment. Of 14 patients who developed extensive local or metastatic disease, 12 did so within 4 years after prostatectomy. The data were analyzed only on 82 patients with a minimum of 4 years' follow-up. Age and presence of a second unrelated primary tumor were important predictors of absolute 4-year survival. While histologic grade (and tumor volume) failed to predict death at 4 years, histologic grade was an important variable but essentially dependent on the extent of tumor involvement.

These authors found that no patient with a well differentiated tumor had clinically progressive cancer while only a third of the patients with high-grade lesions [Hopkins grade 3 or Gleason's total score, 7–10] had progression to locally invasive or metastatic disease. They emphasized that grading was subjective, and that 74% of their lesions were classified as Hopkins grade 2 or

Gleason 5–6. Cantrell et al. (1981) did not describe Hopkins grading system but Jewett et al. had defined it in 1968.

Gleason (1977) has compared his system with other grading systems. His 2–4 are grade I, his 5–7 are grade II, and his 8–10 are grade III. He reported local spread in 34.6% and dissemination in 12.3% of his grades II and III, respectively—indicative of lack of discrimination between his grades II and III.

Pistenma et al. (1979) and Bagshaw (1984) have claimed that when Gleason patterns were less than 5, no positive lymph nodes were present. On the other hand, Olsson (1985) reported nodal involvement in 20% or more of patients with Gleason 2–4 primary lesions. Furthermore, a large proportion (nearly 40%) of patients with Gleason's 8–10 primary tumors do not have lymph node spread.

Smith and Middleton (1985) reported that of patients with well differentiated tumors, 6% had gross and 9% had microscopic lymph node disease.

Experience with CaP subjected to radiation therapy has given similar contradictory results (Barzell et al. 1977; Cupps et al. 1980; Bagshaw 1984).

Perhaps the unreliability of the Gleason system is due to the fact that the NPCP recommended that clinical staging should not be used in establishing a prognostic index. In various pre-NPCP reports Gleason et al. had emphasized that adding the clinical stages to the sum of primary and secondary patterns improved the reliability of the system.

Dissatisfaction with the Gleason system, because it is difficult to master, it is not easily reproducible, and it has limited reliability, has led to further proposals on grading.

Alternative Grading Systems

In 1980, Gaeta et al. proposed a "new approach to grading of CaP." It is essentially a modification of the system mentioned above except that it recognizes two elements: (a) glandular differentiation or lack of it, and (b) the nuclear characteristics of the individual tumor cells. Glands grade I consist of well defined small, medium, or large glands separated by scant stroma. Glands grade II include medium and small glands, less uniform with significant variation of size and configuration and separated by more abundant stroma. Glands grade III include small acini with a significant loss of acinar configuration and with a variable pattern of small or large cells arranged in clusters, clumps, or singly; this group includes any category that has well defined areas of cribriform or scirrhous configuration. Glands grade IV include those with complete or predominant loss of any recognizable organizations, diffusely infiltrating. This category also includes a small number of carcinomas composed of solid and expansile masses.

Nuclear grade I is characterized by nuclear features indistinguishable from normal nuclei; nucleoli, if present, are uniform and inconspicuous. Nuclear grade II includes those tumors with relatively uniform cells with moderately pleomorphic nuclei; there is more irregular chromatin distribution with a looser texture than in grade I, and frequent presence of easily recognizable nucleoli. Nuclear grade III includes those tumors whose cells exhibit nuclear pleomorphism and/or the presence of a single, large, and acidophilic nucleolus, frequently set against a chromatin background disclosing a vesicular character. Nuclear grade IV includes the occasional tumors with unusual mitotic activity and those with bizarre or giant nuclei.

Gaeta et al. found a good correlation between the two parameters. Glandular grade I tumors often had nuclear grade I cells. The final grade was based on the worst of the two. In 169 cases 6 were grade I, 43 grade II, 83 grade III, and 37 grade IV. They had 1 cancer death in 6 grade I, 16 deaths in 43 grade II, 60 deaths in 83 grade III, and 34 deaths in 37 grade IV tumors.

Brawn et al. (1982) proposed a grading system based on differentiation. In grade 1, 75%–100% of the tumor forms glands while 0%–25% does not, except predominantly cribriform–papillary tumors. In grade 2, 50%–75% of the tumor forms glands, while 25%–50% does not; this category includes tumors consisting of 50% or more of cribriform–papillary pattern. In grade 3, 25%–50% of the tumor forms glands, while 50%–75% does not. In grade 4, 0%–25% of the tumor is differentiated (gland-forming), while the remainder is undifferentiated (non-gland-forming). Brawn et al. had a 91% 5-year survival for 84 grade 1 patients, a 60% 5-year survival for 75 grade 2 and 3 patients, and a 15% 5-year survival for 23 grade 4 patients.

In 1980 the World Health Organization (WHO) published the results of the deliberations of its Panel of Experts on Tumors of the Prostate. (Mostofi et al. 1980). After a review of the existing grading system, the Panel essentially endorsed the Mostofi system as this system took into account both differentiation and anaplasia. Differentiation was defined as formation of glands which could be small or large, fused or cribriform (Figs. 2.1–2.3), or undifferentiated (Fig. 2.4).

In a study of almost 1000 patients with CaP using nuclear anaplasia alone, death rates were 1.24 for patients with slight nuclear anaplasia (Fig. 2.5) (9 of 107), 4.51 for those with moderate nuclear anaplasia (Fig. 2.6) (144 of 564), and 14.88 for those with marked anaplasia (Fig. 2.7) (63 of 127). Death rates were expressed as deaths per 1000 patient months using cancer deaths only. Adding stage (1–4) to grades (1–3) gave the following results: in 191 patients with a stage and grade sum of 2–4, death rates were 0.46; in 342 with a sum of 5, the rates were 2.75; in 357 with a sum of 6, the rates were 8.53; and in 97 with a sum of 7, the rates were 25.92.

Schroeder et al. (1982) evaluated the prognostic significance of 12 histologic and cytologic parameters. Each parameter was correlated with the survival data of 346 patients treated by radical prostatectomy. Statistically significant differences in survival rates were found with only two parameters—glandular differentiation and anaplasia as defined by Mostofi.

In 758 patients, Böcking et al. (1982) reported their results of combined histologic and nuclear grading based on the WHO proposals (Mostofi et al. 1980). They distinguished four patterns for histologic grading.

1. Well differentiated adenocarcinoma: Large, well constructed, uniformly round or oval glands lined by a single layered cylindrical epithelium. The epithelial cells still show polarity.
2. Poorly differentiated adenocarcinoma: Smaller glands differing in size and form and sometimes without discernible lumen. The epithelium sometimes seems multilayered. The epithelial cells are cuboidal and without polarity.

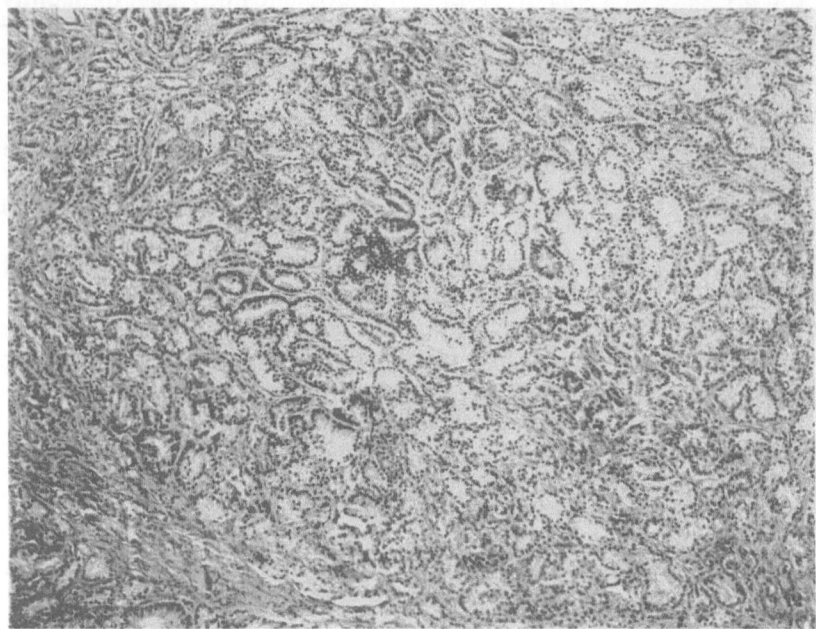

Fig. 2.1. Carcinoma of the prostate, well differentiated. The tumor consists principally of small glands. AFIP Neg. 86-7295; H&E, × 60.

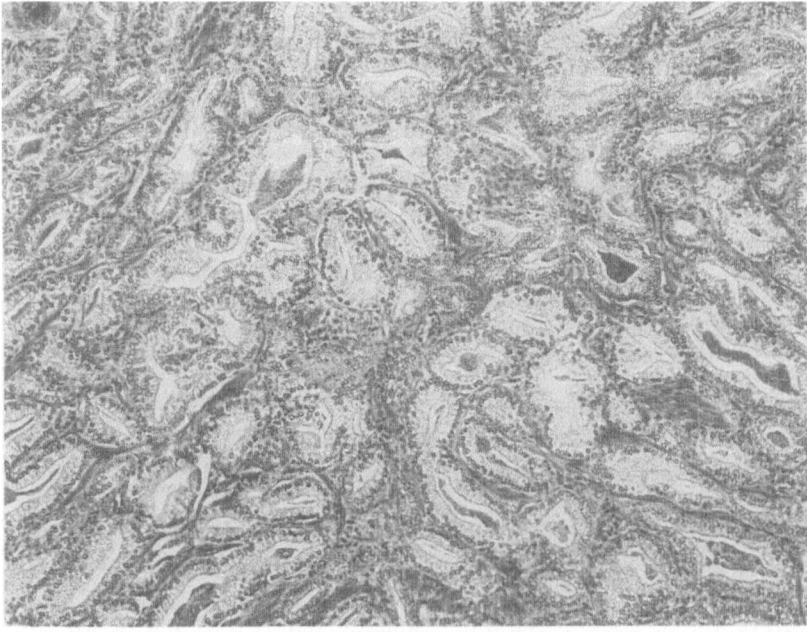

Fig. 2.2. Carcinoma of the prostate, well differentiated. The tumor consists principally of large acini. AFIP Neg. 86-7296; H&E, × 100.

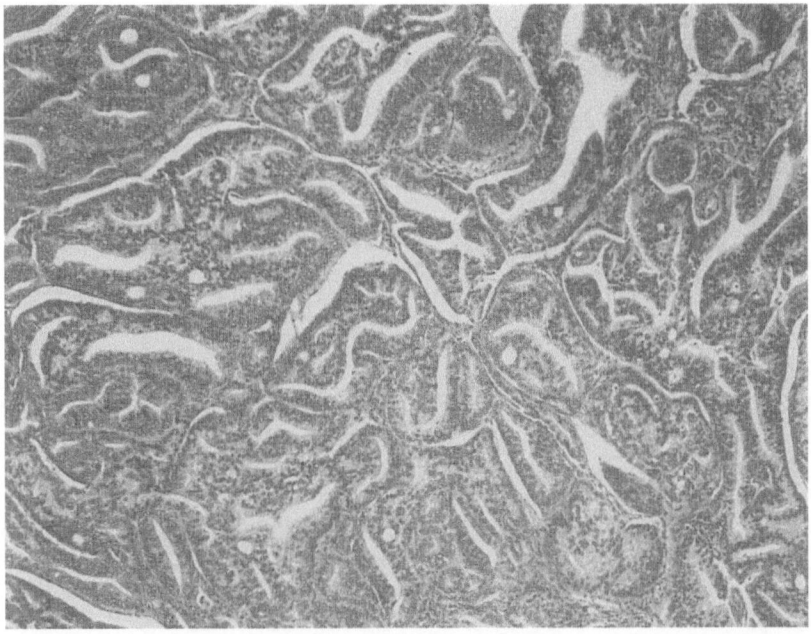

Fig. 2.3. Carcinoma of the prostate, moderately differentiated. The tumor forms glands in glands. AFIP Neg. 86-7297; H&E, × 60.

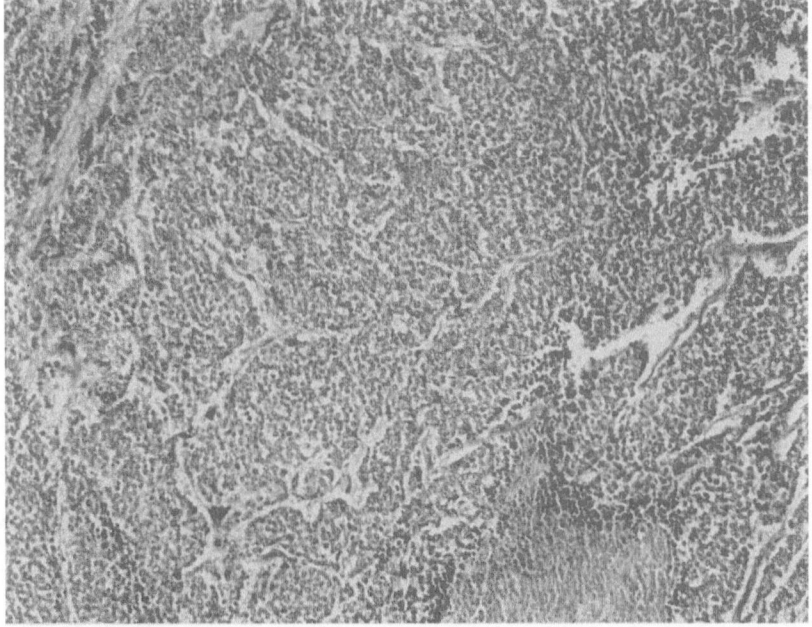

Fig. 2.4. Carcinoma of the prostate, poorly differentiated. The tumor forms solid sheets with rare gland formation. AFIP Neg. 86-7298; H&E, × 100.

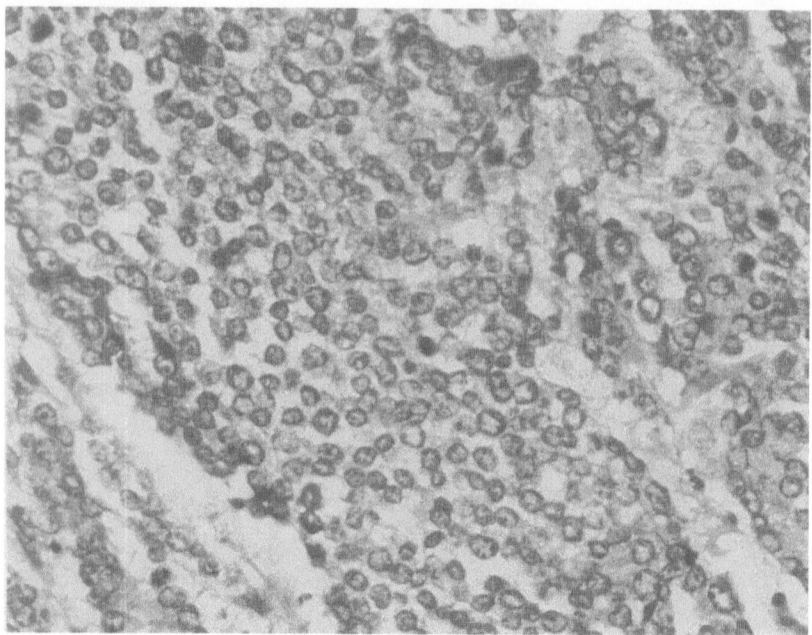

Fig. 2.5. Carcinoma of the prostate, nuclear grade I. The nuclei vary slightly from the normal. AFIP Neg. 86-7299; H&E, × 400.

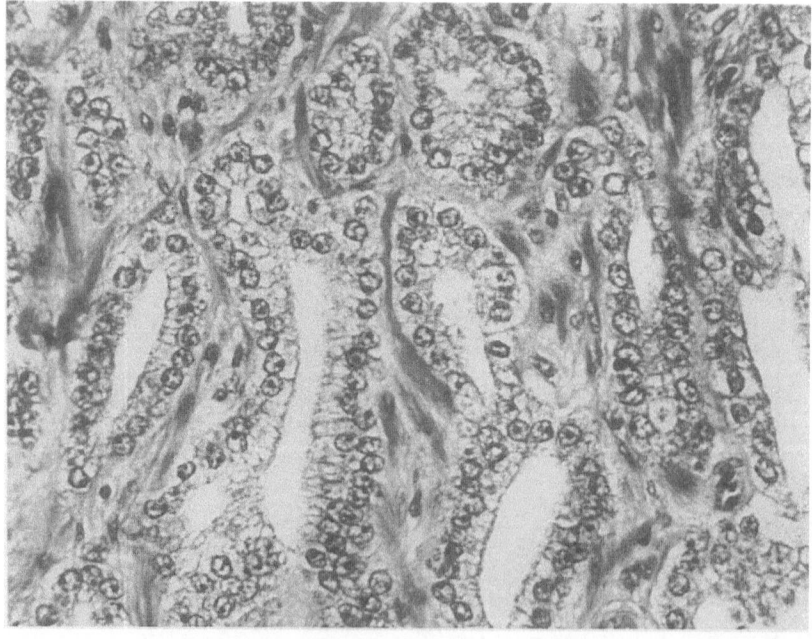

Fig. 2.6. Carcinoma of the prostate, nuclear grade II. The nuclei vary moderately from the normal. AFIP Neg. 86-7300; H&E, × 400.

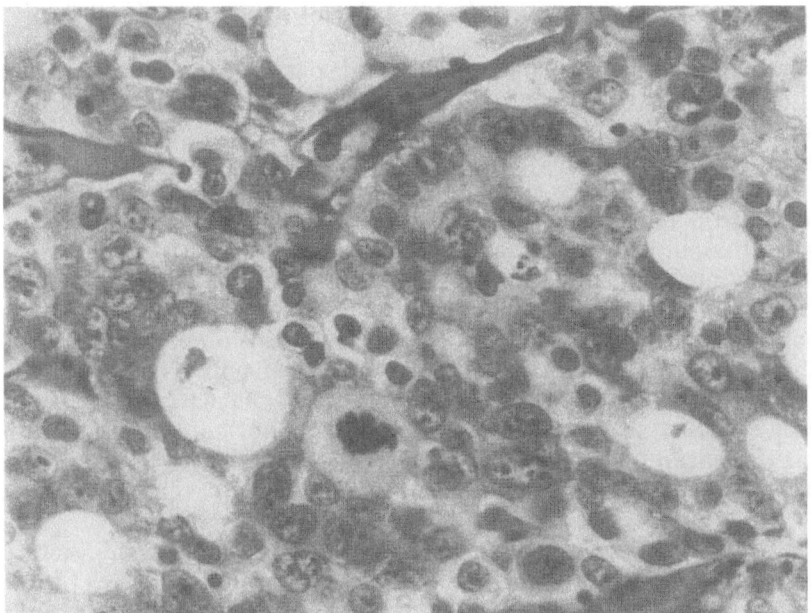

Fig. 2.7. Carcinoma of the prostate. Nuclear grade III. The nuclei vary markedly from the normal. AFIP Neg. 86-7301; H&E, × 400.

3. Cribriform adenocarcinoma: Sieve-like epithelial formations containing no connective tissue, with multiple gland-like lumina (gland in gland) and completely surrounded by stroma.
4. Solid undifferentiated adenocarcinoma: Gland formation is no longer demonstrable, growth is in solid balls or cords of cells or individual cells.

Rating numbers of 1–4 were assigned to these growth patterns in the above order.

Three grades of nuclear anaplasia were distinguished:

1. Mild nuclear anaplasia: Small nuclei of uniform size with no or small nucleoli.
2. Moderate nuclear anaplasia: Medium sized nuclei and nucleoli with moderate variation of nuclear and nucleolar size.
3. Marked nuclear anaplasia: Large nuclei and nucleoli with marked variation of nuclear and nucleolar size.

The combined grade of CaP resulted from adding the rating number of histologic growth pattern to the rating number of nuclear anaplasia. The sum of rating numbers 2–3 corresponded to grade I, 4–5 to grade II, and 6–7 to grade III. Combined grade I was seen in 8%, grade II in 57%, and grade III in 35% of cases. Four percent of those patients were stage A, as staged according to the staging system of Flocks et al (1969), 23% were stage B, 45% stage C, and 18% stage D. Ten percent were incidental carcinomas.

None of the patients with combined grade I CaP but 35% of grade III cases had metastases . Fifty-three percent of patients with grade III carcinoma had metastases at the time of admission.

The survival probability of patients with well differentiated adenocarcinoma, as reported by these authors, was not significantly different from that of healthy age-matched control males, whereas all other histologic grades revealed a significantly decreased probability of survival. The survival probability of patients with slight nuclear anaplasia was significantly lower than that of patients with the other two grades of nuclear anaplasia. The three different combined histologic malignancy grades differed significantly from each other. The survival time was significantly reduced in patients with grade II and III carcinomas. These comments were valid when the probabilities were calculated for patients who had received essentially the same therapy, either hormonal, surgical, or both. Patients with distant metastases and grade III CaP died in 4 years after the diagnosis was made, whereas those with grade II CaP lived an average of 1 year longer.

Böcking et al. (1982) have recorded a remarkable ease of learning and a significant level of reproducibility using the two systems. The same slides of 100 of their cases were graded by three pathologists and one semi-skilled young physician. For instruction the pathologists received, in writing only, the grading system with no verbal feedback (i.e., no tutorial of any type). The person untrained in histologic diagnostic procedures was, in addition, trained by the senior author.

Grading of the same tumor by the author, 3 months later, resulted in the same grade in 87.5% of cases. This intra-observer reproducibility was 85.5% for histologic and 73.5% for cytologic results. In 95% of cases the senior author agreed with the tumor grade that was most often assigned by all the investigators. The other investigators agreed with the grading system results in 86% on an average. When the different grading results were compared against the diagnosis with highest degree of accordance, the mean interobserver reproducibility was 91%. The person especially trained for this grading, although inexperienced in histologic diagnosis, achieved an 87% agreement.

This study has provided a numerical grading system using the WHO–Mostofi system—eliminating the justifiable criticism of its absence in that system.

While Gaeta et al. (1980), Gaeta (1981), and Brawn et al. (1982) did not report on reproducibility in as much detail as Böcking et al., their systems seem to be easily learned and readily reproducible.

Guinan et al. (1982) evaluated three prognostic systems (Gleason classification, Whitmore staging, and Broders grading) in 93 patients. Disease-free survivals correlated with a lower Gleason classification, Whitmore staging, and Broders grades. The correlation between the various systems and disease-free status showed no statistically significant differences between Gleason, Whitmore, or Broders systems and presence of absence of disseminated prostatic carcinoma. The overall accuracy of the Whitmore and Broders systems exceeded that of the Gleason classification. These authors concluded that the Gleason classification system has no prognostic advantage over other commonly employed systems.

In a letter to the Editors, Byar (1983) made some interesting comments on the Guinan et al. report. Cutting the Gleason score between 6 and 7 rather than between 5 and 6, the accuracy rate of the Gleason system would be greater than that reported for the Broders system (85% vs 76%), From the data presented, Byar calculated the sensitivity of the Gleason system to be greater than that of the Broders system (87% vs 62%). This would mean that of patients whose cancers are known to have progressed, a much greater proportion were Gleason's 6–10 than Broders III and IV. On the other hand, the accuracy of the Broders system is greater than the Gleason system in these data because its specificity is greater. This would mean that of those patients who have not yet shown signs of progression (but may later), a higher proportion are Gleason 6–10 than Broders III or IV. Simplified, the Broders system predicted that 68% of the patients' cancers would not progress and so far 65% have not progressed, so the Broders system applied to these data is likely to have greater accuracy for this system alone. Byar noted that in this context sensitivity could be more important than specificity.

Myers et al. (1982) reported preliminary findings on 13 patients with micrometastasis to pelvic lymph nodes treated with radical prostatectomy and pelvic lymphadenectomy but no adjuvant hormonal therapy. The patients were followed until the documented appearance of metastasis to bone or soft tissue. Sections from the initial lesion stained with hematoxylin and eosin and examined under the light microscope revealed that the nucleoli in the primary Gleason pattern were prominent or intermediate (regardless of the Gleason grade) in nine cases and the mean interval to progression was shorter in the group of four patients in whom nucleoli were judged to be not prominent.

The Need for a New Approach in Pathologic Prognostication

This review has demonstrated that the Gleason system is not easily learned, is not easily reproducible even in Gleason's own hands, and does not consistently correlate with clinical and pathologic staging. Its current use in many hospitals is simply because NPCP has required its use. The other systems, based on anaplasia and/or differentiation, are demonstrably easier to learn, easier to reproduce, and have as good, if not better, correlation between clinical behavior and pathologic grading.

Grading, whether based on growth pattern or anaplasia and differentiation, is of limited value. In fact, all grading systems going back to Broders' (1925) have the following deficiencies:

1. They are all subjective to varying degrees—they depend essentially on the mood of the pathologist.
2. In varying degrees they all recognize good tumors and bad tumors, but most of the patients are in the intermediate group.
3. In all grading systems it is assumed that each grade has a monomorphous cell population. There is strong evidence that this is not the case.

4. In their report of the NPCP endorsement of Gleason system, Murphy and Whitmore (1979) pointed out that at the present level of information no grading system reliably predicts the lethal potential of a tumor in an individual patient nor the responsiveness of an individual tumor to various forms of therapy and cautioned against the use of tumor grade in an individual patient as a basis for treatment. These observations, which are often ignored, are as pertinent today (1987) as they were in 1979.

It has been demonstrated that the Gleason system, as presently advocated, is less sensitive and specific than Broders' grading system based on differentiation (Guinan et al. 1982) or the WHO system, based on combined differentiation and anaplasia (Böcking et al. 1982; Epstein et al. 1984).

We concur with Albertsen (1982) that what the urologist needs is reliable information from the pathologist which can help him in the management of the specific patient with CaP. Since the behavior of a tumor in an individual patient is based almost entirely on the interplay between the neoplastic cell and the host (and probably to a lesser extent on what the surgeon does other than the surgical removal of the tumor), the most productive line of approach would seem to be the study of the tumor cell: the nucleus, the nucleolus, the cytoplasm, the nuclear and cell membranes, and the epithelial stromal interaction. Regrettably, the endorsement of the Gleason system by the NPCP has tended to discourage an active role by pathologists in investigating these parameters as the Gleason system of grading CaP has come to be regarded as the finale of pathologists' contribution to the management of patient with CaP. Fortunately, there have been a few exceptions.

In 52 patients with localized and metastatic adenocarcinoma of the prostate, Tannenbaum et al. (1982) measured nucleolar surface area by stereoscopically analyzing pictures obtained by the backscattered electron imaging attachment to a scanning electron microscope. The data were compared with the Gleason grading system. In patients with no evidence of disease 3 years or more after radical prostatectomy, the initial biopsy demonstrated nucleolar surface areas which averaged $1.28 \ \mu m^2$ (range $0.60-2.27 \ \mu m^2$) whereas patients with metastasis or dying of cancer exhibited an average nucleolar surface area of $5.17 \ \mu m^2$ (range $2.49-10.01$). With a single exception in this 52 patient survey, progressive disease was always accompanied by nucleolar surface area measurements larger than $2.40 \ \mu m^2$. There was close correlation in nucleolar surface measurements between the initial biopsy and the radical prostatectomy specimens; in contrast, Gleason grades varied by more than 30% between the initial and final specimens in 70% of the cases. Only 9 of 16 patients with aggressive disease (initial biopsy and radical prostatectomy) ever demonstrated Gleason grades above 6.

Diamond et al. (1982) analyzed the changes in size and shape of tumor nuclei. The shape and morphology of nuclei were determined by computer-assisted image analysis using fixed sections studied at light microscopic level. Prior to undertaking the study they selected ten patients with Hopkins grades 1 and 2 (Jewett et al. 1968) stage B disease.

Four of the ten patients developed metastasis 9 years or less postoperatively, and six lived for over 15 years without evidence of metastatic disease. Multiple sections from each were image analyzed for number of nucleoli per nucleus, nucleolar area as percentage of nucleus, total nucleolar area, nuclear area, nuclear circumference, and nuclear roundness factor. The nuclear roundness factor clearly separated the group of patients with stage B_1 disease without identifiable preoperative metastasis who demonstrated metastasis post-prostatectomy from that group who lived for more than 15 years without evidence of metastatic disease.

The mean nuclear roundness factor of all malignant nuclei was 1.059, whereas the mean roundness factor of all normal epithelial nuclei was 1.034. Comparison of the nuclear roundness factor of cancer nuclei in those who had metastasized and those who were alive and well 14 years later showed a mean roundness factor of 1.069 for the former and 1.047 for the latter. No overlap between the groups for any individual value was seen. In contrast, the mean roundness factor of the normal nuclei was identical for the two groups.

Because of concern regarding the uniformity of tissue fixation and their observation that the nuclear roundness factor of normal tissue varied from patient to patient, they calculated a relative nuclear roundness factor for each patient. The relative nuclear roundness factor was defined as the quotient of the cancer nuclear roundness factor divided by the roundness factor of that patient's normal epithelial nuclear roundness factor measured within the same section. The mean relative nuclear roundness factor of those patients who were alive and well for more than 14 years postoperatively was 1.013. The mean relative roundness factor for those patients who had metastasis was 1.034.

The authors found that while comparison of nuclear areas did demonstrate a difference between malignant and normal prostatic epithelial nuclei, one could not distinguish metastasizing tumors from nonmetastasizing ones. Either absolute or relative nuclear roundness factor did discriminate between the two, but the authors preferred relative nuclear roundness as this took into account the adjacent normal epithelial nuclei.

Epstein et al. (1984) evaluated the nuclear roundness factor and attempted to correlate it to the Gleason system. They selected 19 patients with stage A_2 disease who had received no treatment until clinical progression of the disease was evident. They found that nuclear roundness factor clearly identified those tumors that clinically progressed without treatment and those that did not, in contrast to the Gleason system, which produced significant prognostic overlap. What separated most of these tumors was the quantification and degree of irregularity of a relatively small subpopulation of cancer nuclei among a majority of rounder nuclei.

The advantages of quantitative morphometric shape analysis include accuracy, reproducibility, applicability to needle biopsies, and ability to generate a number that describes the morphology of an individual patient's cancer; in addition, of course, the computer can store and recall data. To date, however, the number of cases studied is small.

Heterogeneity of Cytoplasmic Contents

These studies have focused attention on the heterogeneity of the nucleus. There is another point to consider—the heterogeneity of the cytoplasm.

By light microscopy as many as five different cells may be recognized: clear cells, dark cells, eosinophilic cells, vacuolated cells, and cells with amphophilic cytoplasm. Most, if not all, tumors show at least two, and often more cell types. The clinical significance of this has not been investigated.

Kastendieck and Altenahr (1976) studied 28 histologically proven CaPs ultrastructurally. Five different cell types were found: undifferentiated; embryonic tumor cells; immature tumor cells with a beginning glandular differentiation; highly differentiated glandular tumor cells, functionally deranged glandular tumor cells with cytoplasm overloaded by organelles; and degenerative tumor cells. Typical basal cells could be found in some carcinomas. These authors did not relate the cell type to behavior or response to treatment.

Sinha et al. (1977) compared the ultrastructure features of 22 CaPs (14 untreated, 8 treated with 1–5 mg diethylstilbestrol daily and 30 mg Provera daily for varying lengths of time). The tumors possessed well and poorly differentiated acini and invasive cells. Malignant acini contained numerous columnar (secretory) cells in untreated but few treated patients.

Two distinct basal cells were observed in both groups: type I (light) and type II (dark) cells. In both untreated and treated tumors, type I cells were characterized by having round nuclei with many small aggregates of euchromatin, large nucleoli, and electron-lucent nucleoplasm. Type II cells had highly pleomorphic nuclei, folded nuclear envelope, sometimes deficient in localized areas, euchromatin, many small aggregates of heterochromatin, large pleomorphic nucleoli, and relatively electron-opaque nucleoplasm. Both cells were invasive. CaPs which were or subsequently became refractory to estrogen showed more abundant type II basal cells than did responsive CaPs. Sinha et al. postulated that the type II basal cells as well as some type I basal cells are endocrine unresponsive from the outset.

The heterogeneity of the cytoplasm is best appreciated with application of immunopathology. In studies of several hundred CaPs we have found that all grades of carcinoma have some cells that are negative for prostatic acid phosphatase and prostatic specific antigen, others that are strongly positive, and still others that are weakly positive. Furthermore, some carcinoma cells may be positive for one and negative for the other, positive for both, or negative for both. In histologically undifferentiated tumors (tumors that do not form glands), cells that are identical with H&E stain may be negative, slightly positive, or strongly positive with either one or the other, and sometimes with both of these markers. To date these observations have not been related to the response to therapy or to survival.

Studies of estrogen, androgen, and other receptors have not as yet proven helpful.

Future Perspectives

Since in most instances it is the metastasis that kills the patient and metastases occur as a result of the invasive and metastatic potential of the neoplastic cell, it would seem obvious that we must study the individual cell, and that in each low-grade tumor we must look for, identify, and quantitate the relatively small clone or clones that have aggressive, invasive, and metastatic potential. These clones are often overlooked in low-grade tumors. In the intermediate and high-grade tumors what is needed is the recognition of clones of cells that will respond to a specific form of therapy. There are other features that we need to study but these are the most important. Over-emphasis on grading has resulted in diverting the necessary attention and support that are needed for the study of the CaP cells. Until this is done, we will not be in a position to identify the tumor that could be left alone or given a specific form of therapy designed for that specific cell type.

The introduction of fine needle aspiration, which is commonly used in Europe, especially in Scandinavia, and is being employed in North America, will be the death knell of any diagnostic and grading system that is not based on the cell type as such aspirations rarely include glands, let alone enough tissue to identify the growth pattern of the tumor.

References

Albertsen P (1982) Histologic grading and the practicing urologist. Prostate 3:333–338

Bagshaw MA (1984) Radiotherapy of prostatic cancer: Stanford University experience. In: Kurth KH, Dubruyne FM et al. (eds) Progress and controversies in oncological urology. Alan B. Liss, New York p 493

Barzell W, Bean MA, Hilaris BS, Whitmore WF (1977) Prostatic adenocarcinoma: relationship of grade and local extent to the pattern of metastases. J Urol 118:278–282

Böcking A, Kiehn J, Heinzel-Wach M (1982) Combined histologic grading of prostatic carcinoma. Cancer 50:288–294

Brawn PN, Ayala AA, von Eschenbach AC, Hussey DH, Johnson DE (1982) Histologic grading study of prostatic adenocarcinoma. The development of a new system and comparison with other methods. Cancer 49:113–120

Broders AC (1925) The grading of carcinoma. Minn Med 8:726–730

Byar DP (1983) Grading prostatic cancers. Letter to the editors. Urology 22:462–463

Cantrell BB, DeKlerk DP, Eggleston JC, Boinott JK, Walsh PC (1981) Pathological factors that influence prognosis in stage A prostatic cancer: the influence of extent versus grade. J Urol 125:516–520

Corriere JN, Cornog JL, Murphy JJ (1970) Prognosis in patients with carcinoma of the prostate. Cancer 25:911–918

Cupps RE, Utz DC, Fleming TR, Carson CC, Zincke H (1980) Definitive radiation therapy for prostatic carcinoma: Mayo Clinic experience. J Urol 124:855–859

Diamond DA, Berry SJ, Umbricht C, Jewett HJ, Coffey DC (1982) Computerized image analysis of nuclear shape as a prognostic factor for prostatic cancer. Prostate 3:321–332

Donohue RE, Fauver HE, Whitesel JA, Augspurger RR (1981) Prostatic carcinoma: influence of tumor grade on results of pelvic lymphadenectomy. Urology 17:435–440

Epstein JI, Berry SJ, Eggleston JC (1984) Nuclear roundness factor. A predictor of progression in untreated stage A2 prostatic cancer. Cancer 54:1666–1671

Flocks RH (1969) Carcinoma of the prostate. J Urol 101:741–749

Fowler JE, Whitmore WF (1981) The incidence and extent of pelvic lymph node metastases in apparently localized prostatic cancer. Cancer 47:2941–2945

Gaeta JF (1981) Glandular profiles and cellular patterns in prostatic cancer grading. Urology [Suppl] 17:33–37

Gaeta JF, Asirwatham JE, Miller G, Murphy GP (1980) Histologic grading of primary prostatic cancer: a new approach to an old problem. J Urol 123:689–693

Gleason DF (1966) Classification of prostatic carcinomas. Cancer Chemother Rep 50:125–128

Gleason DF (1977) Histologic grading and clinical staging of prostatic carcinoma. In: Tannenbaum M (ed) Urologic pathology: the prostate. Lea & Febiger, Philadelphia, pp 171–198

Gleason DF, Mellinger GT, The Veterans' Administration Cooperative Urological Research Group (1974) Prediction of prognosis for prostatic adenocarcinoma and combined histological grading and clinical staging. J Urol 111:58–64

Grayhack JT, Assimos DG (1983) Prognostic significance of tumor grade and stage in patients with carcinoma of the prostate. Prostate 4:13–31

Guinan P, Ray V, Totonchi E, Bush I (1982) An evaluation of the Gleason classification system in prostatic carcinoma. In: Proceedings of the 77th Annual Meeting of the American Urological Association, Kansas City, 16–20 May 1982. American Urological Association, Baltimore, 131 (abstr)

Harada M, Mostofi FK, Corle DK, Byar DP, Trump BF (1977) Preliminary studies of histological prognosis in cancer of the prostate. Cancer Treat Rep 61:223–225

Jewett HJ, Bridge RW, Gray SF Jr, Shelly WM (1968) The palpable nodule of prostatic cancer. Results 15 years after radical excision. JAMA 203:403–406

Kastendieck H, Altenahr E (1976) Cyto- and histo-morphogenesis of the prostatic carcinoma. A comparative light and electron microscopic study. Virchows Arch [A] 370:207–224

Kramer SA, Spahr J, Brendler CG, Glenn JR, Paulson DF (1980) Experience with Gleason's histopathologic grading in prostatic cancer. J Urol 124:223–225

Kramer SA, Cline WA, Farnham R, Carson CC, Cox EB, Hinshaw W, Paulson DF (1981) Prognosis of patients with stage D_1 prostatic adenocarcinoma. J Urol 125:817–819

Mellinger GT (1977) Prognosis of prostatic carcinoma. In: Grundmann E, Vahlsieck W (eds) Tumors of the male genital system. Springer, Berlin Heidelberg New York, pp 61–72 (Recent results in cancer research, vol 60)

Mellinger GT, Gleason DF, Bailar J III (1967) The histology and prognosis of prostatic cancer. J Urol 97:331–337

Mostofi FK (1976) Problems of grading carcinoma of prostate. Semin Oncol 3: 161–169

Mostofi FK (1980) Pathology and staging in prostatic carcinoma. In: Proceedings of the 66th Scientific Assembly and Annual Meeting of the Radiological Society of North America, Inc., Oak Brook, Ill. 16–21 November 1980

Mostofi FK, Price EB Jr (1973) Tumors of the male genital system, Fasc 8. Atlas of tumor pathology, 2nd series, Armed Forces Institute of Pathology, Washington DC

Mostofi FK, Sesterhenn I, Sobin LH (1980) International histological classification of prostatic tumors. WHO, Geneva

Murphy GP, Whitmore WF (1979) A report of the workshops on the current status of the histologic grading of prostate cancer. Cancer 44:1490–1494

Myers RP, Neves RJ, Farrow GM, Utz DC (1982) Nucleolar grading of prostatic adenocarcinoma: light microscopic correlation with disease progression. Prostate 3:423–432

Olsson CA (1985) Staging lymphadenectomy should be an antecedent to treatment in localized prostatic carcinoma. Urology [Suppl] 25:4–6

Pistenma DA, Bagshaw MA, Freiha FS (1979) Extended-field radiation therapy for prostatic adenocarcinoma: status report of a limited prospective trial. In: Johnson DE, Samuels ML (eds) Cancer of genitourinary tract. Raven Press, New York, p 229

Prout GR Jr, Heaney JA, Griffin PP, Daly JJ, Shipley WU (1980) Nodal involvement as a prognostic indicator in patients with prostatic carcinoma. J Urol 124:226–231

Schroeder FH, Blom JHM, Hop WJC, Mostofi FK (1982) Grading of prostatic carcinoma—an evaluation of 346 patients. In: Proceedings of the 77th Annual Meeting of the American Urological Association, Kansas City, 16–20 May 1982. American Urological Association, Baltimore, 131 (abstr)

Sinha AA, Blackard CE, Seal US (1977) A critical analysis of tumor morphology and hormone treatments in the untreated and estrogen-treated response and refractory human prostatic carcinoma. Cancer 40:2836–2850

Smith JA, Middleton RG (1985) Implications of volume of nodal metastasis in patients with adenocarcinoma of the prostate. J Urol 133:617–619

Tannenbaum M, Tannenbaum S, DeSandis PN, Olson CA (1982) Prognostic significance of nucleolar surface area in prostatic cancer. Urology 19:546–551

Wilson JWL, Morales A, Bruce AW (1983) The prognostic significance of pathological grading and pathological staging in carcinoma of prostate. J Urol 130:481–483

Chapter 3

Tumor Markers in Prostatic Disease

A. W. Bruce and B. K. Choe

Introduction

One of the current problems in the diagnosis of prostatic cancer is that there is no procedure which can detect early localized disease curable by surgery and that truly localized cancers can only be detected by rectal examination in 10%–20% of patients. Another problem is the variability of the natural history of the disease. Clinically, some tumors remain localized for long periods, producing few, if any symptoms or signs, and others disseminate widely before symptoms are manifested. Due to this, numerous grading systems, as well as highly sophisticated cytometric systems, have been introduced to correlate the morphologic parameters of the cancer cells with their biologic characteristics, such as growth rate and metastatic potential. In addition, various biochemical or immunochemical markers have been researched in the past, and some of the molecular markers of prostatic cancer have found a place in the clinical laboratory (Benson and Coffey 1983; Whitmore 1984).

Tumor markers may be defined as cellular expressions, either structural or molecular, which can identify the proliferative and/or metastatic behavior of the particular tumor. Metabolites or gene products of tumors can serve as markers, if these molecules are tumor specific. In addition, even if certain metabolites or gene products are produced by normal cells as well as by tumor cells, as long as they do not normally appear in the circulation their detection in the serum will signify the breakdown of the normal tissue barrier. Prostatic acid phosphatase and prostate-specific antigen are examples of such molecules. Further, the invasive growth of tumors often disrupts the normal enzyme profile and metabolic pattern of the surrounding tissue cells, compressed by the tumor burden, and these alterations in the adjacent cells may also serve as markers of metastatic behavior. Serum alkaline phosphatase and urine hydroxyproline are examples of such markers and may be useful in the detection of bone metastases of prostatic origin.

In the normal prostate, the boundary between glandular epithelial cells and stromal cells is the basement membrane, a resilient and stable structural barrier with a slow turnover rate. The intact basement membrane does not contain pores large enough for large protein molecules to diffuse through. Ultrastructural studies (Brandes et al. 1964: Kirckheim et al. 1974) have shown that the greater portion of the basement membrane is actually the external wall at the nonluminal outer surface of the plasma membrane of the basal cells.

The hallmark of early malignancy is the absence of basal cells and the loss of basement membrane. Histopathologically, the glands are seen back to back in a glandular arrangement, but there is usually deletion of stromal cells between those glands (Mostofi and Price 1973: Tannenbaum 1977). It is thus possible that molecular markers expressed at a localized stage of the disease become detectable, since the basement membrane may have undergone localized degradation by a compressive effect or by actual invasion by tumor cells. The problem which limits early detection of these markers is the extent of tumor mass synthesizing these molecules, the diffusion process, the half-life of the molecules, and ultimately the assay methods.

In this chapter, an overview will be presented of markers of prostatic cancer that are useful in clinical investigations. Due to the substantial amount of literature in this area, reference will be made, when appropriate, to recent reviews in which further details may be found. We ask the indulgence of our colleagues in Urology: the required brevity of this article has enforced arbitrary choices of references and simplifications.

Prostatic Acid Phosphatase

Prostatic Acid Phosphatase as a Prostatic Cancer Marker

The role of prostatic acid phosphatase (PAPase) as a marker of prostatic cancer was first recognized by Gutman and Gutman in the late 1930s. They demonstrated a marked increase in the enzymatic hydrolysis of the organic phosphates at acidic pH in the serum of prostatic cancer patients. In the 1940s, Huggins and Hodges showed that prostatic cancer was hormonally dependent and that serum acid phosphatase activity was decreased in men with prostatic carcinoma after castration or estrogen treatment. Since then serum acid phosphatase has been extensively evaluated as a marker of prostatic cancer. As acid phosphatases are widely distributed in all human body fluids and tissues, a great deal of effort was directed, during the 1940s and 1950s, toward the discovery of specific substrates or inhibitors which defined acid phosphatases of prostatic origin. L-Tartrate was identified as a specific inhibitor of PAPase (Fishman et al. 1953) and Shulman et al. (1964) discovered an acid phosphatase specific to the prostate. This work became the basis for extensive immunochemical studies and the development of immunoassays during the 1970s.

Human cells contain the genetic information for several acid phosphatases, some coded for by single genes and some by multigene families. The red cell acid phosphatase gene (ACP-1 on chromosome 2) codes for a low molecular weight (15 000–20 000 daltons) protein with distinctive catalytic characteristics. The lysosomal acid phosphatase gene (ACP-2 on chromosome 11) codes for a 90 000-to 100 000-dalton protein synthesized by most differentiated cells and stored in the lysosomes. The genetic arrangement of this locus is complex, since most cells, such as megakaryocytes, granulocytes, lymphocytes, osteoclasts, and epithelial cells of the liver and kidney, express more than one acid phosphatase isoenzyme. Serum acid phosphatase is made up of a mixture of acid phosphatases from several cell types (Brock and Mayo 1978).

Human PAPase is unique in a number of ways:

1. It is immunochemically distinct from lysosomal isoenzymes and is not synthesized by other epithelial cells of nonprostatic origin.
2. It is synthesized and secreted as a result of androgen stimulation, and its synthesis ceases after antiandrogen treatment.
3. It does not appear in the circulation without disruption of the boundary between epithelial cells and glandular epithelial cells and stroma. When cancer cells arise and proliferate in the prostate, most of them appear to retain their differentiated functions, including the expression of steroid hormone receptors and the production of PAPase. As cancer cells proliferate, however, loss of polarity of the epithelium and organelles and invasion of the basement membrane and lymphatic channels by the tumor ultimately lead to a leakage of PAPase into the general circulation. Serum PAPase level should, therefore, serve as an indicator of the invasive behavior of the prostatic carcinoma cells.

Biochemical and Immunochemical Characteristics

Prostatic acid phosphatase has been purified from both the prostate and seminal plasma. PAPase is a glycoprotein with a molecular weight of about 100 000, consisting of two identical subunits of approximately 50 000 daltons each. The carbohydrate content accounts for 7%–10% of the molecular weight. Due to the heterogeneity of this carbohydrate moiety, PAPase can be separated into several electrophoretic variants, with isoelectric points (pI) between 4.2 and 5.5 on isoelectric focusing. No enzymatic or antigenic differences have been recognized among the electrophoretic variants of PAPase. Most of the enzymatic activity and antigenicity of native PAPase is lost upon dissociation into its subunits. The biochemical and antigenic characteristics of PAPase have been reviewed (Lin et al. 1980; Ostrowski 1980; Choe and Rose 1982).

Antiserum raised against purified PAPase exhibits immunologic reactivity only with PAPase of prostate tissue extract, and not with extracts from other tissues. Recently, Lee et al. (1982) generated murine monoclonal antibodies against PAPase, and identified three different antigenic determinants on the PAPase molecule. Lillehoj et al. (1982) also produced murine monoclonal antibodies which identified three nonoverlapping antigenic determinants on one domain of PAPase. Structural studies have also revealed that the PAPase molecule may consist of three domains, one of which may contain the active site of the enzyme, as well as the antigenic determinant that cross-reacts with lysosomal acid phosphatase (Choe et al. 1982).

Serum Level

Enzymatic Methods

Until a decade ago, normal ranges of acid phosphatase activity in serum or plasma depended on the substrate used; therefore, a wide range of normal values was described in the literature. This has compromised the comparison of published data. In most automated assay systems presently in use, α-naphthol phosphate or thymophthalein monophosphate has been used as a substrate and L(+)-tartrate as the inhibitor. The technical aspects of the various biochemical assays of acid phosphatase activity have been discussed previously (Bodansky 1972; Sodeman and Batsakis 1977; Prellwitz and Ehrenthal 1982).

A large number of reports have been published concerning the clinical significance of acid phosphatase activity levels in the serum of patients with carcinoma of the prostate. Normal ranges of serum acid phosphatase activity and the percentage of prostatic cancer patients with elevated serum levels are summarized in Tables 3.1 and 3.2.

Table 3.1. Normal ranges of serum acid phosphatase activity

Total	Tartarate-inhibitable	Substrate	Source
0.5–5.0 King-Armstrong U/dl	0–0.5 King-Armstrong U/dl	Phenylphosphate	Fishman et al. (1953)
1.2–2.5 King-Armstrong U/dl	0–0.6 King-Armstrong U/dl	Phenylphosphate	Murphy et al. (1969)
1–2.5 IU/ml		α-Naphthylphosphate	Bruce et al. (1979)
0–0.8 IU/l		Thymolphthalein-monophosphate	Pontes et al. (1978)

Table 3.2. Total and tartarate-inhibitable acid phosphatase activity in the sera of prostatic cancer patients[a]

Patient category	Total acid phosphates (%)	Tartarate-inhibitable acid phosphatase (%)
Benign hyperplasia	2–7	0
Cancer confined to prostate	5–10	5–12
Cancer beyond capsule	10–30	2.4–40
Cancer with bone metastases	60–90	48–90

[a]Data compiled from: Nesbit et al. 1951; Fishman et al. 1953; Mathes et al. 1956; Nobles et al. 1957; Cook et al. 1962; Murphy et al. 1969; Townsend 1977.

Immunologic Methods

In 1960, Flocks and his group produced antibodies against human prostatic tissue. Subsequently, Shulman et al. (1964) described PAPase as the tissue-specific antigen of the prostate. Interest was then focused on the purification and antigenicity of human PAPase, and attempts were made to develop immunologic assays for the enzyme. There are two types of PAPase assays—competitive binding assays and binding assays. Radioimmunoassays are examples of competitive binding assays while counter immunoelectrophoresis, the solid phase immunoadsorbent assay, enzyme immunoassay, and the sandwich type enzyme immunoassay utilize binding assay technology. Details of these methods have been reviewed (Choe and Rose 1982; Chu 1981).

Clinical Application

Specificity and Sensitivity

The clinical application of PAPase immunoassays has been discussed in depth elsewhere (Bruce and Mahan 1982; Prellwitz and Ehrenthal 1982). We will summarize previously discussed data, in addition to reviewing some of the more recent findings.

The normal range of PAPase values obtained by immunologic assays (Table 3.3), are somewhat variable due to technologic and methodologic differences among investigators. Presently, several commercial kits are available, and comparison of assay results has become more meaningful. The value of immunologic assays in relation to enzymatic assays becomes evident from examination of the specificity and sensitivity of each method. Specificity refers to the percentage of normal values in patients without disease while sensitivity is defined as the percentage of elevated values among patients with disease. A few investigators (Foti et al. 1977; Griffiths 1980; Lee et al. 1980; Bruce et al. 1979) compared immunologic assays with enzymatic methods and the results are summarized in Table 3.4. For those patients with benign prostatic hyperplasia (BPH) or nonprostatic cancers, the specificity for the two types of assay is quite similar. However, according to the data shown in Table 3.4 the sensitivity of immunoassays is higher than that of enzymatic assays. This claim continues to be the subject of some controversy.

Table 3.3. Normal values of serum prostatic acid phosphatase determined by radioimmunoassay

Method	No. of patients	Normal range	Source
Double antibody	385	0.8–6.5 ng/ml	Choe et al. 1980
Solid-phase	200	0.5–7.2 ng/0.1 ml	Cooper et al. 1978 Foti et al. 1977
Double antibody	226	0.75–4.45 ng-ml	Mahan and Doctor 1979
Double antibody	194	1.0–5.0 ng/ml	Prellwitz and Ehrenthal 1982
Double antibody	53	1.0–10.0 ng/ml	Vihko et al. 1978
Double antibody	212	1.5–5.7 ng/ml	New England Nuclear Kit
Solid-phase	197	0–2.0 ng/ml	Mallinckrodt Kit

PAPase Levels vs Stage and Grade of the Prostatic Cancer

For stage A and B disease, the immunologic assays are more sensitive than the enzymatic assays (Table 3.4). Further, when the normal levels are raised to exclude 99.5% of normal men and 95% of the BPH patients, few false-positive values have been observed with stage A and B disease (e.g., Griffiths 1980). Although immunologic assays may detect some patients with intracapsular tumors, Schacht et al. (1984) have stated that false-positives are a major limitation to this test. It would seem that the interpretation of an elevated level of PAPase in apparently localized disease remains very controversial. In clinical

Table 3.4. Specificity and sensitivity of immunologic vs enzymatic assays of acid phosphatase in prostatic diseases

(A) Specificity (percentage of patients with normal PAPase value in the absence of the evidence of prostatic carcinoma)[a]

Total prostatectomy		Benign hyperplasia		Nonprostatic cancer	
I[b]	E[b]	I	E	I	E
100	100	89–91	92–97	86–94	86–100

(B) Sensitivity (percentage of patients with elevated PAPase value with confirmed diagnosis of prostatic carcinoma)[a]

Clinical stage							
A		B		C		D	
I	E	I	E	I	E	I	E
12–74	5–50	32–79	13–15	47–77	23–31	86–92	57–74

[a]Data compiled from: Foti et al. 1977; Griffiths 1980; Lee et al. 1980a; Bruce et al. 1982; Bruce et al. to be published.
[b]I, immunologic assay; E, enzymatic assay.

stage C disease, however, enzymatic assays show the serum PAPase level to be elevated in approximately 23%–31% of patients, while immunologic methods reveal an elevated level in 47%–77%. In stage D disease, 57%–74% of men have increased levels of PAPase by enzymatic assay, whereas 86%–92% of men show elevation by radioimmunoassay. The data compiled by Bruce et al. (to be published) and Bruce and Mahan (1986) clearly indicate that the serum PAPase levels increase with stage (e.g., Table 11.4 in Bruce and Mahan 1986).

Controversy exists regarding the relationship between PAPase secretion and the grade of the primary tumor. In the analysis of PAPase, using our own radioimmunoassay and two commmercial kits (e.g., Table 11.5 in Bruce and Mahan 1986), we found elevated levels associated with primary tumors showing poorly differentiated histologic patterns (range: 7–48 ng/ml for poorly differentiated, 15–100 ng/ml for moderately differentiated, and 12–100 ng/ml for well differentiated). However, large tumors are generally anaplastic and it is necessary to consider not only the grade of the primary tumor but also the metastatic state and the tumor burden.

The role of PAPase immunoassay in the identification of micrometastases seems to require further correlative studies. The prediction of pelvic lymph node involvement, with elevated PAPase as the only index of dissemination, has indicated a 60% incidence using enzymatic assays and an 85% incidence using radioimmunoassay, while the incidence of positive nodes with normal PAPase levels was 22% and 28% respectively (Chatal et al. 1982; Whitesel et al. 1982). Wilson et al. (1983), however, reported poor correlation between PAPase and the presence of positive regional lymph nodes. In Whitesel's series, 79% of patients with persistently elevated PAPase levels had metastases, regardless of the clinical stage of the tumor. It is not clear why patients with lymphatic, soft tissue, and bony metastases frequently exhibit normal serum activities of total and tartrate-labile phosphatases and normal immunoassay values. Probably, in these cases, poorly differentiated tumor cell subpopulations have evolved among the original tumor cell population through the presently unknown mechanisms of tumor cell heterogeneity. It has also been shown by immunoperoxidase techniques that metastatic cells vary markedly in their ability to synthesize PAPase (Mahan et al. 1980). The measurement of bone marrow levels of PAPase has no advantages over serum values due to the fact that its circulation is constantly equilibrated with the general circulation of the blood.

Monitoring and Screening

Several groups have shown that serum PAPase levels are adequate as a monitoring parameter of therapeutic response in prostatic cancer (Killian et al. 1981; Bruce and Mahan 1986; Scardino 1982). If an elevated PAPase level returns to normal as a result of therapy, survival is prolonged. A decrease of 50% in PAPase level results in longer survival times, but the prognosis is not as good as is seen with a decrease to normal levels. A stable or rising PAPase level is an indicator of treatment failure.

Current evidence also indicates that PAPase levels have little value as a screening tool for prostatic cancer in the general population (Cooper and Finkle 1980; Watson and Tang 1980; Fleishman et al. 1982; Bruce and Mahan 1986).

Immunohistology

Immunohistologic application of anti-PAPase antibodies has been useful in identifying PAPase-secreting cells in tissues. Since the prostatic glandular epithelial cells are virtually the only cells producing this enzyme, these antibodies may be useful in identifying metastatic prostatic cancer cells in tissue biopsies. Immunofluorescence (Pontes et al. 1977), the immunoperoxidase method (Jobsis et al. 1978), and the peroxidase–antiperoxidase method (Li et al. 1980) have been used. Li et al. (1980) identified metastatic lesions in all 20 prostatic cancer patients with known primary disease and metastatic lesions in bone marrow, lymph nodes, and lung. In a series of studies done by Yam et al. (1981), this technique yielded a positive result in 114 of 120 deparaffinized prostatic tissue sections, indicating a sensitivity of 96.3%.

In another study (Yam et al. 1983), 21 of 22 bone marrow biopsies of patients with known metastatic prostatic carcinoma showed positive staining; the only patient showing no activity had only two small tumor foci. Finally, of 27 patients with metastatic disease and primary cancer of unknown origin, 14 eventually had positive staining of the metastatic cells, including lesions in the lung, bone, lymph nodes, and large intestine. Adenoid cystic carcinoma of the prostate originates from periurethral glands or metaplastic urethral mucosa and does not synthesize PAPase. Kuhajda and Mann (1984) reported a case of adenoid cystic carcinoma of the prostate and distinguished it from prostatic adenocarcinoma by immunohistologic staining for PAPase and PA. One limitation of the immunohistologic study of PAPase-producing cells is that PAPase secretion often parallels the degree of anaplasia of the tumor. PAPase synthesis is absent in cells of poorly differentiated cancers (Bates et al. 1982; Lippert et al. 1982; Pontes et al. 1982; Yam et al. 1983). In addition to this, background staining of tissues may make interpretation of the result difficult. Within these limitations, the immunohistologic method for detection of PAPase is useful in identifying metastatic prostatic cancer cells in tissue.

Recently, Goldberg and Deland (1984) used radiolabeled anti-PAPase antibodies for nuclear imaging of metastatic prostatic cancer. Human monoclonal antibodies to PAPase have been produced in our laboratory (Yamaura et al. 1985), and their application to the nuclear imaging of tumors is in progress.

Commentary

The development of immunologic assays for PAPase had been expected to become a major tool in the detection of localized adenocarcinoma of the prostate. The sentiment among urologists, however, has been one of disappointment due to the shortcomings of the immunoassays. Technically, PAPase immunoassays have two main additional requirements: (a) the availability of high affinity antibodies that can increase the detection level and (b) increased specificity of the antibody (PAPase has three domains each antigenically unique and shared with other acid phosphatases). These technical requirements are resolvable.

However, a more fundamental problem lies in the biology of early prostatic cancer. PAPase will appear in the general circulation only when the normal membrane barrier has disappeared or has been damaged. The absence of basal cells (basal cells contribute a part of the basement membrane) is the hallmark of malignancy, and this change signifies the structural alteration of the basal membrane (the boundary between the gland and the stroma). Therefore, it is likely that the leakage of PAPase will depend on whether the tumor follows an invasive or an expansive course. Anti-PAPase immunohistology will continue to be useful in the identification of metastatic cancer cells of prostatic origin, and loss of the expression of PAPase in prostatic cancer cells may be useful as an indicator of loss of the androgen sensitivity of these cells.

In summary, it is felt that:

1. PAPase measurements (both enzymatic and immunologic) will continue to be used in the staging of patients with adenocarcinoma of the prostate. At present, controversy remains regarding the value of immunologic methods in assessing apparent localized disease owing to a significant percentage of false-positive findings. However, a clear relationship between an elevated PAPase value and the presence of micrometastases has not been defined. Elevation of PAPase by enzymatic methods probably indicates metastatic spread, whereas raised immunologic values may still be associated with localized disease.

2. Response to therapy may be monitored by assessment of PAPase. The final word on the respective values of enzymatic and immunologic methods of assay remains to be said. At present, continuing careful assessment of both methods appears warranted.

Prostate-Specific Antigen

Biochemical and Immunochemical Characteristics

In 1979, Wang et al. discovered an antigenic protein unique to human prostate and designated it prostate-specific antigen (PA) (Wang et al. 1982). The function of this protein is unknown to date. PA is a glycoprotein of molecular weight

34 000, with carbohydrate accounting for about 7% of the total molecular weight. After resolution in sodium dodecylsulfate-polyacrylamide gel electrophoresis (SDS-PAGE), purified PA was found to consist of a single neutral polypeptide with an isoelectric point of 6.9 and a sedimentation coefficient of 3.1 S. PA is a major secretory protein of human prostate. There are, apparently, no significant differences in the PA concentration, per gram of tissue or per milligram of DNA, found in normal prostate, BPH, and prostatic carcinoma tissues. The concentration of PA in seminal plasma ranges from 0.41 to 1.78 mg/ml. Higher concentrations are occasionally found in some individuals. PA is a tissue-specific antigen of the prostate; it has never been demonstrated in other tissues, such as urethra, bladder, seminal vesicles, testis, kidney, liver, stomach, pancreas, or colon. The details of purification and biochemical and immunochemical characterization of PA have been reviewed by Wang et al. (1982).

The specificity of PA has been confirmed by polyclonal antibodies (Wang et al. 1982) in competitive binding and immunohistochemical studies. These antibodies reacted with prostatic tissue (normal, cancerous, or metaplastic) but not with a variety of other normal and malignant tissues. Immunohistologic studies have suggested that expression of PA by those cells appears to be correlated with their degree of cytologic differentiation (Papsidero et al. 1983). Frankel et al. (1982) have produced three monoclonal antibodies to PA (1F3, 2G7, and 1C5). By cross-binding and cross-blocking analysis with these antibodies, two nonoverlapping epitopes on PA molecules have been defined.

Immunoassays and Their Application

The finding of Kuriyama et al. (1980) that serum concentrations of PA were significantly elevated in patients with advanced prostatic cancer suggested its potential usefulness as a tumor marker. Their sandwich-type enzyme-linked immunosorbent assay (ELISA) has a laboratory sensitivity of 0.1 ng of PA per milliliter, with a working range of 0.1–10 mg/ml. Frankel et al. (1982) also developed a sandwich-type RIA with sensitivity and specificity similar to that of ELISA.

There is a correlation between mean serum concentrations of PA and stage of prostatic cancer. Stages A, B, C, and D are associated with mean concentrations of 4.8, 5.0, 10.1, and 24.2 ng/ml, respectively. Unfortunately, serum PA levels in patients with stage A and B disease are similar to levels in patients with BPH, and significantly higher than those of normal controls and patients with nonprostatic diseases. The rates of detection of PA in patients with prostatic cancer were 63% (5/8), 79% (27/34), 77% (43/56), and 86% (296/344) for stages A, B, C, and D, respectively. Furthermore, PA seems to be a potential marker for monitoring recurrence and development of metastases, as well as response to therapy (Kuriyama et al. 1981).

Diagnosis with Multiple PAPase and PA Immunoassays

Kuriyama et al. (1982) have reported the results of simultaneous assays of PAPase and PA in the staging of prostatic cancer. In many patients serum PAPase levels do not correlate with PA levels. The regulation of gene expression of these two antigens is totally unknown at present; however, one reason for the discordant variation of these two markers may be their different molecular weights. PA is a relatively small protein (34 000 daltons), whereas native PAPase molecules are quite large (100 000 daltons). PA molecules may diffuse through the basement membrane even without the breakdown of normal tissue boundaries. This probably accounts for the frequent elevation of serum PA levels among BPH patients, whereas PAPase levels are not increased so frequently in these patients.

Using a cut-off of 15.5 ng/ml for PAPase (mean of normal controls + 3 SD) and 7.5 ng/ml for PA (mean of BPH group + 2 SD), the simultaneous assay detected elevation of either of these markers in the sera of 58% (7/12) of patients with stage A, 58% (21/36) with stage B, 68% (19/28) with stage C, and 91% (106/116) with stage D prostatic cancer. Detection frequencies for PAPase and PA were 33% and 25%, 42% and 28%, 64% and 36%, and 73% and 64%, for stages A, B, C, and D prostatic cancer, respectively. None of the controls showed elevation of either marker. Simultaneous assays were found to have a clinical sensitivity of 80% and a specificity of 96%, and currently appear to yield the most reliable information for stage A and B disease.

Commentary

Since the PA molecules (mol. wt. 34 000) are smaller than the PAPase molecules (mol. wt. 100 000), their leakage into the general circulation can occur prior to the appearance of PAPase. The simultaneous assay of these two markers will increase the specificity and sensitivity of either single assay. Simultaneous assay of the PAPase and PA may thus be the method of choice for the diagnosis of localized adenocarcinoma of the prostate and for the earliest detection of micrometastases.

Other Markers of Metastatic Prostatic Cancer

Alkaline Phosphatase

Alkaline phosphatase is widely distributed in diverse tissue cells—bone, the hepatobiliary tract, intestinal mucosa, and the placenta. It is located intracellularly in the microsomal fraction and in the plasma membrane. There are four known isoenzymes: bone, liver, intestinal, and Regan, or tumor, isoenzyme. Regan isoenzyme resembles placental alkaline phosphatase. During adolescence, the bone isoenzyme is predominant but in adults the majority of serum alkaline phosphatase is of liver or gastrointestinal mucosal origin.

Since osteoblasts are a rich source of alkaline phosphatase, an elevation of the enzyme associated with prostatic cancer is usually related to bone or liver metastases. Ninety-one percent of prostatic cancer patients with radiographically documented metastases to bone showed elevation of total serum alkaline phosphatase levels. The majority of these were positive for the bone isoenzyme (Wajsman et al. 1978). Even though total serum alkaline phosphatase levels were normal in stage C patients, Wajsman et al. (1978) found that 44% of these patients showed elevation of the bone isoenzyme. Apparently an increase in the level of the bone isoenzyme may be evidence of bone metastases. Serial measurements of bone alkaline phosphatase may also be of value in monitoring the response of patients with bone metastases to treatment (Wajsman et al. 1978; Grayhack and Wendel 1979; Pontes et al. 1981). The Regan isoenzyme is elevated in 18%–20% of patients with advanced prostatic cancer (Slack et al. 1981; Schmidt et al. 1982). Consistently elevated levels of the liver isoenzyme may also reflect metastases of prostatic cancer (Killian et al. 1981).

Urinary Hydroxyproline

Two-thirds of the body's hydroxyproline is found in the collagen matrix of bone, and the rest in nonosseous collagen; therefore urinary hydroxyproline may be a useful marker for bony metastases of prostatic cancer (Bishop and Fellows 1977). It would appear that its value as a marker of bone metastases is comparable to radionuclide bone scans and to acid and alkaline phosphatase measurements. Since bone scan activity is based on the calcium metabolism of bone, and urinary excretion of hydroxyproline reflects changes in the bone matrix, these two tests complement one another. Urinary hydroxyproline levels have been used to monitor the progression of disease and response to hormonal therapy and chemotherapy in patients with advanced prostatic cancer (Moopan et al. 1980). Recently, Hopkins et al. (1983) introduced a spot test for urinary hydroxyproline, giving results comparable to the 24-hour urine method.

Other Enzyme Markers

An elevation of serum levels of lactic dehydrogenase (LDH) isoenzymes IV and V is associated with advanced prostatic cancer (Dennis and Prout 1963). Serum ribonuclease levels have also been found to be elevated in approximately 70% of prostatic cancer patients (Catalona et al. 1973; Chu et al. 1977). More than 70% of patients also showed increased creatine kinase isoenzyme BB (Silverman et al. 1979). Elevation of levels of these isoenzymes appears to be related to the disruption of cellular organization that accompanies neoplastic growth. Isoenzyme profiles may be useful in the investigation of disease course of individual patients; currently, however, these isoenzymes are rarely utilized in clinical urology as prostatic cancer markers.

Commentary

Although the radionucleotide bone scan is the standard procedure for the confirmation of bone metastases of prostatic cancer, both alkaline phosphatase and urinary hydroxyproline are also useful auxiliary investigative methods.

Other Potential Antigenic Markers of Prostatic Cancer

Urinary Prostatic Cancer Antigen

Edwards et al. (1982), using two-dimensional electrophoresis, identified a protein, PCA-1, with a molecular weight of 40 000, in the urine of 16 of 17 prostate cancer patients, but not in the urine of 22 control subjects. This protein was also detected in BPH and prostate tumor tissue extracts. Development of assays for this protein and assessment of its role as a tumor marker are presently being carried out.

Monoclonal Antibody-Defined Antigens

It is now accepted that malignant tumors are composed of diverse cell populations which show considerable heterogeneity in a variety of properties, such as morphology, chromosome markers, cell surface antigens, invasiveness, and metastatic capacity. Monoclonal antibodies have been developed in an effort to study the antigenic changes in the tumor cells indicative of invasive and metastatic behavior. To date, three different laboratories have generated murine monoclonal antibodies that recognize prostate-specific antigens (Ware et al. 1982; Frankel et al. 1982; Starling et al. 1982, 1984). However, the roles of these monoclonal antibody-defined antigens as tumor markers have not yet been established.

Ware et al. (1982) described a prostate-specific antigen of mol. wt. 54 000, defined by their monoclonal antibody alpha pro 3, which appears to be a prostatic epithelial cell differentiation antigen. Starling et al. (1982, 1984) described two prostate-specific antigens defined by their monoclonal antibodies 83.21 and 6.2, which may be other urogenital epithelial cell differentiation antigens. Frankel et al. (1982) generated a series of monoclonal antibodies which appeared to be specific either to prostatic cells (epithelium or stroma) or to epithelial cells in general (polyepithelial antibodies). Their epithelium-specific antibodies, 35 and 24, appear to define other prostatic differentiation antigens. At present it is not clear why hybridoma technique predominantly identifies these differentiation antigens; however, it is conceivable that they may represent major antigens expressed in the cells and tissues employed by the investigators in question. The search for antigenic markers for invasive cancers continues.

Commentary

A search for morphologic markers for invasive tumors resulted in histopathologic grading of prostatic cancer. In recent years, attempts have been made to analyze quantitatively the sizes, shapes, and intracellular structures of the tumor cells and to correlate these parameters with their biologic behaviour. Among these cytometric approaches are stereology (Bartsch and Rohr 1982), morphometry (Kurth et al. 1982: Diamond et al. 1982), and flow cytometry (Benson and Coffey 1983). Perhaps the most impressive technique is the evaluation of the relative nuclear roundness of the prostatic cancer cells (Diamond et al. 1982). In theory, monoclonal antibodies to tumor cell surface antigens also have potential comparable to these cytometric approaches. If monoclonal antibodies which identify marker antigens associated with invasive behavior of prostatic cancer become available, application of those antibodies may provide more effective histopathologic grading and nuclear imaging of metastatic cancers than do cytometric approaches. However, such expectations have not been fulfilled by the monoclonal antibodies currently available.

Summary and Perspectives

PAPase is the oldest marker of prostatic cancer still in use, and assays for this enzyme are important in the clinical staging of the disease. Enzymatic and immunoassays of PAPase are sufficiently sensitive and specific for the detection of elevated serum levels of the enzyme. Another equally useful marker is PA. The sensitivity and specificity of assays of this protein are high. The use of PA as a tumor marker complements the use of PAPase. In some prostatic cancer patients, PA levels are elevated without a detectable increase in serum PAPase levels. As discussed, the appearance of PAPase or PA in the circulation signifies the breakdown of the normal tissue boundary between glandular epithelium and stromal cells; therefore the presence of either marker in the circulation may be an early sign of metastases. However, the possibility that an elevation of serum levels of either protein may be associated with localized tumor growth cannot be dismissed at present.

Both PAPase and PA have been found to be useful in identifying metastatic cancers of prostatic origin by immunohistopathologic studies of sections of tumor biopsies. Radiolabeled antibodies against PAPase and PA may be useful in the future for nuclear imaging of prostatic cancer and for the delivery of chemotherapeutic drugs.

Tumor markers (PAPase, PA) also play a role in staging patients with adenocarcinoma of the prostate and have been found to be useful in monitoring response to therapy and the early detection of clinical failure.

Other markers of prostatic cancer which are presently being investigated include the polyamines, creatine kinase BB, LDH V/I ratio, CEA, prostacyclin, and ribonuclease. They are present in the circulation of prostatic cancer patients and are produced by tumor cells. Alkaline phosphatase is expressed at relatively high levels by osteoblasts; therefore appearance of this enzyme in high levels in the general circulation has been used in the clinical identification and confirmation of bone metastasis of prostatic cancer.

Acknowledgement. We are indebted to Susan Burton for her many hours of assistance with the preparation of this manuscript.

References

Bartsch G, Rohr HP (1982) Stereology—a new method to assess normal and pathological growth of the prostate. In: Jacobi GH, Hohenfellner R (eds) Prostate cancer. Williams & Wilkins Co., Baltimore, pp 433–459

Bates RJ, Chapman CM, Prout GR Jr, Ling CW (1982) Immunohistochemical identification of prostatic acid phosphatase: correlation of tumor grade with acid phosphatase distribution. J Urol 127:574–580

Benson MC, Coffey DS (1983) Prostate cancer research: current concepts and controversies. Semin Oncol 1:323–330

Bishop MC, Fellows GJ (1977) Urine hydroxyproline excretion: a marker of bone metastasis in prostatic carcinoma. Br J Urol 49:711–716

Bodansky O (1972) Acid phosphatase. Adv Clin Chem 15:43–147

Brandes D, Kirchheim D, Scott WW (1964) Ultrastructure of the human prostate: normal and neoplastic. Lab Invest 13:1541–1566

Brock DJH, Mayo O (1978) The biochemical genetics of man, 2nd edn. Academic Press

Bruce AW, Mahan DE (1982) The role of prostatic acid phosphatase in the investigation and treatment of adenocarcinoma of the prostate. Ann NY Acad Sci 309:110–121

Bruce AW, Mahan DE (1986) Acid phosphatase: its estimation and clinical significance. In: Blandy JP, Lytton B (eds) The prostate (BIMR Urology). Butterworth, Surrey pp 147–162

Bruce AW, Mahan DE, Morales A, Clark AF, Belville WD (1979) An objective look at acid phosphatase determinations. Br J Urol 51:213–217

Catalona WJ, Chretien P, Matthews W et al. (1973) Serum ribonuclease in urologic cancer. Relation to host immunocompetence. Urology 1:577–581

Chatal JP, Daver A, Fleury-Govern MC et al. (1982) The value of prostatic acid phosphatase (PAP) in predicting lymph node metastases in patients undergoing pelvic lymphadenectomy for prostatic cancer (abstract No. 235). American Urological Association Annual Meeting, Kansas City

Choe BK, Rose NR (1982) Prostatic acid phosphatase: a marker for human prostatic adenocarcinoma. In: Busch H, Yeoman LC (eds) Tumor markers. Methods in Cancer Research. 19:199–232. Academic Press, New York

Choe BK, Pontes EJ, Dong MK, Rose NR (1980) Double antibody immunoenzyme assay for human prostatic acid phosphatase. Clin Chem 26:1854–1859

Chu TM (ed) (1981) Biochemical markers for cancer. Marcel Dekker, New York

Chu TM, Wang MC, Kuciel R (1977) Enzyme markers in human prostatic carcinoma. Cancer Treat Rep 61:193–200

Cook WB, Fishman WH, Clard BG (1962) Serum acid phosphatase of prostatic origin in the diagnosis of prostatic carcinoma. Clinical evaluation of 2408 tests by the Fishman-Lerner method. J Urol 88:281–287

Cooper JF, Finkle WD (1980) Current experience with radioimmunoassay techniques for prostatic acid phosphatase. Prostate 1:441–450

Cooper JF, Foti A, Herschman H, Finkle W (1978) A solid phase radioimmunoassay for prostatic acid phosphatase. J Urol 119:388–391

Dennis LJ, Prout GR (1963) Lactic dehydrogenase in prostatic cancer. Invest Urol 1:101–111

Diamond DA, Berry SJ, Jewett HJ et al. (1982) A new method to assess metastatic potential of human prostatic cancer: relative nuclear roundness. J Urol 128:729–734

Edwards JJ, Anderson NG, Tollaksen SL, Von Eschenbach AC, Guevara J Jr (1982) Proteins of human urine: II. Identification by two dimensional electrophoresis of a new candidate marker for prostatic cancer. Clin Chem 28:160–163

Fishman WH, Dast RM, Bonner CD, Leadbetter WF, Lerner F, Homburger F (1953) A new method for estimating serum acid phosphatase of prostatic origin applied to the clinical investigation of cancer of the prostate. J Clin Invest 32:1034–1044

Fleishmann J, Catalona W, Fair W et al. (1982) Lack of value of radioimmunoassay for prostatic acid phosphatase as a screening test for early prostate cancer (abstract No. 233). American Urological Association Annual Meeting, Kansas City

Foti AG, Cooper JR, Herschmann H, Melvaez RR (1977) Detection of prostatic cancer by solid-phase radioimmunoassay of serum prostatic acid phosphatase. N Engl J Med 297:1357–1361

Frankel AE, Rouse RV, Wang MC, Chu TM, Herzenberg LA (1982) Monoclonal antibodies to human prostate antigen. Cancer Res 42:3714–3718

Goldberg DM, Deland FH (1984) Clinical studies of prostatic cancer imaging with radiolabeled antibodies against prostatic acid phosphatase. Urol Clin North Am 11:277–281

Grayhack JT, Wendel EF (1979) Carcinoma of the prostate. In Kendall AR, Karafin L (eds) Urology, vol 2. Harper and Row, Hagerstown, pp 1–32

Griffiths JC (1980) Prostate-specific acid phosphatase: reevaluation of radioimmunoassay in diagnosing prostatic disease. Clin Chem 26:433–436

Hopkins SC, Nissenkorn I, Palmieri GMA, Ikard M, Moinuddin M, Soloway MS (1983) Serial spot hydroxyproline/creatinine ratios in metastatic prostatic cancer. J Urol 129:319–323

Jobsis AC, DeVries GP, Anhold RRH, Sanders GTB (1978) Demonstration of prostatic origin of metastases. An immunohistochemical method for formaline-fixed embedded tissue. Cancer 41:1788–1793

Killian CS, Vargas FP, Pontes EJ et al. (1981) The use of serum isoenzymes of alkaline and acid phosphatase as possible quantitative markers of tumor loan in prostate cancer. Prostate 2:187–206

Kirckheim D, Brandes D, Bacon RL (1974) Fine structure and cytochemistry of human prostatic carcinoma. In: Brandes D (ed) Male accessory sex organs: structure and function in mammals. Academic Press, New York, pp 397–405

Kuhajda FP, Mann RB (1984) Adenoid cystic carcinoma of the prostate, a case report with immunoperoxidase staining for prostate-specific acid phosphatase and prostate-specific antigen. Am J Clin Pathol 81:257–260

Kuriyama M, Wang MC, Papsidero LD et al. (1980) Quantitiation of prostate-specific antigen in serum by a sensitive enzyme immunoassay. Cancer Res 40:4658–4662

Kuriyama M, Wang MC, Lee CL et al. (1981) Use of human prostate-specific antigen in monitoring prostate cancer. Cancer Res 41:3874–3876

Kuriyama M, Wang MC, Lee CL et al. (1982) Multiple marker evaluation in human prostate cancer with the use of tissue-specific antigens. J Natl Cancer Inst 68:99–104

Kurth KH, Binder A, ten Kate FJW (1982) Prostate cancer: value of histophotometric tissue diagnosis. In: Jacobi GH, Hohenfellner R (eds) Prostatic cancer. Williams & Wilkins, Baltimore, pp 461–470

Lee CL, Killian CS, Murphy GP, Chur TM (1980) A solid phase immunoadsorbent assay for serum prostatic acid phosphatase. Clin Chim Acta 101:209–216

Lee CL, Li CY, Jou YH, Murphy GP, Chu TM (1982) Immunochemical characterization of prostatic acid phosphatase with monoclonal antibodies. Ann NY Acad Sci 309:52–61

Li CY, Lam KWK, Yam LT (1980) Immunohistochemical diagnosis of prostatic cancer with metastasis. Cancer 46:706–712

Lillehoj HS, Choe BK, Rose NR (1982) Monoclonal antibodies to human prostatic acid phosphatase: probes for antigenic study. Proc Natl Acad Sci (USA) 79:5061–5065

Lin MF, Lee CL, Wojcieazyn JW, Wang MC, Valenzuela LA, Murphy GP, Chu TM (1980) Fundamental biochemical and immunological aspects of prostatic acid phosphatase. Prostate 1:415–425

Lippert MC, Bensimon H, Javadpour N (1982) Immunoperoxidase staining of acid phosphatase in human prostatic tissue. J Urol 128:1114–1116

Mahan DE, Doctor BPA (1979) A radioimmune assay for human prostatic acid phosphatase level in prostatic disease. Clin Biochem 12:10–17

Mahan DE, Bruce AW, Manley PN, Franchi L (1980) Immunohistochemical evaluation of prostatic carcinoma before and after radiotherapy. J Urol 124:488–491

Mathes G, Richmond SG, Sprunt DS (1956) Use of L-tartrate in determining prostatic serum acid phosphatase. Report of 514 cases. J Urol 75:143–150

Moopan MU, Wax SH, Kim H, Wang JC, Tobin MS (1980) Urinary hydroxyproline excretion as a marker of osseous metastasis in carcinoma of the prostate. J Urol 123:694–696

Mostofi FK, Price EB Jr (1973) Malignant tumors of the prostate. In: Tumors of the male genital system. Atlas of tumor pathology. Armed Forces Institute of Pathology, Washington, pp 218–225

Murphy GP, Reynoso G, Kenny GM, Gaeta JG (1969) Comparison of total and prostatic fraction serum acid phosphatase levels in patients with differentiated and undifferentiated prostatic carcinoma. Cancer 23:1309–1314

Nesbit RM, Baum WC, Mich AA (1951) Serum phosphatase determination in diagnosis of prostatic cancer. A review of 1150 cases. JAMA 145:1321–1324

Nobles ER Jr, Kerr WS Jr, Dutoit CH, Rourke GM (1957) Serum prostatic acid phosphatase levels in patients with carcinoma of the prostate. JAMA 164:2020–2025

Ostrowski W (1980) Human prostatic acid phosphatase: physiochemical and catalytic properties In: Spring-Mills E, Hafaz ESE (eds) Male accessory sex glands. Elsevier/North-Holland Biomedic, Amsterdam, pp 197–213

Papsidero LD, Croghan GA, Wang MC et al. (1983) Monoclonal antibody (F5) to human prostate antigen. Hybridoma 2:139–147

Pontes JE, Choe BK, Rose NR, Pierce JM Jr (1977) Indirect immunofluorescence for identification of prostatic epithelial cells. J Urol 117:459–463

Pontes JE, Choe BK, Rose NR, Pierce JM (1978) Bone marrow acid phosphatase in staging of prostatic cancer: how reliable is it? J Urol 119:772–776

Pontes JE, Choe BK, Rose NR, Ercole C, Pierce JM Jr (1981) Clinical evaluation of immunological methods for detection of prostatic acid phosphatase. J Urol 126:363–365

Pontes JE, Chu TM, Slack N, Karr J, Murphy GP (1982) Serum prostatic antigen measurement in localized prostatic cancer: correlation with clinical course. J Urol 128:1216–1218

Prellwitz W, Ehrenthal W (1982) Serum and bone marrow acid phosphatase as a diagnostic marker in prostatic cancer. In: Jacobi GH, Hohenfellner R (eds) Prostatic cancer. Williams & Wilkins, Baltimore pp 129–162

Scardino P (1982) Serum acid phosphatase assays and other tumour markers of prostatic cancer. In: Prostate cancer videoconference guide book. American Urology Association Office of Education, pp 109–113

Schacht MJ, Garnett JE, Grayhack JT (1984) Biochemical markers in prostatic cancer. Urol Clin North Am 11:253–267

Schmidt JD, Slack NH, Chu TM, Murphy GP (1982) Placenta-like isoenzymes of alkaline phosphatase in prostatic cancer. J Urol 127:457–459

Shulman S, Mamrod L, Gonder MJ, Soanes WA (1964) The detection of prostatic acid phosphatase by antibody reactions in gel diffusion. J Immunol 93:474–480

Silverman LM, Dermer GB, Zwieg MH, Van Steirteghem AC, Tokes ZA (1979) Creatinine kinase BB: a new tumor associated marker. Clin Chem 25:1432–1435

Slack NH, Chu TM, Wajsman LZ, Murphy GP (1981) Carcinoplacental isoenzyme (Regan) in carcinoma of the prostate. Cancer 47:146–151

Sodeman TM, Batsakis JG (1977) Acid phosphatase in urologic pathology. In: Tannebaum M (ed) Urologic pathology. The prostate. Lea and Febiger, Philadelphia, pp 129–139

Starling JJ, Seig SM, Beckett ML, Schellhammer PF, Ladaga LE, Wright GL Jr (1982) Monoclonal antibodies to human prostate and bladder tumour-associated antigens. Cancer Res 42:3084–3089

Starling JJ, Beckett ML, Wright G Jr (1984) Monoclonal antibodies to prostate adenocarcinoma antigens. In: Wright GL (ed) Monoclonal antibodies and cancer, Marcel Dekker, New York, pp 253–286

Tannenbaum M (1977) Histopathology of the prostate gland. In: Tannenbaum M (ed) Urologic pathology—the prostate. Lea and Febiger, Philadelphia, pp 303–397

Townsend RM (1977) Enzyme tests in diseases of the prostate. Ann Clin Lab Sci 7:254–261

Vihko P, Sajanti E, Janne O, Peltonen L, Vihko R (1978) Serum prostate-specific acid phosphatase development and validation of a specific radioimmunoassay. Clin Chem 24:1915–1919

Wajsman Z, Chu JM, Bross D et al. (1978) Clinical significance of serum alkaline phosphatase isoenzyme levels in advanced prostatic carcinoma. J Urol 199:244–246

Wang MC, Kuriyama M, Papsidero LD, Loor RM, Valenzeula LA, Murphy GP, Chu TM (1982) Prostate antigen of human cancer patients. In: Busch H, Yeoman LC (eds) Tumor markers. Methods in Cancer Research 19:179–197. Academic Press, New York

Ware JL, Paulson DE, Parks SF, Webb KS (1982) Production of monoclonal antibody of aPro 3 recognizing a human prostatic carcinoma antigen. Cancer Res 42:1215–1222

Watson RA, Tang DB (1980) The predictive value of prostatic acid phosphatase as a screening test for prostatic cancer. N Engl J Med 303:497–499

Whitesel JA, Donohue RE, Mani JH et al. (1984) Acid phosphatase: influence on the management of carcinoma of the prostate. J Urol 131:70–72

Whitmore WFJ (1984) Natural history and staging of prostate cancer. Urol Clin North Am 11:205–220

Wilson JWL, Morales A, Bruce AW (1983) The prognostic significance of histological grading and pathological staging in carcinoma of the prostate. J Urol 130:481–483

Yam LT, Janckila AJ, Lam KW et al. (1981) Immunohistochemistry of prostatic acid phosphatase. Prostate 2:97–107

Yam LT, Winkler CF, Janckila AJ et al. (1983) Prostatic cancer presenting as metastatic adenocarcinoma of undetermined origin: immunodiagnosis by prostatic acid phosphatase. Cancer 51:283–287

Yamaura N, Makino M, Walsh LJ, Bruce AW, Choe BK (1985) Production of monoclonal antibodies against prostatic acid phosphatase by in vitro immunization of human spleen cells. J Immunol Meth 84:105–116

Chapter 4

Hormone Receptors in Prostatic Cancer

B.G. Mobbs and J.G. Connolly

Introduction

During the last decade, the clinical use of steroid hormone receptor assays has become an accepted part of the management of a number of diseases of hormone target organs. In breast cancer, and to a lesser extent in endometrial cancer, the concentrations of receptors for estrogen and progestin in the malignant tissue are regarded as prognostic factors in early disease, and as predictive factors for the value of endocrine treatment for patients with advanced disease (Knight et al. 1980; McGuire and Clark 1983). In acute lymphocytic leukemia, the cellular concentration of glucocorticoid receptors appears to be an indicator of prognosis and response to glucocorticoid therapy (Costlow et al. 1982). The assay of androgen receptor (AR) in cultured genital skin fibroblasts can assist in the diagnosis and selection of treatment of benign conditions such as androgen resistance syndromes (Bardin and Wright 1980). It is therefore somewhat disappointing that studies of the application of AR assays to the management of prostatic carcinoma, which is known to be an androgen-sensitive disease in the majority of cases, have met with very limited success. Some of the reasons for this are inherent in the nature of the disease and are discussed below. Nevertheless, the research involved in the development of these assays, together with that into related areas of the biochemistry of human and animal prostatic tissue, has added much to our knowledge of the basic mechanisms involved in the control of prostatic growth.

Factors Limiting Biochemical Investigation on Human Prostate

Tissue Acquisition

A major difficulty in any type of biochemical investigation of the prostate is that of obtaining suitable tissue for study. With regard to carcinoma, many patients presenting with this disease already have metastatic involvement, and in such cases, primary tumor tissue is not resected unless the gland is causing obstructive symptoms. If surgery is performed, it is usually by transurethral resection (TUR). There are two schools of thought regarding the use of tissue thus obtained for biochemical investigation. Some investigators believe that TUR tissue cannot provide valid data owing to the damage caused by the cauterizing current. However, there is evidence from organ culture and metabolic studies that selected TUR material is viable (Bard and Lasnitzki 1977; Sanefugi et al. 1982; Habib et al. 1985b). Data from Albert et al. (1982) show that the type of current and the loop size used are of importance in conserving receptor proteins. They observed no significant difference in mean cytosol or nuclear AR values when these were considered separately between specimens obtained by open operation and specimens obtained by TUR using a large loop and a high frequency current. However, the mean total (i.e., cytosol and nuclear) receptor levels were significantly lower in the TUR specimens. The use of a coagulating current and a small loop further decreased the receptor concentrations. These experiments were carried out on benign prostatic hypertrophic (BPH) tissue. When TUR is used to obtain malignant tissue, which occurs predominantly near the periphery of the gland, a further difficulty may be caused by "dilution" of the malignant tissue in the chips with nonmalignant tissue from the periurethral region. It is clear that if tissue obtained by TUR is to be used, it must be selected very carefully.

While needle biopsy is commonly used to obtain tissue for diagnostic purposes, it does not usually yield sufficient tissue for accurate biochemical analysis (Blankenstein et al. 1982). Multiple needle biopsies from the same area of a single gland have been used for this purpose (Walsh and Hicks 1979), but this procedure may not be acceptable in all centers. It is also important to monitor the histopathology of the biopsies in order to ensure that they contain unadulterated tumor tissue. Cold punch-resected specimens have been used as a source of tissue in a few centers (Donnelly et al. 1983; Kitano et al. 1983). A further source of prostatic carcinoma tissue may be provided by involved lymph nodes: these may yield pure tumor tissue with insignificant stromal content, but may be less well differentiated than the primary tumor.

The availability of normal human prostatic tissue with which to compare carcinoma tissue has been equally limited. Since some degree of BPH is so common, occurring in 50% of men over the age of 50 and increasing in incidence with age (Walsh 1984), normal prostatic tissue has usually been obtained from younger men undergoing cystoprostatectomy, at autopsy, or from brain-dead donors kept on life-support systems until shortly before excision of the tissue. Apparently normal tissue from the peripheral region of glands removed by open prostatectomy for BPH in older patients has also been used. The use of autopsy specimens has been questioned by Walsh et al. (1983), since they found that the slow cooling of tissue from body temperature resulted in reduction of 5α-dihydrotestosterone (DHT) levels in the tissue, compared with similar tissue removed surgically and cooled rapidly.

Tissue Heterogeneity

Possible "dilution" of malignant tissue with benign and/or normal tissue has already been mentioned. Prostatic carcinomas may consist of a mixture of glandular components which display varying degrees of differentiation and which may also vary in biochemical differentiation. It follows that histologic control of the tissue under study is of great importance in evaluation of the results. The normal gland has a complex regional anatomy (McNeal 1981; Tisell and Salander 1975): carcinoma arises in the area termed the peripheral zone by McNeal. When studying the normal gland it is therefore important to be able to identify the origin of the tissue used.

Relationship Between Androgen Receptor Content and Response to Endocrine Manipulation

Cytosol Androgen Receptor[1]

Early attempts to relate AR content with the course of disease after hormonal manipulation were based on assay of free cytosol receptor (i.e., receptor not bound by endogenous steroid), as is the practice in breast cancer. Experimental work on the rat ventral prostate had established DHT, a metabolite of testosterone, as the natural ligand for AR in the prostate (Fang et al. 1969; Rennie and Bruchovsky 1972): therefore radiolabeled DHT was initially used as ligand for the assays on human tissue. However, this steroid binds with almost equally high affinity to the sex steroid transport protein sex hormone binding globulin (SHBG), which is present in considerable concentrations in human prostate extracts (Rosen et al. 1975) and which is increased in concentration after estrogen treatment (Mobbs et al. 1975). In order to discriminate the binding of ^{3}H-DHT to AR from binding to SHBG, a variety of methodologic strategems were adopted. These included physical separation by sucrose density

---

1. Recent evidence (Jensen 1984) suggests that the terms "cytosol" and "nuclear" receptor may not reflect the true localization of receptor within the cell in vivo, but represent the distribution in subcellular fractions after tissue homogenization under the conditions used in the majority of steroid receptor assays. For convenience these terms will be retained throughout this chapter, but it is realized that they may refer to different physiochemical states of the receptor molecule rather than to cellular localization. "Cytosol" receptors refers to that fraction extractable with low ionic strength buffers; "nuclear" receptor, to that fraction not extracted under these conditions. Thus, nuclear "translocation" may reflect a change in molecular conformation and ability to bind to nuclear components with high affinity, rather than a transfer of receptor from one compartment to another.

gradient centrifugation, gel electrophoresis, Sephadex chromatography, and protamine sulfate precipitation, and/or differential competition for the two binding proteins by cyproterone acetate (Menon et al. 1977; Krieg et al. 1979; Mobbs et al. 1977, 1978; Geller et al. 1975). However, attempts to relate free cytosol AR assayed by these methods to previously untreated patients' response to hormonal therapy were unsuccessful (Wagner 1980).

In the rat ventral prostate, which has been widely used as a model for the investigation of androgen action, it was found that in the intact animal, the majority of cytosol AR sites are occupied by endogenous androgen, and that a large proportion of total cellular sites are located in the nuclear fraction (Bruchovsky et al. 1975; Blondeau et al. 1975). If circulating testosterone levels are lowered by treatment such as castration, a redistribution of receptor takes place: nuclear receptor is released into the cytosol fraction, and most receptor sites are freed from endogenous androgen. In one study, therefore, free cytosol AR was assayed in prostatic carcinoma specimens *after* serum testosterone levels had been lowered by endocrine manipulation, and the results were examined in relation to the response of the patients to the hormonal treatment (Mobbs et al. 1980a). It was found that the best responses occurred in the middle of the range of values obtained: patients with very low cytosol AR concentrations were unresponsive, but those with exceptionally high concentrations were also unresponsive. Some of these latter patients were in relapse after long-term treatment with synthetic estrogens and most of these high binding tumors were poorly differentiated. There have been other reports of exceptionally high free cytosol AR concentrations in poorly differentiated and/or hormone-insensitive carcinomas (Krieg et al. 1979; Kirdani et al. 1984). A partial explanation for this may be the lack of endogenous ligand available for binding to AR (see below). There is also some evidence from animal models that estrogen treatment can induce AR synthesis. Clinical evidence suggests that AR present in tumors of patients who have relapsed after orchiectomy and/or estrogen treatment is still able to reactivate the cancer if circulating testosterone is restored (Fowler and Whitmore 1981).

An improvement in methodology was brought about by the introduction of the synthetic androgen methyltrienolone (R1881), which is bound by AR with high affinity but is not bound significantly by SHBG. Moreover, this steroid is not metabolized during incubation. Also, in order to prevent degradation of receptor, stabilizers such as thiol reducing agents, protease inhibitors, and sodium molybdate were added to buffers used for homogenization and/or incubation. These modifications are particularly important during "exchange" assays, in which endogenous ligand is replaced by the radioactively labeled ligand during incubations carried out for longer times and/or at higher temperatures than in the free site assay. Using these modifications, Ekman et al. (1979) reported a good correlation of clinical response to hormonal treatment with the capacity of tumor cytosol to bind R1881. However, these results are difficult to interpret as many of the specimens contained a low ratio of malignant to nonmalignant tissue. Also it is known that R1881 binds to progesterone receptors (PgR) as well as to AR, and it is now customary to compete out binding to PgR by including excess triaminolone acetonide in the incubation medium (Zava et al. 1979). A number of investigators have assayed total AR in normal and/or prostatic carcinoma cytosols using this method, and the results obtained are listed in Table 4.1. As the values are expressed in a variety of ways, it is not always possible to make comparisons between different studies. When the results are expressed in terms of cytosol protein, it appears that the mean concentration of cytosol AR in carcinoma tissue is higher than that in normal tissue. However, this difference is probably due to the greater cellularity in the carcinoma tissue, as it is not observed when the results are expressed on the basis of DNA content. Nevertheless, it is clear that there are wide variations between individual tissue specimens. No correlation was observed between total cytosol AR and histologic tumor grade or between cytosol AR and response to hormonal therapy in the three studies in which this was examined (Trachtenberg and Walsh 1982; Brendler et al. 1984; Gonor et al. 1984). Longer follow-up of the patients in the latter study (Gonor et al. 1984) suggested that cytosol AR may be able to discriminate between patients with short- and long-term survival: however, these authors stress that due to the small number of patients in their study, corroboration is needed (Fentie et al. 1986).

Table 4.1. Concentration (mean ± SEM) of total cytosol AR in normal and untreated malignant human prostatic tissue

Reference	Normal	Carcinoma
	Expressed as fmol/mg cytosol protein	
Walsh and Hicks (1979)		29 ± 26^a
Shimazaki et al. (1981)	8.8 ± 0.8	22.1 ± 2.8
Ekman et al. (1982)	12 ± 3^a (peripheral region)	
Donnelly et al. (1983)	15.2 ± 1.6	21.2 ± 3.0
	Expressed as fmol/mg DNA	
Trachtenberg et al. (1982a)	259 ± 133 (young subjects)	
Trachtenberg and Walsh (1982)		154 ± 134
Ekman et al. (1982)	367 ± 25^a (peripheral region)	
Barrack et al. (1983)	387 ± 26 ——————— NS ——————— 364 ± 26	
Brendler et al. (1984)		Good responders 319 ± 109 ⎫ NS Poor responders 139 ± 14 ⎭
	Expressed as fmol/g tissue	
Donnelly et al. (1984)	586 ± 75	665 ± 119
Gonor et al. (1984)		Good responders 1427 ± 437 ⎫ NS Poor responders 671 ± 232 ⎭

NS, no significant difference between means.
[a] Mean ± SD rather than mean ± SEM.

Androgen Metabolism and Receptor Activity

An important distinction between the mechanisms of estrogen and of androgen action in their respective target organs is that the principal circulating estrogen, estradiol, is not metabolized before binding to its receptor protein, whereas the main circulating androgen, testosterone, has a considerably lower affinity for AR than DHT, its 5α-reduced metabolite. Much of the data available on androgen metabolism in the prostate has been derived from investigations on benign hypertrophic tissue and is therefore beyond the scope of this review: for this information, the reader is referred to Bruchovsky et al. (1980), Habib et al. (1981), Hudson et al. (1983), and Krieg (1984). Although studies on normal human glands are limited, 5α-reductase activity has been found to be high (although usually not as high as in BPH tissue), and the concentration of the 5α-reduced metabolites of testosterone greatly exceeds that of testosterone itself (Hudson et al. 1983; Krieg 1984; Belis 1980; Vihko et al. 1981; Bruchovsky et al. 1980).

DHT has a higher affinity for AR than any other natural androgen, and is therefore considered to be the true intracellular hormone, while testosterone can be considered a pro-hormone. Thus the requirements for androgen sensitivity are firstly, a sufficient concentration of AR, and secondly, the ability to generate the ligand (DHT) by the 5α-reduction of testosterone. If production of DHT is impaired, less AR will be bound and translocated to the nuclear fraction. In general, the 5α-reductase activity in untreated carcinoma specimens has been found to be similar to, or less than that in normal tissue (Bruchovsky et al. 1980; Hudson et al. 1983; Krieg 1984). Nevertheless, DHT concentrations, although very variable, often exceed those in normal tissue (Geller et al. 1979; Vihko et al. 1981; Krieg 1984). The activity of 3α(β)-hydroxysteroid dehydrogenase, the enzyme responsible for the further metabolism of DHT to 3α(β)-androstanediol, is often lower in malignant than in normal tissue, and this may explain the net accumulation of DHT in spite of reduced 5α-reductase activity (Bruchovsky et al. 1980; Hudson 1982; Krieg 1984). However, there is evidence that poorly differentiated and/or metastatic carcinoma has reduced levels of both 5α-reductase and DHT (Jenkins and McCaffery 1974; Kliman et al. 1978; Morfin et al. 1979; Belis and Tarry 1981; Habib et al. 1985a). This would be expected to result in a high ratio of cytosol to nuclear AR, and a high proportion of cytosol AR which is unbound by endogenous DHT. In a study in which both total and unbound cytosol AR were assayed in a series of nine untreated prostatic carcinomas with a malignant component of 65%–100%, it was in fact found that both the absolute concentration of bound sites and (where significant concentrations were present) the proportion of bound sites were related to the degree of differentiation of the tumor (Mobbs et al. 1980b; Table 4.2). Data on a relationship between degree of differentiation and the relative concentrations of AR in the cytosol and nuclear fractions are scant, but it is of interest that Shain et al. (1980) observed high cytosol to nuclear AR ratios in three moderately or poorly differentiated carcinomas, one of which was metastatic. However, this study was carried out with ^{3}H-R1881 as ligand in the absence of triamcinolone acetonide, so that some PgR may have been included.

Table 4.2. Relationship between degree of differentiation and bound cytosol AR in prostatic carcinoma

Patient No.	% malignant component	Degree of differentiation	Total cytosol AR concentration (fmol/mg DNA)	Concentration of bound AR (fmol/mg DNA)	% bound sites
1a[a]	70	W	1520	1383	91
2	65	M–W	970	824	85
3	70	M–W	580	406	70
4	80	P–W	670	462	69
5	80	P and W	360	134	37
1b[a]	80	P–M	90	0	0
6	95	P–M	54	54	100
7	100	P–M	330	96	23
8	100	P	880	97	11

W, M, P: well, moderately, and poorly differentiated.
[a]Specimens 1a and 1b were taken from the same patient 15 months apart.

Nuclear Androgen Receptor

It is clear from the foregoing discussion that total or unbound cytosol AR concentrations are unlikely to be useful for the prediction of the androgen sensitivity of prostatic carcinoma. With hindsight, it now seems obvious that the AR concentrations in the nuclear fraction are more likely to indicate the degree of biochemical differentiation and probable response to hormonal manipulation.

In interpreting the data available on nuclear AR concentrations, it is necessary to be aware that receptor in this fraction appears to be present in a number of different molecular states, which vary in their extractability. The conventional assay of nuclear AR is based on the binding capacity of a high ionic strength extract of the nuclear fraction. This is termed the salt-extractable AR, and represents 80% of the total nuclear AR when the tissue is homogenized in the presence of a thiol-reducing agent such as dithiothreitol (Barrack et al. 1983). However, in the absence of these agents, a large proportion of nuclear AR is resistant to salt extraction. Part of this salt-resistant fraction is also resistant to extraction with DNAase, and is termed the nuclear matrix fraction: in rat ventral prostate this represents 50%–70% of the total nuclear AR (Barrack 1983). The significance of the matrix-bound sites is controversial (see discussion in Rennie et al. 1983a). The sites appear to have identical characteristics to those of the other nuclear sites, apart from their tight association with the matrix. However, it has been suggested that the matrix-bound sites may be associated with the small percentage of DNA tightly attached to the matrix, and that this DNA may itself be associated with genes concerned with the regulation of hormone-stimulated events (Barrack 1983).

Some recent data on androgen receptor values obtained from nuclear fractions of normal and malignant human prostatic tissue are listed in Table 4.3. It is of interest that Barrack et al. (1983) observed a significant difference between the concentration extracted by salt in cancer tissue (227±20 fmol/mg DNA) and the same fraction in normal tissue (157±17 fmol/mg DNA), although total nuclear AR concentrations were similar in both types of tissue. These authors found that the ratio of salt-extractable to salt-resistant AR was approximately 2:1 in the cancer tissue, but 1:1 in normal and BPH tissue, suggesting that the interaction between the receptor and the nuclear acceptor sites may be altered in malignant tissue. The mean nuclear AR content observed by Trachtenberg and Walsh (1982) in the primary tumors of patients with metastatic disease (207±168 fmol/mg DNA) was considerably lower than the mean found by the same investigators in the nuclei of normal tissue (703±133 fmol/mg DNA) (Trachtenberg et al. 1982a).

Four studies have been carried out in which the nuclear AR concentration of prostatic carcinomas has been related to response to hormonal manipulation. The results indicate that nuclear AR content is likely to be useful as a partial indicator of androgen sensitivity, but that it may be necessary to supplement it with other indicators. In a series of 32 patients Ghanadian and his colleagues (1981) found that 10 of 13 patients whose tumors contained nuclear AR concentrations of more than 500 fmol/mg DNA responded to endocrine therapy for at least 2 years. All of ten patients whose tumors contained less than 500 fmol/mg DNA relapsed within 2 years. The relationship between nuclear AR and response was less striking at 6 months. A relationship between AR values and response was also reported by Trachtenberg and Walsh (1982). In a series of

Table 4.3. Nuclear AR concentration (mean ± SEM) in normal and malignant human prostate

Reference	Salt-extractable	Salt-resistant	Total
	Normal		
	Expressed as fmol/mg DNA		
Trachtenberg et al. (1982a) (5)[a]	703 ± 133	–	703 ± 133[b] (young subjects)
Barrack et al. (1983) (7)	157 ± 17	170 ± 28	327 ± 27
	Expressed as fmol/g tissue		
Donnelly et al. (1984) (3)	38 ± 21	325 ± 139	–
	Malignant		
	Expressed as fmol/mg DNA		
Trachtenberg and Walsh (1982) (23)	207 ± 168	–	207 ± 168[b]
Barrack et al. (1983) (11)	227 ± 20	128 ± 13	355 ± 23

[a]Numbers in parentheses represent number of specimens assayed.
[b]Extracted in the presence of dithiothreitol: a small proportion of nuclear AR may have remained salt resistant and would therefore not be included in this total.

23 patients, significantly higher mean duration of response and mean survival times were observed for patients whose tumors contained more than 110 fmol/ mg DNA than for those whose tumors contained lower concentrations. There was considerable overlap in response times in these two groups, suggesting that nuclear AR may be a valuable factor for prognosis and indicator for treatment, but must be supplemented by other information.

These conclusions are confirmed by two other studies in which salt-extractable and salt-resistant nuclear AR were assayed separately (Table 4.4). Gonor et al. (1984) observed significantly higher mean values for both fractions and for total nuclear AR in tumors which became stable or regressed following treatment than in tumors which progressed. On the other hand, Brendler et al. (1984) observed a significant difference only in the salt-extractable fraction. Where the grade of differentiation was examined in relation to the AR content, no relationship was found (Trachtenberg and Walsh 1982; Brendler et al. 1984; Gonor et al. 1984). In all these studies, there was considerable overlap in the nuclear AR concentrations (or fractions thereof) between the good and the poor responders. There have therefore been attempts to establish other markers of androgen sensitivity.

Table 4.4. Nuclear AR concentrations (mean ± SEM) in prostatic carcinoma in relation to response to hormonal manipulation

Reference	Salt-extractable	Salt-resistant	Total
Brendler et al. (1984)	*Expressed as fmol/mg DNA*		
Good responders (9)[a]	198 ± 21 $P<0.05$	73 ± 9 NS	271 ± 27 $P>0.05<0.1$
Poor responders (7)	139 ± 14	68 ± 9	207 ± 20
Gonor et al. (1984)	*Expressed as fmol/g tissue*		
Good responders (7)	193 ± 53 $P<0.05$	611 ± 192 $P<0.05$	803 ± 219 $P<0.05$
Poor responders (6)	45 ± 17	119 ± 34	164 ± 41

NS, no significant difference between means.
[a]Numbers in parentheses represent number of specimens assayed.

Other Potential Biochemical Markers of Androgen Sensitivity

It has been suggested by some investigators that the DHT content of prostatic tissue might indicate its androgen sensitivity. Geller et al. (1984) found that hormonally manipulated stage D patients whose tumors contained DHT concentrations above 2.5 ng/g tissue had better responses than those whose tumors contained less than 2.0 ng/g. No correlation was observed between cytosol or nuclear AR concentrations and DHT concentration. Belis and Tarry (1981) also reported that in stage D patients there was a correlation between duration of response to hormonal manipulation and the DHT content of their tumor tissue. These authors also observed a relationship between DHT concentration and tumor grade, but not with tumor stage. These results were not confirmed by Brendler et al. (1984), who could find neither a significant difference in the testosterone or DHT content of tumor tissue from good and poor responders to hormonal manipulation nor a relationship between DHT content and tumor grade. However, these investigators have devised a multiple index using five biochemical variables, which gave a better discrimination between good and poor responders than any one variable alone. The variables were salt-extractable nuclear AR, prostate-specific acid phosphatase, and three enzymes involved with androgen metabolism, viz. 5α-reductase, $3\alpha(\beta)$-hydroxysteroid oxidoreductase, and 17β-hydroxysteroid oxidoreductase (Brendler et al. 1985).

Histochemical Indicators of Androgen Sensitivity

Because of the limitations described on pp. 64–65, it is doubtful whether any biochemical test, including AR assay, will have as wide an application in the management of prostatic carcinoma as estrogen and progesterone assays do in the management of breast cancer. Development of a reliable histochemical procedure permitting visualization of a marker for androgen sensitivity would be a valuable supplement to the biochemical methods in use, in that it would make it possible to discriminate between the malignant and the nonmalignant components in the specimen under examination. It would also be applicable to small samples, such as are obtained by needle biopsy. The histochemical localization of AR itself has been attempted using fluorescent conjugates of testosterone, DHT, or R1881 (Pertschuk et al. 1984; Naito et al. 1981): the value of this approach is controversial because of the low affinity and poor specificity of the fluorescent ligands for AR (e.g., Berns et al. 1984). In the event that antibody to AR becomes available, analogous to the monoclonal antibodies to estrogen receptor (ER) which have been produced (Greene et al. 1984), it would be possible to visualize AR with more confidence. However, such an antibody is likely to react with the total cellular AR. As described above, cytosolic AR is not necessarily related to androgen sensitivity: thus it would be necessary to raise an antibody to that fraction of the AR which is defined as nuclear in the biochemical assay, or even to a subfraction of this, such as the salt-extractable nuclear AR. Alternatively, it might be possible to apply this technique after differential extraction procedures had been applied to tissue sections.

Another approach to the localization of AR at the cell level is that of autoradiography. With the availability of radioactive androgens with very high specific activity, it is possible to inject physiologic doses into experimental animals followed by localization of the androgen (presumably bound to AR) in frozen tissue sections (Weaker and Sheridan 1983). As well as the androgen administration by injection, such experiments require very long exposure (several months) of the autoradiographic film and are impractical for clinical use. It has been found possible to localize radioactive estradiol in breast carcinoma tissue sections by autoradiography after incubation of the tissue with the labeled hormone (Buell and Tremblay 1983); this avoids the necessity for injection and may reduce the time necessary for exposure. This approach has been used to localize ^{3}H-DHT binding sites in human and experimental rat prostatic carcinoma. Localization of ^{3}H-DHT was observed primarily in acinar epithelial cells in the human tissue, and also in extra-acinar epithelioid cells in the rat tumors (Beckman et al. 1985).

In breast carcinoma, it has been found that a marker for the functional integrity of ER, i.e., PgR, is a better prognostic factor and indicator of hormonal sensitivity than ER itself (McGuire and Clark 1983). Similarly, in prostatic carcinoma, a marker for functional AR may be a more useful indicator of androgen sensitivity than AR itself. Such an approach at the biochemical level was discussed on p. 71. Of the biochemical variables mentioned there, prostate-specific acid phosphatase (PSAP) is probably the most promising with regard to the development of a potential immunohistochemical test for the detection of androgen sensitive cells. A significant correlation has been observed between concentrations of PSAP and DHT in the epithelium of BPH tissue (Bolton et al. 1981), and at least one study has indicated that PSAP staining in carcinoma specimens may be related to response to hormonal therapy (Pontes et al. 1981). All histochemical methods have the potential for problems in tissue sampling, and the acquisition of quantitative data by these methods is difficult. Histochemical and biochemical methods may therefore best be considered as complementary approaches for the evaluation of androgen sensitivity in prostatic carcinoma.

Is the Prostate a Target Organ for Estrogen?

The action of pharmacologic doses of estrogen in the control of prostatic growth is thought to be mainly indirect, by the exertion of a negative feedback effect on the secretion of gonadotropins. Local effects, such as the inhibition of 5α-reductase activity (Briggs and Briggs 1973; Jenkins and McCaffery 1974; Orestano et al. 1974; Tan et al. 1974) and the partial inhibition of androgen binding to AR by high concentrations of estradiol (but not synthetic estrogens) (Mobbs et al. 1980a), have been observed, but it is not known whether these effects have a therapeutic role in the treatment of prostatic carcinoma. There is a good deal of evidence from animal models that exogenous estrogen can modulate prostatic growth, either of the fibromuscular component (Mawhinney and Neubauer 1979) or (in the dog) in the development of glandular hyperplasia (Cochran et al. 1981). In several animal systems, estrogen treatment has been reported to result in increases in prostate cytosol AR concentrations (Ip et al. 1980; Bouton et al. 1981; Frenette et al. 1981). In some, castration did not result in similar increases, as would be expected if the changes were due merely to redistribution of AR secondary to reduced testosterone levels (Bouton et al. 1981; Frenette et al. 1982). In the dog, estrogen treatment of castrated animals also resulted in increased nuclear AR levels (Trachtenberg et al. 1982b).

There is circumstantial evidence that endogenous estrogens might be involved in the etiology of BPH in man. Skoldefors et al. (1978) have reported higher estrogen levels in the blood and urine of patients with BPH than in controls, and Seppelt (1978) has demonstrated a correlation between the amount of stroma in BPH tissue and plasma and urinary estrogen concentrations. A further study indicated that estrogen (particularly estradiol) appears to be concentrated in the nuclei of the stromal component of BPH (Kozak et al. 1982). In carcinoma, it is of interest that Belis and Tarry (1981) observed that the concentrations of estradiol and estrone in prostatic carcinoma tissue decreased with increasing tumor grade. Mean concentrations of both estrogens in the tissue were above their mean concentrations in plasma (Belis 1980), but even in well differentiated carcinomas the estrogen concentration was approximately 100-fold less than that of DHT (Belis and Tarry 1981). A recent report by Rose et al. (1984) notes that estradiol (but not estrone) concentrations in the prostatic fluid of prostatic carcinoma patients were significantly higher than in that of control subjects of similar age. Concentrations of both estrogens were often higher in the prostatic fluid than in serum of the same subjects. There was no significant difference in the plasma estradiol or estrone concentrations between patients and controls. The significance of these observations remains to be demonstrated. It has already been mentioned that in some patients with prostatic carcinoma, long-term estrogen treatment was associated with much higher concentrations of unbound cytosol AR than would be expected from redistribution and "empty-ing" of receptor (Mobbs et al. 1983). Whether this increase was brought about by the estrogen treatment or whether it reflects progression of the tumor to a state in which AR regulation has broken down is not clear.

Estrogen Receptor in the Prostate

If the prostate is to be considered an estrogen target organ, it would be expected to contain ER and, in analogy with female target organs, estrogen treatment would be expected to induce PgR. ER has been observed in rat, dog, and baboon prostate (Armstrong and Bashirelahi 1978; Ginsberg et al. 1980; Robinette et al. 1978; Dube et al. 1979; Hawkins et al. 1980; Karr et al. 1978), and in experimental prostatic tumors in the rat (Heston et al. 1979; Markland and Lee 1979). In nonmalignant prostatic tissue from human subjects the presence of ER has been more controversial. In the cytosol, ER has usually been undetectable or observed in low concentrations, usually less than 20 fmol/mg cytosol protein (Kirdani et al. 1984; Bashirelahi et al. 1979; Auf and Ghanadian 1982; Murphy et al. 1980; Ekman et al. 1983; Donnelly et al. 1983). There are few recent data on the frequency of occurrence and concentration of ER in prostatic carcinoma: the reports that have been published indicate that ER occurs in 40%–100% of specimens, in concentrations similar to those in normal tissue. Ekman et al. (1983) observed both high affinity sites, corresponding to the classical receptor, and another class of sites with lower affinity for estradiol. Both types of site were observed in cytosol and in nuclear salt-extractable and salt-resistant fractions. The mean values for the high affinity sites in normal peripheral prostate and in carcinoma cytosol were less than 10 fmol/mg protein, and total nuclear ER values were less than 40 fmol/mg DNA. Similar concentrations of high affinity sites in normal and carcinoma tissue were observed by Murphy et al. (1980) and by Donnelly et al. (1983): however, these investigators did not report evidence for the presence of lower affinity sites. It is of interest that, when a sensitive enzyme immunoassay using monoclonal antibody to ER was used to quantitate ER in prostatic tissue, its presence could be demonstrated only in normal peripheral tissue, and not in BPH or cancer specimens. No ER could be demonstrated in any prostatic specimens using monoclonal antibody for ER in an immunohistochemical technique (Ekman et al. 1983). However, using autoradiography, Beckman et al. (1985) have observed uptake of ^{3}H-estradiol by extra-acinar epithelioid cells in prostatic carcinoma tissue after incubation in labeled medium.

Progesterone Receptor in the Prostate

In female target organs, the presence of significant quantities of PgR indicates estrogenic activity—indeed in breast carcinoma, as mentioned above, PgR concentrations are considered by many to be a better indicator of estrogen sensitivity than ER, since PgR synthesis depends on the functional activity of the latter. It is therefore of interest that PgR has been detected in BPH tissue by a number of investigators, sometimes in considerable quantities (Gustafsson et al. 1978; Ekman et al. 1982; Bashirelahi et al. 1983a; Schneider et al. 1984). In the cytosol, concentrations up to 150 fmol/mg cytosol protein have been reported. In one study, the concentration in the stromal and epithelial components were similar when expressed in terms of cytosol protein, but when expressed in terms of DNA content, i.e., when differences in cellularity were taken into account, the concentration in the stroma was considerably higher than that in the epithelium (Sirrett 1983). The few reports available on the PgR content of normal and malignant prostatic tissue indicate that concentrations are usually below 20 fmol/mg cytosol protein (Gustafsson et al. 1978; Ekman et al. 1979; Ekman et al. 1982). However, it is of interest that the highest value reported (180 fmol/mg cytosol protein) was observed in a carcinoma specimen from a patient who had been treated with massive doses of Honvol (diethylstilbestrol diphosphate) (Bashirelahi et al. 1983b). This raises the question of induction of PgR in prostatic tissue in patients treated with estrogen, as occurs in female target organs. Such induction would be difficult to establish unequivocally in man, but it has been observed in the dog (Frenette et al. 1982) and in the R3327 experimental prostatic carcinoma in the rat (Ip et al. 1980; Mobbs and Johnson 1985a). This tumor has been widely used as a model for human prostatic carcinoma, as it has a similar enzyme profile, contains androgen and estrogen receptors, and its growth can be retarded by castration and estrogen treatment. However, as a fraction of the cell population is not androgen sensitive, the tumor eventually relapses from hormonal control, and growth is resumed (Isaacs et al. 1978). In this model, we have demonstrated much higher concentrations of progestin-specific binding in tumors from diethylstilbestrol-treated rats than from untreated controls (Mobbs and Johnson 1985a). This binding protein has the characteristics of a progestin receptor, and the concentration is positively linearly related to the amount of DES ingested and to nuclear ER concentrations in the same tumors (Mobbs and Johnson 1985b, 1986).

It is interesting to speculate on the significance of PgR in male androgen target tissue. The mean concentration of progesterone in normal and hyperplastic human prostate has been reported to be similar to or higher than the mean concentration of testosterone in the same specimens (Hammond 1978; Belis 1980). Progestins are known to act as antiandrogens, both by the inhibition of 5α-reductase, for which progesterone is a better substrate than testosterone (Rennie et al. 1983b), and to some extent by competing with DHT for AR (Mobbs et al. 1980a). In the presence of significant amounts of PgR, however, progesterone might be sequestered by the receptor and prevented from playing its antiandrogenic role. PgR might thus act as a modulator of androgen metabolism.

It might be possible to exploit the presence of PgR in carcinoma tissue, particularly in patients who have been treated with estrogen, by using it as a target for a cytotoxic drug conjugated with a progestin. Since the ability of estrogen to induce PgR may well be independent of its antiandrogenic effect, this therapeutic approach might be applicable in patients whose tumors have relapsed from antiandrogenic control. The effectiveness of such an approach might depend on the tissue distribution of PgR: if it is present largely in the stromal component rather than in the glandular epithelium, the effectiveness would be limited. No information is yet available on the distribution of PgR in prostatic carcinoma tissue.

Receptors for Prolactin and Other Polypeptide Hormones

As long ago as 1946, Huggins and Russell demonstrated that hypophysectomy combined with castration resulted in a more complete atrophy of the dog prostate than castration alone. Grayhack observed a similar phenomenon in the rat (1963), and subsequent experimental work suggested that prolactin could promote growth and function of the prostate by modulating the uptake and utilization of androgen. This work has been recently reviewed by Jacobi (1982). Still more recently, Grayhack, Lee and their colleagues have shown that the mechanism by which prolactin retards regression of the lateral prostate after castration is not mediated by androgen receptors (Assimos et al. 1984) but is due rather to the inhibition of proteolytic degradation, probably by altering the interaction between proteolytic enzymes and their substrates (Smith et al. 1985).

The concept of the prostate as a target organ for prolactin is supported by demonstration of binding sites for this hormone. In human tissue, sites have been demonstrated biochemically (Keenan et al. 1979; Leake et al. 1983) and immunohistochemically (Witorsch 1979; Sibley et al. 1981; Purnell et al. 1982). Localization occurred in the glandular epithelium of benign and malignant tissue and was usually observed in the apical cytoplasm of the epithelial cells, but in a few cases appeared to be nuclear. In the investigation by Purnell et al. (1982), it was observed that staining occurred most frequently in poorly differentiated carcinomas. Staining was intensified by preincubation of the tissue with exogenous prolactin. In another study, staining was observed only after the application of exogenous lactogenic hormone: endogenous hormone could not be detected (Witorsch 1979).

The possibility that prolactin may exert a stimulatory influence on the prostate has raised concerns that it may be a factor in the progression of carcinoma, particularly in patients who have been treated with estrogens and/or with antihypertensive agents such as reserpine (Harper et al. 1976; Jacobi 1982). Both these treatments are known to increase serum prolactin levels. However, clinical evidence that alterations in circulating prolactin levels alter the course of the disease is conflicting (Jacobi 1982; Newball and Byar 1973).

Very few data are available on binding sites for polypeptide hormones other than prolactin in the prostate. Sibley et al. (1981, 1984) demonstrated some immunohistochemical staining with antibodies to FSH, LH, and growth hormone. FSH was localized primarily in the epithelium, growth hormone in the stroma, and slight diffuse staining for LH was observed. When the tissue was preincubated with growth hormone, staining for the latter was also observed in epithelial cells. The significance of these results is not yet clear.

Conclusions

The prostate is clearly under very complex hormonal control: during the last decade, the investigation of hormone receptors has indicated that the neoplastic human gland may be a target organ for the direct action of several components in this complex system. We now have a clearer conception of the role of AR as one of the elements which determine androgen sensitivity: where satisfactory tissue samples can be obtained, nuclear AR content can be used as a predictive factor in prognosis and as an indicator for treatment, preferably in combination with other markers for androgen sensitivity. Understanding of the mechanism of AR action has resulted in the development of antiandrogenic drugs which block androgen action by competing with dihydrotestosterone for AR sites. Such drugs provide an alternative to orchiectomy and avoid the side-effects associated with estrogen treatment. The clinical implications of the presence of receptors for estrogen, progesterone, prolactin, and other polypeptide hormones still remain to be explored.

References

Albert J, Geller J, Nachtsheim DA (1982) The type of current frequency used in transurethral resection of the prostate (TURP) affects the androgen receptor. Prostate 3:221–224

Armstrong EG, Bashirelahi N (1978) Determination of the binding properties of estradiol-17β within the cytoplasmic and nuclear fractions of rat ventral prostate. J Steroid Biochem 9:507–513

Assimos D, Smith C, Lee C, Grayhack JT (1984) Action of prolactin in regressing prostate: independent of action mediated by androgen receptors. Prostate 5:589–595

Auf G, Ghanadian R (1982) Characterization and measurement of cytoplasmic and nuclear oestradiol-17β-receptor protein in benign hypertrophied human prostate. J Endocrinol 98:305–317

Bard DR, Lasnitzki I (1977) The influence of oestradiol on the metabolism of androgen by human prostatic tissue. J Endocrinol 74:1–9

Bardin CW, Wright W (1980) Androgen receptor deficiency: testicular feminization, its variants, and differential diagnosis. Ann Clin Res 12:236–242

Barrack ER (1983) The nuclear matrix of the prostate contains acceptor sites for androgen receptors. Endocrinology 113:430–432

Barrack ER, Bujnovsky P, Walsh PC (1983) Subcellular distribution of androgen receptors in human normal, benign hyperplastic and malignant prostatic tissues: characterization of nuclear salt-resistant receptors. Cancer Res 43:1107–1116

Bashirelahi N, Kneussel ES, Vassil TC, Young JD, Sanefugi H, Trump B (1979) Measurement and characterization of estrogen receptors in the human prostate. In: Murphy GP, Sandberg AA (eds) Prostate cancer and hormone receptors. Alan R Liss, New York, pp 65–84

Bashirelahi N, Felder CC, Young JD (1983a) Characterization and stabilization of progesterone receptors in human benign prostatic hypertrophy. J Steroid Biochem 18:801–809

Bashirelahi N, Young JD, Shida K, Yamanaka H, Ito Y, Harada M (1983b) Androgen, estrogen and progesterone receptors in peripheral and central zones of human prostate with adenocarcinoma. Urology XXI:530–535

Beckmann WC, Mickey DD, Fried AF (1985) Autoradiographic localization of estrogen and androgen target cells in human and rat prostatic carcinoma. J Urol 133:724–728

Belis JA (1980) Methodologic basis for the radioimmunoassay of endogenous steroids in human prostatic tissue. Invest Urol 17:332–336

Belis JA, Tarry WF (1981) Radioimmunoassay of tissue steroids in adenocarcinoma of the prostate. Cancer 48:2416–2419

Berns EMJJ, Mulder E, Rommerts FFG et al. (1984) Fluorescent androgen derivatives do not discriminate between androgen receptor-positive and -negative human tumor cell lines. Prostate 5:425–437

Blankenstein MA, Bolt-de Vreis J, Foekens JA (1982) Nuclear androgen receptor assay in biopsy-size specimens of human prostatic tissue. Prostate 3:351–359

Blondeau JP, Corpechot C, le Goascogne C, Baulieu EE, Robel P (1975) Androgen receptors in the rat ventral prostate and their hormonal control. Vitam Horm 33:319–344

Bolton NJ, Lahtonen R, Vihko P, Kontturi M, Vihko R (1981) Androgen and prostate specific acid phosphatase in whole tissue and in separated epithelium from human benign prostatic hypertrophic glands. Prostate 2:209–416

Bouton MM, Pornin C, Grandadam JA (1981) Estrogen regulation of rat prostate androgen receptor. J Steroid Biochem 15:403–408

Brendler CB, Isaacs JT, Follansbee AL, Walsh PC (1984) The use of multiple variables to predict response to endocrine therapy in carcinoma of the prostate: a preliminary report. J Urol 131:694–700

Brendler CB, Follansbee AL, Isaacs JT (1985) Discrimination between normal, hyperplastic and malignant human prostatic tissues by enzymatic profiles. J Urol 133:495–501

Briggs MH, Briggs M (1973) Effects of ethinylestradiol and cyproterone acetate on androgen metabolism by human prostate gland. J Clin Endocrinol Metab 36:600–604

Bruchovsky N, Lesser B, Van Doorn E, Craven S (1975) Hormonal effects on cell proliferation in rat prostate. Vitam Horm 33:61–100

Bruchovsky N, Callaway T, Lieskovsky B, Rennie PS (1980) Markers of androgen action in human prostate: potential use in the clinical assessment of prostatic carcinoma. In: Wittliff JL, Dapunt O (eds) Steroid receptors and hormone-dependent neoplasia. Masson, New York, pp 121–131

Buell RH, Tremblay G (1983) The localization of ^{3}H-estradiol in estrogen receptor-positive human mammary carcinoma as visualized by thaw-mount autoradiography. Cancer 51:1625–1630

Cochran RC, Ewing LL, Niswender GD (1981) Serum levels of follicle stimulating hormone, luteinizing hormone, prolactin, testosterone, 5α-dihydrotestosterone, 5α-androstane-3α,17β-diol, 5α-androstane-3β,17β-diol, and 17β-estradiol from male beagles with spontaneous or induced benign prostatic hyperplasia. Invest Urol 19:142–147

Costlow ME, Pui C-H, Dahl GV (1982) Glucocorticoid receptors in acute lymphocytic leukemia. Cancer Res 42:4801–4806

Donnelly BJ, Lakey WH, McBlain WA (1983) Estrogen receptor in human benign prostatic hyperplasia. J Urol 130:183–187

Dube JY, Lesage R, Tremblay RR (1979) Estradiol and progesterone receptors in dog prostate cytosol. J Steroid Biochem 10:459–466

Ekman P, Snochowski M, Zatterberg A, Hogberg B, Gustafsson J-A (1979) Steroid receptor content in human prostatic carcinoma and response to endocrine therapy. Cancer 44:1173–1181

Ekman P, Barrack ER, Walsh PC (1982) Simultaneous measurement of progesterone and androgen receptors in human prostate: a microassay. J Clin Endocrinol Metab 55:1089–1099

Ekman P, Barrack ER, Greene GL, Jensen EV, Walsh PC (1983) Estrogen receptors in human prostate: evidence for multiple binding sites. J Clin Endocrinol Metab 57:166–176

Fang S, Anderson KM, Liao S (1969) Receptor proteins for androgens. On the role of specific proteins in selective retention of 17β-hydroxy-5α-androstane-3-one by rat ventral prostate in vivo and in vitro. J Biol Chem 244:6584–6595

Fentie DD, Lakey WH, McBlain WA (1986) Applicability of nuclear androgen receptor quantification to human prostatic adenocarcinoma. J Urol 135:167–173

Fowler JE, Whitmore WF (1981) The response of metastatic adenocarcinoma of the prostate to exogenous testosterone. J Urol 126:372–375

Frenette G, Dube JY, Tremblay RR (1982) Effect of hormone injections on levels of cytosolic receptors for estrogen, androgen and progesterone in dog prostate. J Steroid Biochem 17:271–276

Geller J, Cantor T, Albert J (1975) Evidence for a specific dihydrotestosterone-binding cytosol receptor in the human prostate. J Clin Endocrinol Metab 41:854–862

Geller J, Albert J, Loza D (1979) Steroid levels in cancer of the prostate—markers of tumor differentiation and adequacy of anti-androgen treatment. J Steroid Biochem 11:631–636

Geller J, de la Vega DJ, Albert J, Nachtsheim DA (1984) Tissue dihydrotestosterone levels and clinical response to hormonal therapy with patients with advanced prostate cancer. J Clin Endocrinol Metab 58:36–40

Ghanadian R, Auf G, Williams G, Davis A, Richards B (1981) Predicting the response of prostatic carcinoma to endocrine therapy. Lancet II:1418

Ginsberg M, Jung-Testas I, Baulieu EE (1980) Specific high-affinity oestradiol binding in rat ventral prostate. J Endocrinol 87:285–292

Gonor SE, Lakey WH, McBlain WA (1984) Relationship between concentrations of extractable and matrix-bound nuclear androgen receptor and clinical response to endocrine therapy for prostatic adenocarcinoma. J Urol 131:1196–1201

Grayhack J (1963) Pituitary factors influencing growth of the prostate. Natl Cancer Inst Monogr 12:189–199

Greene GL, Sobel NB, King WJ, Jensen EV (1984) Immunochemical studies of estrogen receptors. J Steroid Biochem 20:51–56

Gustafsson J-A, Ekman P, Pousette A, Snochowski M, Hogberg B (1978) Demonstration of a progestin receptor in human benign prostatic hyperplasia and prostatic carcinoma. Invest Urol 15:361–366

Habib FK, Tesdale AL, Chisholm GD, Busuttil A (1981) Androgen metabolism in the epithelial and stromal components of the human hyperplasic prostate. J Endocrinol 91:23–32

Habib FK, Busuttil A, Robinson RA, Chisholm GD (1985a) 5α-Reductase activity in human prostate cancer is related to the histological differentiation of the tumour. Clin Endocrinol 23:431–438

Habib FK, Smith T, Robinson R, Chisholm GD (1985b) Influence of surgical techniques on receptor level and 5α-reductase activity of the human prostate gland. Prostate 7:287–292

Hammond GL (1978) Endogenous steroid levels in the human prostate from birth to old age: a comparison of normal and diseased tissues. J Endocrinol 78:7–19

Harper ME, Peeling WB, Cowley T et al. (1976) Plasma steroid and protein hormone concentrations in patients with prostatic carcinoma, before and during oestrogen therapy. Acta Endocrinol 81:409–426

Hawkins GF, Trachtenberg J, Hicks LL, Walsh PC (1980) Androgen and estrogen receptors in the canine prostate. J Androl 5:234–243

Heston WDW, Menon M, Tananis C, Walsh PC (1979) Androgen, estrogen and progesterone receptors of the R3327 H Copenhagen rat prostatic tumor. Cancer Lett 6:45–50

Hudson RW (1982) Studies of the cytosol 3α-hydroxysteroid dehydrogenase of human prostatic tissue: comparison of enzyme activities in hyperplastic, malignant and normal tissues. J Steroid Biochem 16:373–377

Hudson RW, Moffitt PM, Owens WA (1983) Studies of the nuclear 5α-reductase of human prostatic tissue: comparison of enzyme activities in hyperplastic malignant and normal tissues. Can J Biochem Cell Biol 61:750–755

Huggins C, Russell PS (1946) Quantitative effects of hypophysectomy on testis and prostate of dogs. Endocrinology 39:1–7

Ip MM, Milholland RJ, Rosen J (1980) Functionality of estrogen receptor and tamoxifen treatment of R3327 Dunning rat prostate adenocarcinoma. Cancer Res 40:2188–2193

Isaacs JT, Heston WDW, Weissman RM, Coffey DS (1978) Animal models of the hormone-sensitive and -insensitive prostatic carcinomas, Dunning R-3327-H, R3327-HI, and R-3327-AT. Cancer Res 38:4353–4359

Jacobi GH (1982) Experimental rationale for the investigation of antiprolactins as palliative treatment for prostate cancer. In: Jacobi GH, Hohenfeller R (eds) International perspectives in Urology 3: Prostate cancer. Williams and Wilkins, Baltimore, pp 419–431

Jenkins JS, McCaffery VM (1974) Effect of oestradiol-17β and progesterone on the metabolism of testosterone by human prostatic tissue. J Endocrinol 63:517–526

Jensen EV (1984) Intracellular localization of estrogen receptors: implications for interaction mechanism. Lab Invest 51:487–488

Karr JP, Sufrin G, Kirdani RY, Murphy GP, Sandberg AA (1978) Prostatic binding of estradiol-17β in the baboon. J Steroid Biochem 9:87–94

Keenan EJ, Kemp ED, Ramsay EE, Garrison LB, Pearse HD, Hodges CV (1979) Specific binding of prolactin by the prostate gland of rat and man. J Urol 122:43–46

Kirdani RY, Pontes EJ, Murphy GP, Sandberg AA (1984) Correlation of estrogen and androgen receptor status in prostatic disease measured by high pressure liquid chromatography. J Steroid Biochem 20:401–406

Kitano T, Usui T, Yasukawa A, Nakahara M, Nihira H, Miyachi Y (1983) Androgen receptor in electroresected and cold punch-resected specimens. Urology XXI:119–122

Kliman B, Prout GR, Maclaughlin RA, Daly JJ, Griffin PP (1978) Altered androgen metabolism in metastatic prostate cancer. J Urol 119:623–626

Knight WA, Osborne CK, Yochmowitz MG, McGuire WL (1980) Steroid hormone receptors in the management of breast cancer. Ann Clin Res 12:202–207

Kozak I, Bartsch W, Krieg M, Voigt KD (1982) Nuclei of stroma: site of highest estrogen concentration in human benign prostatic hyperplasia. Prostate 3:433–438

Krieg M (1984) Biochemical endocrinology of human prostatic tumors. In: Bresciani F, King RJB, Lippman M, Namer M, Raynaud J-P (eds) Progress in cancer research and therapy, vol 32. Raven Press, New York, pp 425–452

Krieg M, Bartsch W, Janssen W, Voigt KD (1979) A comparative study of binding, metabolism and endogenous levels of androgens in normal, hyperplastic and carcinomatous human prostate. J Steroid Biochem 11:615–624

Leake A, Chisholm GD, Habib FK (1983) Characterization of the prolactin receptor in human prostate. J Endocrinol 99:321–328

Markland FS, Lee L (1979) Characterization and comparison of the estrogen and androgen receptors from the R-3327 rat prostate adenocarcinoma. J Steroid Biochem 10:13–20

Mawhinney MG, Neubauer BL (1979) Actions of estrogen in the male. Invest Urol 16:409–420

McGuire WL, Clark GM (1983) The prognostic role of progesterone receptors in human breast cancer. Semin Oncol 10:2–6

McNeal JE (1981) The zonal anatomy of the prostate. Prostate 2:35–49

Menon M, Tananis CE, McLoughlin MG, Lippman ME, Walsh PC (1977) The measurement of androgen receptors in human prostatic tissue utilizing sucrose density gradient centrifugation and a protamine precipitation assay. J Urol 117:309–312

Mobbs BG, Johnson IE (1985a) Characterization of estrogen-induced progestin binding in cytosol of the R3327 prostatic carcinoma of the rat. J Steroid Biochem 22:57–62

Mobbs BG, Johnson IE (1985b) Relationships between estrogen intake, serum testosterone, and tumor androgen, estrogen, and progesterone receptor levels in diethylstilbestrol-treated rats bearing the R3327 prostatic adenocarcinoma. Prostate 7:293–304

Mobbs BG, Johnson IE (1986) Quantitative relationships between cytosol and nuclear estrogen and progesterone receptors in the R3327 prostatic carcinoma of rats treated with diethylstilbestrol. Prostate 8:255–264

Mobbs BG, Johnson IE, Connolly JG (1975) In vitro assay of androgen binding by human prostate. J Steroid Biochem 6:453–458

Mobbs BG, Johnson IE, Connolly JG, Clark AF (1977) Evaluation of the use of cyproterone acetate competition to distinguish between high-affinity binding of [³H]-dihydrotestosterone to human prostate cytosol receptors and to sex hormone-binding globulin. J Steroid Biochem 8:943–949

Mobbs BG, Johnson IE, Connolly JG (1978) Androgen receptor assay in human benign and malignant prostatic tumor cytosol using protamine sulphate precipitation. J Steroid Biochem 9:289–301

Mobbs BG, Johnson IE, Connolly JG (1980a) Androgen receptors and treatment of prostatic cancer. In: Schroder FH, de Voogt HJ (eds) Steroid receptors, metabolism and prostatic cancer. Excerpta Medica Amsterdam, pp 225–239

Mobbs BG, Johnson IE, Connolly JG (1980b) The effect of therapy on the concentration and occupancy of androgen receptors in human prostatic cytosol. Prostate 1:37–51

Mobbs BG, Johnson IE, Connolly JG, Thompson J (1983) Concentration and cellular distribution of androgen receptor in human prostatic neoplasia: Can estrogen treatment increase androgen receptor content? J Steroid Biochem 19:1279–1290

Morfin RF, Charles J-F, Floch HH (1979) $C_{19}O_2$-steroid transformations in the human normal, hyperplastic and cancerous prostate. J Steroid Biochem 11:599–607

Murphy JB, Emmott RC, Hicks LL, Walsh PC (1980) Estrogen receptor in the human prostate, seminal vesicle, epididymis, testis, and genital skin: a marker for estrogen-responsive tissues. J Clin Endocrinol Metab 50:938–948

Naito H, Ito H, Wakisaka M, Kambegawa A, Shimazaki J (1981) Histochemical observation of R1881 binding protein in human benign prostatic hypertrophy. Invest Urol 18:337–340

Newball HH, Byar DP (1973) Does reserpine increase prolactin and exacerbate cancer of prostate? Case control study. Urology II:525–529

Orestano F, Klose K, Rubin A, Knapstein P, Altwein JE (1974) Testosterone metabolism in benign prostatic hypertrophy. Suppression by diethylstilbestrol and gestonerone capronate. Invest Urol 12:151–156

Pertschuk LP, Macchia RJ, New York Prostate Cancer Binding Site Study Group (1984) Histochemical androgen binding assay in prostatic cancer. J Urol 131:1096–1098

Pontes JE, Rose NR, Ercole C, Pierce JM (1981) Immunofluorescence for prostatic acid phosphatase: clinical applications. J Urol 126:187–189

Purnell DM, Hillman EA, Heatfield BM, Trump BF (1982) Immunoreactive prolactin in epithelial cells of normal and cancerous human breast and prostate detected by the unlabelled antibody peroxidase–antiperoxidase method. Cancer Res 42:2317–2324

Rennie PS, Bruchovsky N (1972) In vitro and in vivo studies on the functional significance of androgen receptors in rat prostate. J Biol Chem 247:1546–1554

Rennie PS, Bruchovsky N, Chang H (1983a) Isolation of 3S androgen receptors from salt-resistant fractions and nuclear matrices of prostatic nuclei after mild trypsin digestion. J Biol Chem 258:7623–7630

Rennie PS, Bruchovsky N, McLoughlin MG, Batzold FH, Dunstan-Adams EE (1983b) Kinetic analysis of 5α-reductase isoenzymes in benign prostatic hyperplasia (BPH). J Steroid Biochem 19:169–173

Robinette CL, Blume CD, Mawhinney MG (1978) Androphilic and estrophilic molecules in canine prostate glands. Invest Urol 15:425–431

Rose DP, Laakso K, Sotaranta M, Wynder E (1984) Hormone levels in prostatic fluid from healthy Finns and prostatic cancer patients. Eur J Cancer 20:1317–1319

Rosen V, Jung I, Baulieu EE, Robel P (1975) Androgen-binding proteins in human benign prostatic hypertrophy. J Clin Endocrinol Metab 41:761–770

Sanefugi H, Heatfield BM, Trump BF, Young SD (1982) Studies on carcinogenesis of human prostate. II. Long-term explant culture of normal prostate and benign prostatic hyperplasia: light microscopy. J Natl Cancer Inst 69:751–756

Schneider SL, Pontes E, Greco JM, Murphy GP, Sandberg AA (1984) Characterization of 7–8S progestin binding protein in human prostate using vertical tube rotor. J Steroid Biochem 20:715–723

Seppelt U (1978) Correlation among prostate stroma, plasma estrogen levels and urinary estrogen excretion in patients with benign prostatic hypertrophy. J Clin Endocrinol Metab 74:1230–1235

Shain SA, Boesel RW, Lamm DL, Radwin HM (1980) Cytoplasmic and nuclear androgen receptor content of normal and neoplastic human prostate and lymph node metastases of human prostatic adenocarcinoma. J Clin Endocrinol Metab 50:704–711

Shimazaki J, Hikage T, Sato R, Kodama T, Ito H (1981) Measurement of androgen receptor in cytosols from normal, benign hypertrophic and cancerous human prostates. Endocrinol Jpn 28:725–734

Sibley PEC, Harper ME, Boyce BG, Peeling WP, Griffiths K (1981) The immunocytochemical detection of protein hormones in human prostatic tissues. Prostate 2:175–185

Sibley PEC, Harper ME, Peeling WB, Griffiths K (1984) Growth hormone and prostatic tumors: localization using a monoclonal human growth hormone antibody. J Endocrinol 103:311–315

Sirrett DAN (1983) Progestin binding in benign hyperplastic prostatic tissue. J Steroid Biochem 19:163–167

Skoldefors H, Blomstedt B, Carlstrom K (1978) Serum hormone levels in benign prostatic hyperplasia. Scand J Urol Nephrol 12:111–114

Smith C, Assimos D, Lee C, Grayhack JT (1985) Metabolic action of prolactin in regressing prostate: independent of androgen action. Prostate 6:49–59

Tan SY, Antonipillai, Pearson Murphy BE (1974) Inhibition of testosterone metabolism in the human prostate. J Clin Endocrinol Metab 39:936–941

Tisell L-E, Salander H (1975) The lobes of the human prostate. Scand J Urol Nephrol 9:185–191

Trachtenberg J, Walsh PC (1982) Correlation of prostatic nuclear androgen receptor content with duration of response and survival following hormonal therapy in advanced prostatic cancer. J Urol 127:466–471

Trachtenberg J, Bujnovsky P, Walsh PC (1982a) Androgen receptor content of normal and hyperplastic human prostate. J Clin Endocrinol Metab 54:17–21

Trachtenberg J, Hicks LL, Walsh PC (1982b) Androgen and estrogen receptor content in spontaneous and experimentally induced canine prostatic hyperplasia. J Clin Invest 65:1051–1052

Vihko R, Bolton N, Hammond GL, Lahtonen R (1981) Steroids in normal and diseased human prostatic tissue. In: Fotherby K, Pal SB (eds) Hormones in normal and abnormal tissues. Walter de Gruyter, Berlin New York, pp 523–539

Wagner RK (1980) Lack of correlation between androgen receptor content and clinical response to treatment with diethylstilbestrol (DES) in human prostate carcinoma. In: Schroder FH, de Voogt HJ (eds) Steroid receptors, metabolism and prostatic cancer. Excerpta Medica, Amsterdam, pp 190–197

Walsh PC (1984) Human benign prostatic hyperplasia: etiological considerations. In: Kimball FA, Buhl AE, Carter DB (eds) New approaches to the study of benign prostatic hyperplasia. Alan R Liss, New York, pp 1–25

Walsh PC, Hicks LL (1979) Characterization and measurement of androgen receptors in human prostatic tissue. In: Murphy GP, Sandberg AA (eds) Prostate cancer and hormone receptors. Alan R Liss, New York, pp 51–63

Walsh PC, Hutchins GM, Ewing LL (1983) Tissue content of dihydrotestosterone in human prostatic hyperplasia is not supranormal. J Clin Invest 72:1772–1777

Weaker F, Sheridan PJ (1983) Autoradiographic localization of ^{3}H-dihydrotestosterone in the reproductive organs of baboons. Acta Anat 115:244–251

Witorsch R (1979) The application of immunoperoxidase methodology for the visualization of prolactin binding sites in human prostate tissue. Human Pathol 10:521–532

Zava DT, Landrum B, Horwitz KB, McGuire WL (1979) Androgen receptor assay with [^{3}H] methyltrienolone (R1881) in the presence of progesterone receptors. Endocrinology 104:1007–1012

Chapter 5

Imaging Techniques in the Diagnosis and Pelvic Staging of Prostatic Cancer

P. N. Bretan and R. D. Williams

Introduction

The initial diagnosis of prostatic cancer has typically relied on digital rectal examination which is, compared with other screening modalities, a noninvasive, cost effective, and highly reliable screening technique (Guinan et al. 1980; Chodak and Schoenberg 1984). Despite these advantages, over 50% of cases of prostatic cancer are diagnosed only after the disease has progressed beyond curability. Because earlier detection would allow institution of curative therapy, the search for imaging modalities capable of detecting intraprostatic lesions and delineating local extension has been extensive. This review focuses both on current imaging methods and on those likely to be useful in the future for the diagnosis and pelvic staging of prostatic cancer.

Ultrasonography

Watanabe pioneered the use of transrectal sonographic evaluation of the prostate and produced the first clinically useful scans in 1968. Subsequently, many reports have documented the use of ultrasound for prostate imaging by transrectal (TRU), transabdominal (TAU), and transurethral (TUU) approaches. While each technique has its proponents, TRU is most often used in screening and staging prostatic cancer (Fig. 5.1).

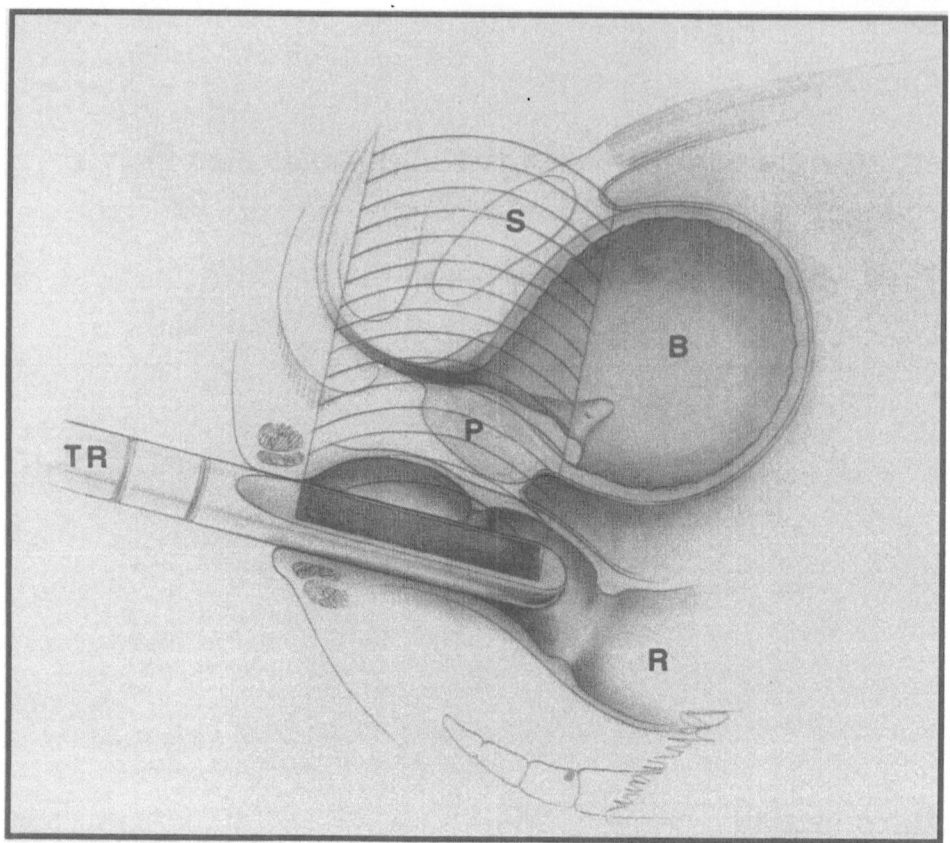

Fig. 5.1. Anatomic relationships identified by TRU: *TR*, 5-mHz rectal probe; *R*, rectum; *B*, bladder; *P*, prostate; *S*, symphysis pubis.

Although utrasound techniques have advanced and the contrast resolution of the prostate and its immediate surroundings have improved, the accuracy of TRU in diagnosing prostatic cancer has varied markedly among investigators. Initially, Watanabe et al. (1977) reported a high prevalence of incidental prostatic cancer among otherwise normal elderly men. Harada et al. (1980) used high resolution TRU equipment with gray-scale and radial techniques to differentiate normal prostates from those containing benign hypertrophy and carcinoma. In a study of 167 patients, they reported the accuracy to be 79%, 97%, and 86% respectively. Brooman et al. (1981) used a specially constructed chair (Aloka), previously described by Watanabe, in the TRU screening for prostatic cancer in 200 patients and reported a false-negative rate of 4% with a false-positive rate of 32%. Although many of these early studies involved patients with known carcinoma of the prostate, the lack of pathologic confirmation raised questions as to the reliability of sonography in differentiating prostatic cancer from other prostatic lesions. Until recently the only sign considered reliable for the diagnosis of prostatic cancer was a capsular breach of heterogeneous internal echo patterns of hyperechoic density as compared with normal prostate. Brooman et al. (1981) described the capsular breach as an area where there was either an apparent absence of the capsule or irregular echo-dense areas which extended through the capsule. By 1983 TRU had emerged as the most accurate noninvasive imaging method of assessing intra- and periprostatic abnormalities, despite the absence of absolute pathologic correlation with sonographic findings. Fritzche et al. (1983) and Velthoven et al. (1984) reviewed their experience in diagnosing prostatic cancer using TRU and reported the sensitivity to range from 80% to 90% and the specificity from 60% to 77%.

In 1984 Spirnak and Resnick reviewed the global experience with TRU prostatic imaging and summarized the typical sonographic findings for specific prostatic lesions. Benign prostatic hyperplasia (BPH) reveals a diffusely enlarged gland contained by a well defined capsule which is circumferentially continuous. BPH also has an increased anterior–posterior diameter and contains multiple fine homogeneous echoes that fade with increased attenuation (Fig. 5.2). Prostatic cancer produces asymmetric enlargement with areas of increased echogenicity (hyperechoic) within the prostate which do not fade with increased attenuation. Sonic shadows can also be produced by prostatic cancer. Finally, their review indicates that prostatitis, similar to prostatic cancer, produces multiple areas of increased echogenicity within the prostatic substance that tend to be more central yet can also produce sonic shadowing. Based on these criteria TRU was unable to distinguish the increased echogenicity of prostatic calculi, infarction, or prostatitis from cancer, contributing to the consistently reported 30%–40% false-positive rate of prostatic cancer diagnosis. Thus TRU was not considered capable of unequivocally diagnosing prostatic cancer and was not considered adequate for prostatic cancer screening.

Subsequent improvements in ultrasound technology, including real-time, linear array transducers and longitudinal scanning, have substantially enhanced its ability to image the prostate accurately. Concurrently, the use of ultrasound to accurately guide fine-gauge biopsy needles directly into suspected prostatic lesions by the transperineal route was developed (Fornage et al. 1983; Rifkin et al. 1983). New concepts in the anatomy of the prostate encouraged more precise interpretation of prostatic sonographic images. In an autopsy study McNeal (1972) determined that the prostate, rather than being divided into lobes as previously thought, comprises zones corresponding to developmental and acquired changes. Importantly, cancer of the prostate was shown to occur most often in the peripheral zone, which is a thin rim of tissue essentially only present posteriorly, laterally, and apically. BPH is found only in the central zone. Thus although prostatic cancer can secondarily involve the central zone, it is usually found close to the rectal surface of the prostate. Although this finding is not surprising, it has improved the overall interpretation of sonographic imaging. Based on these newer findings, it is predictable that TAU would be less sensitive for prostatic cancer as it images the anterior prostate and central zone better than the peripheral zone. Similarly, TRU probes having a short focal point should prove to be the most accurate for imaging the peripheral zone.

Recent reports of studies utilizing newer technology and anatomic information have suggested that prostatic cancer, rather than being hyperechoic as previously described, actually is hypoechoic to echopenic (Figs. 5.3, 5.4). These studies have finally correlated pathologic abnormalities of the prostate with sonographic patterns. Egender et al. (1984) studied ten cadaver prostates by ultrasound and concluded that cancer was echopenic: this finding supported

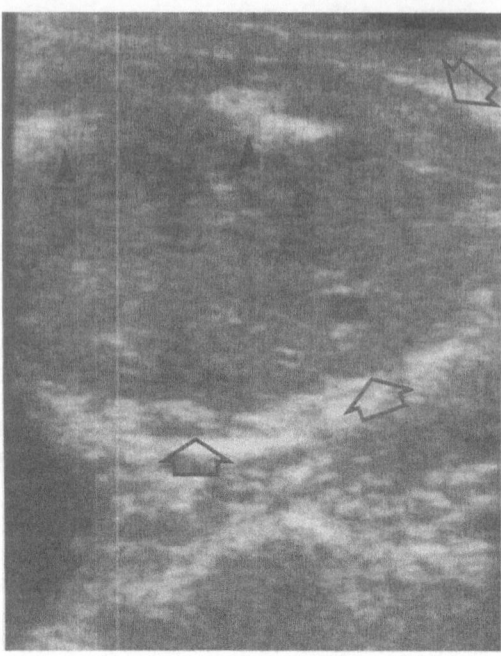

Fig. 5.2. TRU of BPH. Preoperative TRU of 100-g prostate removed via suprapubic prostatectomy. Prostate is diffusely enlarged. Capsule is well formed (*open arrows*). Multiple fine homogeneous echoes fade with increased attenuation (*black arrows*).

Fig. 5.3. TRU of hypoechoic lesion typical of prostatic cancer (*arrows*).
▼

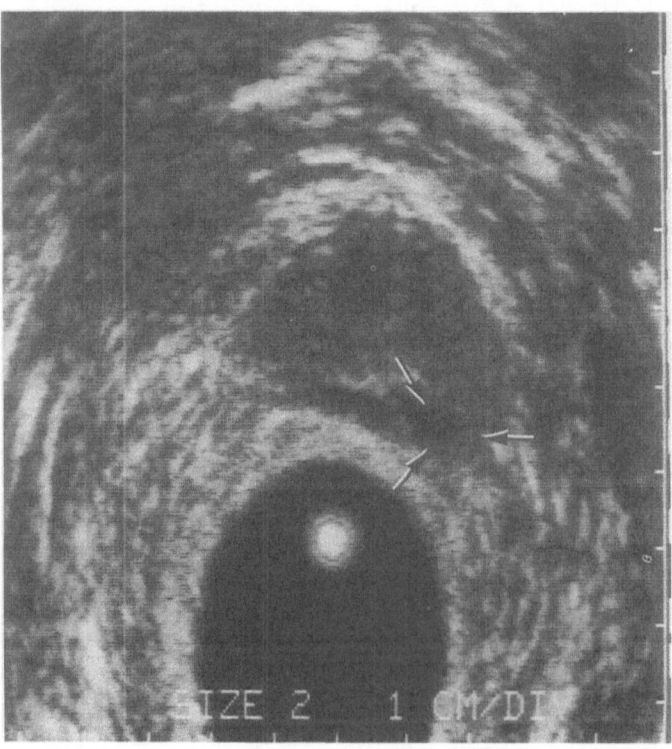

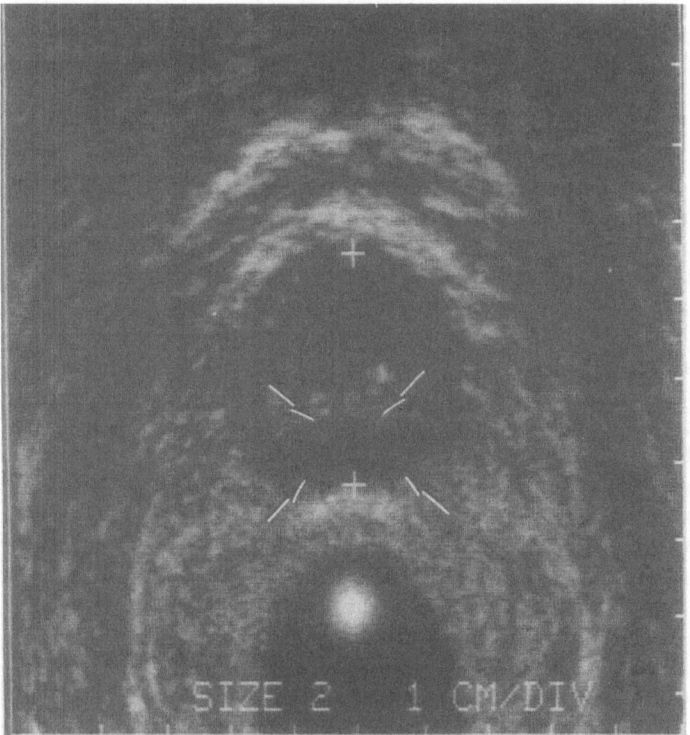

Fig. 5.4. TRU of large echopenic prostatic cancer (*arrows*).

their in vivo experience which had shown that over 70% of patients with prostatic cancer had echopenic lesions. Dähnert and co-workers, in a very convincing study, examined the prostates of 52 patients by TRU prior to radical prostatectomy. They examined 44 of the same prostates by direct ultrasonic scanning in a water bath immediately after prostatectomy and then submitted each specimen for complete histologic sectioning (2- to 3-mm intervals) (Dähnert et al. 1986). They found that BPH had a variable and irregular hypoechoic pattern in the central zone while prostatic cancer showed asymmetry, a tumor bulge posteriorly, and, in 76% of the cases, cancerous lesions which were either hypoechoic (54%) or echopenic (22%). They found no cases where the cancer was echogenic. It is important to realize that only clinical stage A and B patients were included in this study and that the authors observed that as a tumor grows and becomes more extensive, it may shift from hypoechoic to hyperechoic, perhaps accounting for some of the discrepancy in the literature. Finally, in a study of 45 patients who underwent transperineal prostatic biopsy with TRU guidance, Lee et al. (1986) found that normal peripheral zone tissue had a homogeneous isoechoic pattern but that prostatic cancer uniformly had a hypoechoic pattern which was confirmed by pathology in 78% of their cases. Biopsy of hyperechoic lesions demonstrated BPH. The use of linear scanning which allowed the biopsy needle to be accurately placed by direct visualization within the suspected lesion was considered critical to their success.

Not all authors agree with these sonographic findings, however. Burks et al. (1986) and Rifkin et al. (1986) found that more than 60% of patients studied by TRU-guided perineal biopsy had hyperechoic lesions; however, both studies lacked pathologic confirmation of the biopsy site, and hypoechoic lesions in Burks et al.'s study had a higher incidence of cancer than did hyperechoic lesions.

Despite the controversy surrounding the sonographic characteristics of prostatic lesions, it does appear that more specific and accurate criteria for the diagnosis of prostatic cancer have emerged. Whether this new information will increase the specificity of ultrasound studies and therefore be useful for the screening and local staging of prostatic cancer remains to be seen.

TAU and TUU have not been found to be particularly helpful for evaluation of prostatic cancer although TAU has been shown to be accurate in the estimation of prostatic volume (Bartsch et al. 1982) and TUU is a promising approach to evaluating the depth of penetration of bladder tumors (Gammel-guard and Holm 1980).

TRU has been shown to be useful in the treatment follow-up of prostatic cancer patients. For example, Carpenter and Schroder (1984) studied 66 patients whose prostate was examined by TRU before and after treatment for prostatic cancer by castration or pelvic radiotherapy. In hormonally treated cases an early decrease in prostatic volume indicated a favorable prognosis. In irradiated patients TRU did not provide an accurate prediction of prognosis, perhaps due to radiation changes affecting the sonographic image. Finally, TRU has been used successfully in guiding the transperineal placement of radiation seeds for treatment of primary prostatic cancer or local recurrence (Holm et al. 1983).

In summary, only recently have ultrasound criteria been described that will allow accurate differentiation of benign from malignant prostatic lesions. Further study will be required to document sonographic correlation with pathologic diagnosis in a larger number of patients before TRU will be accepted as a reliable screening and local staging technique.

Computed Tomography

Computed tomographic imaging (CT) is a major improvement over conventional X-ray imaging for the diagnosis and staging of pelvic malignancies. There are, however, few studies which correlate pathologic stage with the clinical stage predicted by CT. While CT provides the best spatial resolution of any current imaging modality, it is incapable of either defining lobes or anatomic zones within the prostate, or differentiating normal from abnormal histology of the prostate. Moreover, CT is incapable of detecting intracapsular prostatic cancer. Detection of capsular penetration and/or seminal vesicle involvement of prostatic carcinoma by CT has an accuracy rate ranging from 31% to 73% in reported series (Golimbu et al. 1981; Morgan et al. 1981; Weinerman et al. 1982; Emory et al. 1983).

The normal prostate, as imaged by CT (Fig. 5.5), is symmetric and surrounded by a rim of pelvic fat. Tumor extension is predicted by an

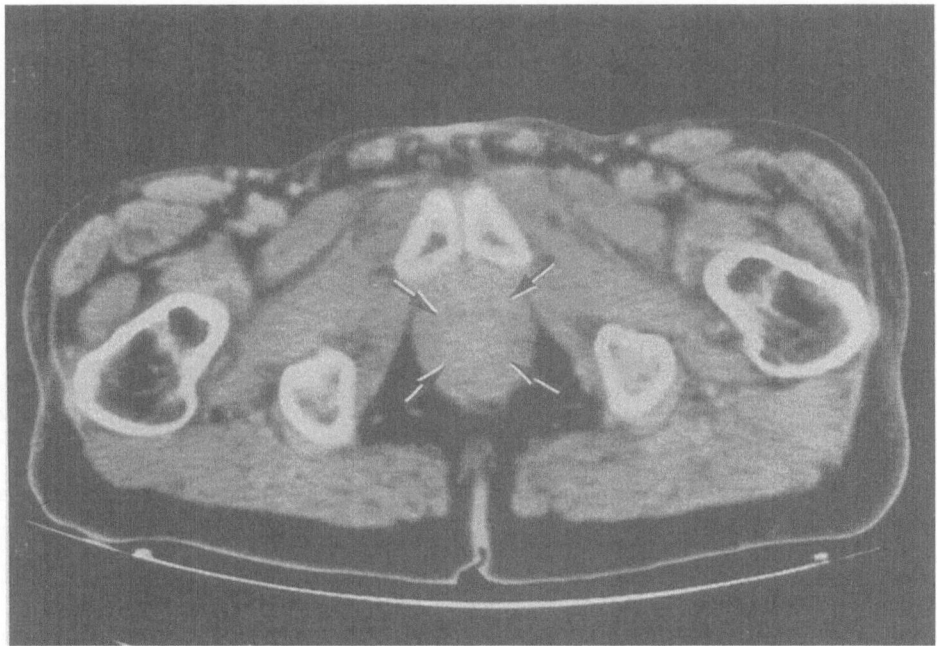

Fig. 5.5. CT of normal prostate (*arrows*)—transaxial image.

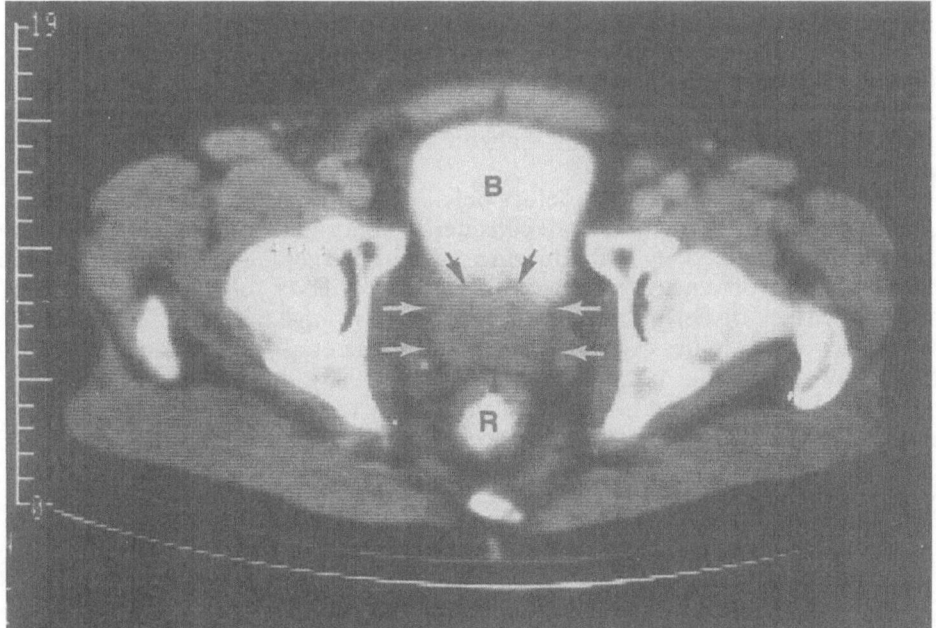

Fig. 5.6. CT of stage B$_2$ prostatic cancer—transaxial image. Note false-positive periprostatic haziness (*long arrows*). The prostate is identified by *short arrows*. *R*, rectum; *B*, bladder.

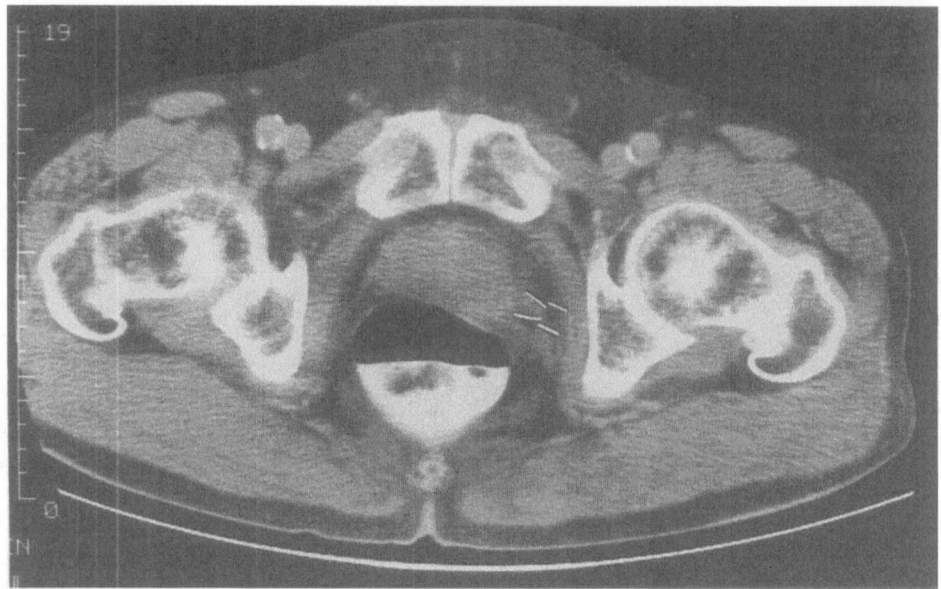

Fig. 5.7. CT of stage C prostatic cancer—transaxial image. Note asymmetry of prostate and apparent extension on the *left* (*arrows*).

interruption in the normal prostatic contour (Figs. 5.6, 5.7), asymmetric enlargement, or periprostatic tissue plane haziness. These radiographic findings are not specific for tumor and can be caused by inflammation or scar tissue from prior pelvic surgery, which would account for the low accuracy rates in reported studies. Denonvilliers' fascia is an important anatomic boundary but it is observed by CT in only half of the patients with a nonmalignant prostate. This limits its usefulness in predicting malignant transcapsular extension or seminal vesicle involvement.

CT imaging can be used to detect pelvic lymph node metastases; however, only nodes larger than 1.5 cm are considered abnormal. Intranodal abnormalities are not detected by CT. Because nodal enlargement is nonspecific and microscopic involvement is undetectable, CT specificity for nodal extension is poor. Accuracy of detecting tumorous nodes has ranged from 31% to 93% in several reported studies (Walsh et al. 1980; Levine et al. 1981; Shankagiri et al. 1982; Sawczuk et al. 1983; Denkhaus et al. 1983). Many of these studies, however, were done with CT scanners inferior by today's standards. Weinerman et al. (1983) have reported a 74% accuracy in pelvic lymph node staging in patients with confirmatory pathologic staging of prostatic cancer using dynamic (rapid sequence) CT.

Recently we reviewed nine patients who had pelvic CT using a current generation scanner prior to radical prostatectomy and pelvic lymphadenectomy (complete pathologic staging) and found the accuracy of CT diagnosis and staging of prostatic cancer to be 22% and 56% respectively (Williams et al. 1986). Although the study was limited, it confirmed our impression that CT is not capable of detecting intracapsular prostatic malignancy and is less accurate than a careful rectal examination for detection of local extension (periprostatic or seminal vesicle involvement). Although CT of the pelvis is not recommended in the routine staging of prostatic cancer, patients with high-grade, large volume, or locally extensive tumors have a greater than 50% probability of nodal involvement and thus may benefit from the study. In these patients, CT-guided needle aspiration cytology of enlarged pelvic lymph nodes could obviate the morbidity of surgical staging.

In summary, pelvic CT is not capable of detecting intracapsular prostatic cancer and thus is not useful for prostatic cancer screening. CT is capable of detecting local extension of prostatic cancer but the specificity is too low to recommend the study routinely. Finally, although CT can detect enlarged tumorous pelvic lymph nodes, its use is only recommended in those patients with a high probability of nodal extension.

Magnetic Resonance Imaging

Magnetic resonance imaging (MRI) relies on the abundance and relative position of protons (hydrogen ions) within living tissues to provide images with precise anatomic detail in multiple planar projections. In addition MRI may provide the simultaneous collection of physiologic and biochemical information. The ability of MRI to depict accurately human pathologic anatomy is related to the difference in proton relaxation parameters between normal tissues and pathologic tissues, such as tumors. A major reason for these differences may be the accumulation of water in pathologic tissues, causing a corresponding increase in proton density and relaxation values. Discussion of the physical principles of MRI are beyond the scope of this presentation but may be found in several excellent reviews (Pykett 1982; Budinger and Lauterbur 1984; Williams and Hricak 1984; Smith 1985).

The advantages of MRI, compared with conventional radiologic techniques, are: (a) soft tissue contrast resolution is superior; (b) direct multiplanar imaging without loss of resolution is routinely available; (c) ionizing radiation is not used; (d) lack of signal in flowing blood allows precise depiction of vascular and perivascular anatomy; and (e) bone and nonferrous surgical clip artifact is negligible. Disadvantages include: (a) inability to detect tissue calcium; (b) lack of suitable contrast agents; (c) contraindication for pacemaker patients; (d) degradation of images by cardiac, respiratory, or bowel motion; and (e) claustrophobia in a small percentage (less than 5%) of patients when placed in the magnet.

Pelvic MRI appears particularly promising because there is relatively little respiratory motion or bowel motion artifact in the pelvis and unlike CT, the MR characteristics of the small amount of pelvic fat (high intensity signal) make organ differentiation in the pelvis much easier. The use of coronal and sagittal images, as well as conventional transaxial images, allows more precise anatomic data acquisition, such as tumor volume measurement and prediction of tumor extension beyond organ confines.

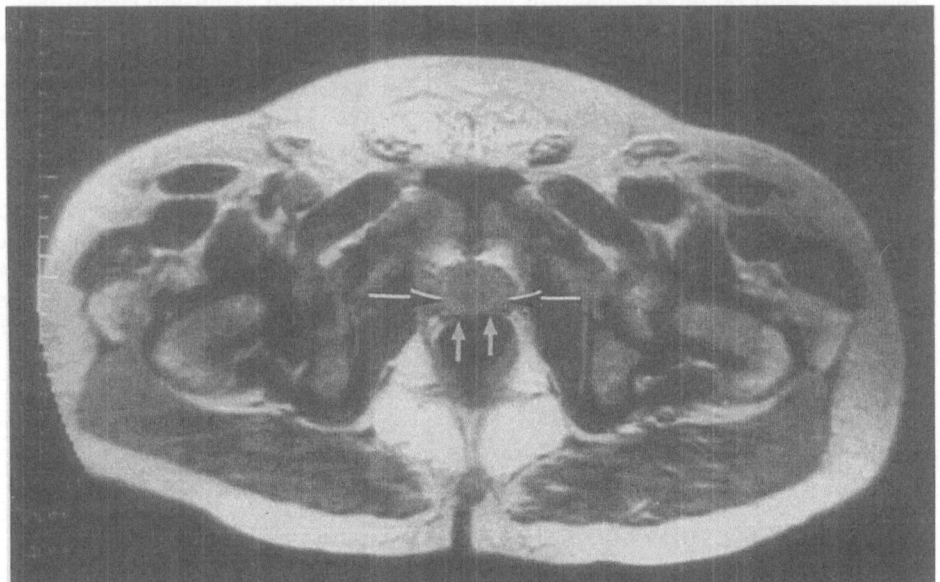

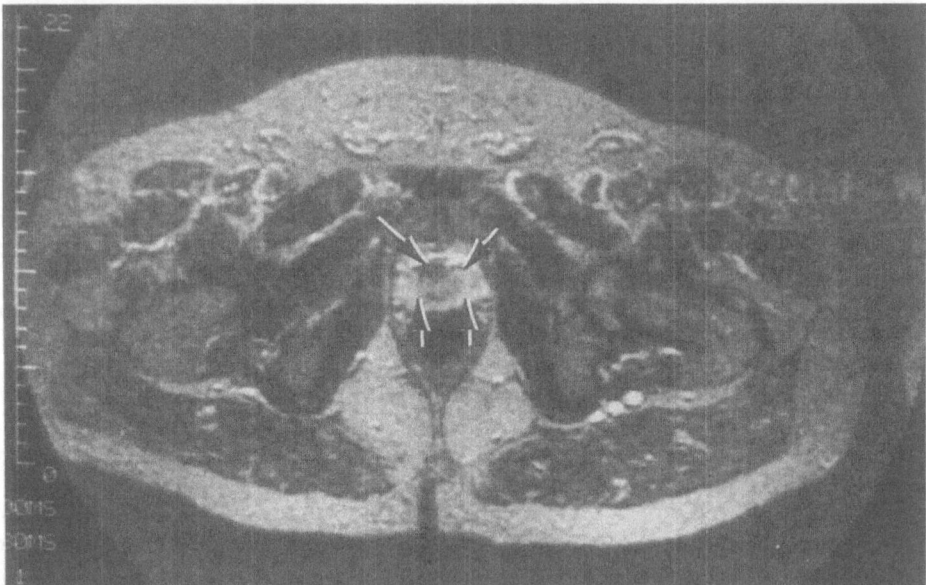

Fig. 5.8a. T$_1$-weighted MRI—transaxial image of normal prostate. Note peripheral zone (*long arrows*) and Denonvilliers' fascia (*short arrows*). **b** T$_2$-weighted MRI—transaxial image of normal prostate. Note peripheral zone (*short arrows*) and central zone (*long arrows*).

Prostatic anatomy is better seen on MRI than with any other modality. The normal prostate has a homogeneously distributed medium intensity signal on T$_1$-weighted images (Williams and Hricak 1984; Demas et al. 1985; Poon et al. 1985). The superior tissue contrast achieved with MRI allows definition of the anatomic zones of the prostate (Williams and Hricak 1984; Williams et al. 1986). The central zone is best seen using spin-echo sequences and has a lower intensity than that of the nearby peripheral zone (Fig. 5.8a, b). The transitional zone is imaged in continuity with the urethra as a region of higher intensity than either the central or peripheral zones. The anatomic boundaries of the prostate are best identified by examination of all three planes. Separation of the bladder and prostate is best imaged on either coronal or sagittal scans (Fig. 5.9). Denonvilliers' fascia is clearly seen as a low intensity line between the rectum and prostate and the seminal vesicles are seen well on both sagittal and axial images.

Benign prostatic hyperplasia (Fig. 5.10) images as an enlarged gland with a uniformly homogeneous medium intensity signal similar to normal prostate (Steyn and Smith 1982; Bryan et al. 1983, 1984; Williams and Hricak 1984; Demas et al. 1985; Poon et al. 1985). Multiplanar images allow accurate volumetric measurements and clear depiction of intravesical extension of the benign tumor. In patients with nodular hyperplasia, only occasionally can a distinction be made between nodular and non-nodular areas. Sagittal scans are particularly valuable in depicting the length of the prostate. This may be important in determining the operative approach in selected patients but is not usually of greater benefit than routine rectal examination.

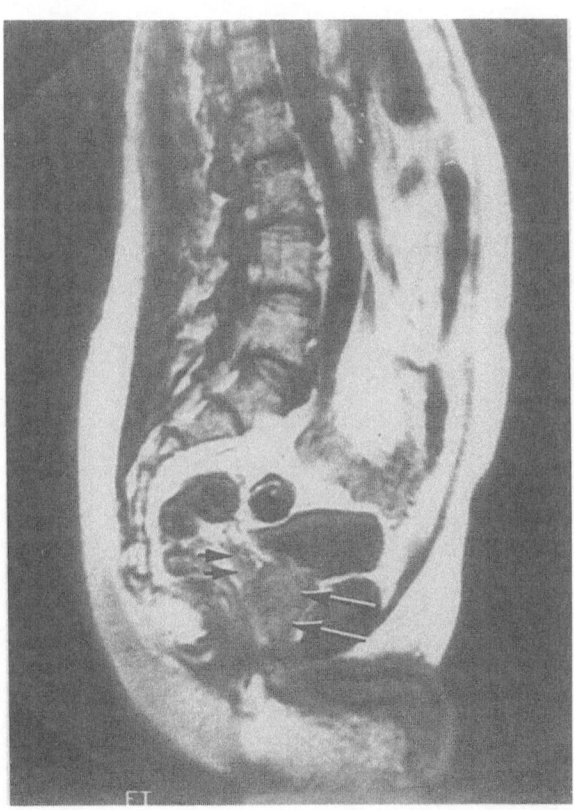

Fig. 5.9. T$_1$-weighted MRI—sagittal image of normal prostate (*long arrows*) and seminal vesicle (*short arrows*).

MRI has shown a regular gland of homogeneous intensity in the only two patients with acute prostatitis reported (Bryan et al. 1984). Chronic prostatitis has revealed an inhomogeneous medium signal intensity with scattered areas of increased signal. These latter findings parallel those seen in patients with prostatic carcinoma, and thus the specificity of MRI in the diagnosis of prostatic cancer is low.

To date MR images on more than 50 patients with prostatic cancer in various stages have been reported. Few of these studies have included pathologic confirmation of the abnormal areas on MRI or correlation with ultrasound or CT scans. In our experience using a 0.35 Tesla (T) MR imager, prostates containing adenocarcinoma showed a homogeneous medium signal intensity laced with focal (usually multiple) areas of higher intensity signal in the area of the peripheral zone (Fig. 5.11) (Williams and Hricak 1984; Demas et al. 1985; Williams et al. 1986). Seminal vesicle involvement was detected by increased intensity signals within the seminal vesicles and obliteration of the bladder – seminal vesicle angle on sagittal images (Fig. 5.12). Extension of tumor outside the prostate was also determined on coronal and axial images, being detected by an obliteration of the capsular margin and high intensity extension into the levator ani. These changes were best appreciated by using more than one planar projection.

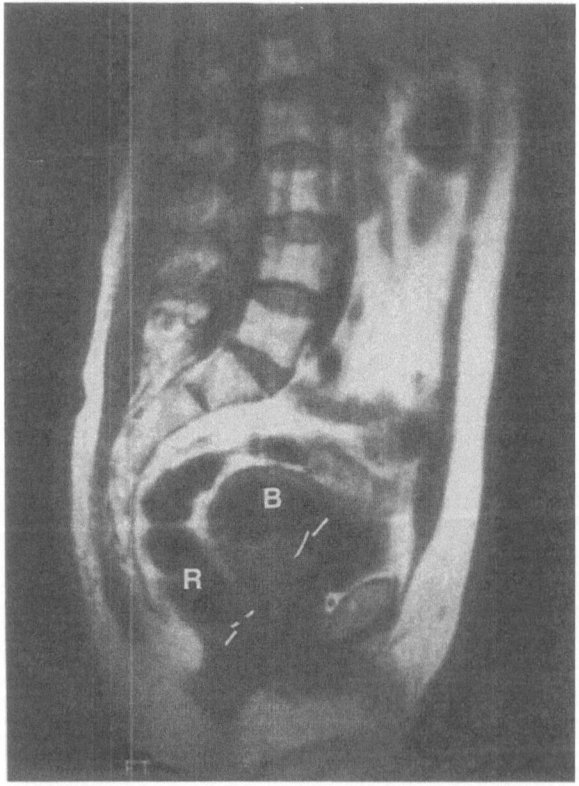

Fig. 5.10. T_1-weighted MRI—sagittal image of BPH. Prostate (*arrows*); *R*, rectum; *B*, bladder.

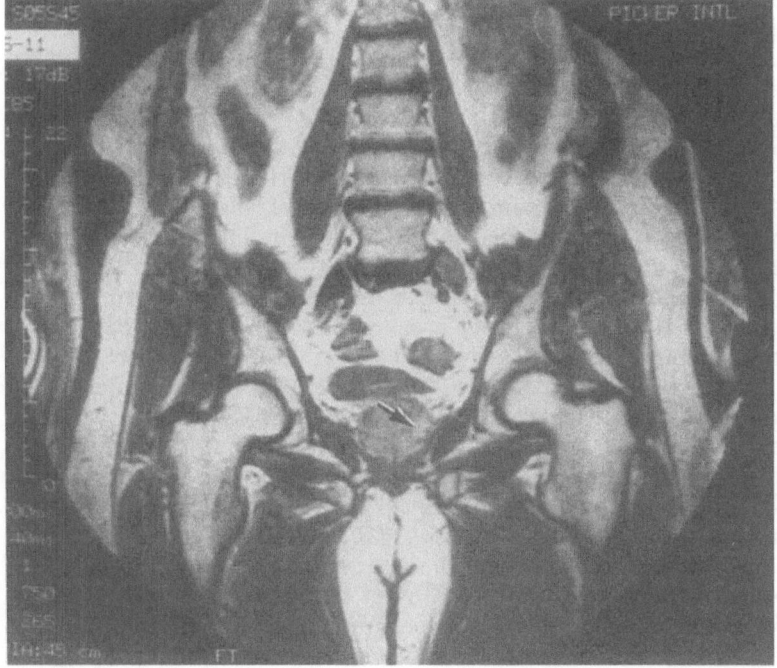

Fig. 5.11. T$_1$-weighted MRI—coronal image of stage B$_1$ prostatic cancer (*arrow*).

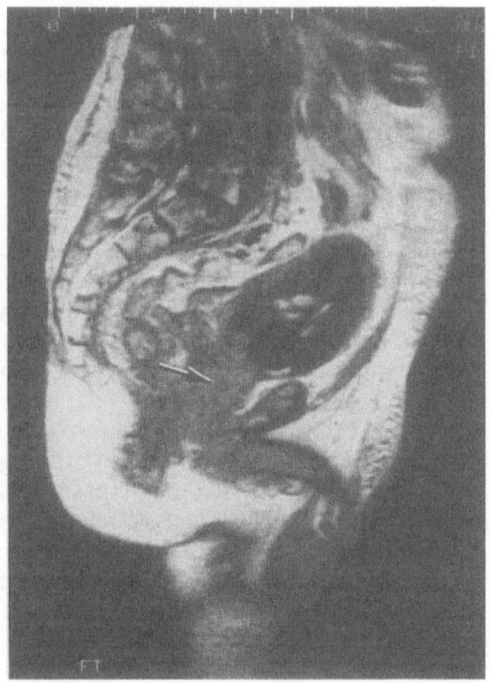

Fig. 5.12. T$_1$-weighted MRI—sagittal image of stage C prostatic cancer. Note heterogeneous signal and loss of bladder–seminal vesicle angle X (*arrow*).

Buonocore et al. (1984) used a 0.86-T MR imager to examine eight patients with known cancer of the prostate. Their studies confirmed our finding of a heterogeneous signal, which was more obvious on T_2-weighted images. Seminal vesicle involvement in two patients also showed a high intensity signal on T_2-weighted images. Bryan et al. (1983) reviewed four patients with prostatic cancer imaged by MR. High intensity areas were demonstrated within the prostate, but the authors described no staging information. Smith (1985) examined prostatic MR images using a resistive 0.08-T magnet and showed cancer to have a more granular image than BPH but similar relaxation times. Steyn and Smith (1982) imaged five patients with prostatic cancer and compared their MRI scans with those of 20 patients with BPH and three with prostatitis. The cancer patients had higher intensity areas within the prostatic substance. However, in one patient no lesion was detected and in three of the BPH patients and two of the prostatitis patients, inhomogeneous scans were falsely interpreted as cancer. Bryan et al. (1984) reported inhomogeneous MRI scans in prostatic cancer patients; however, a few BPH patients had similar findings. In addition, they found similar inhomogeneous results in patients with chronic prostatitis. Poon et al. (1985) studied 25 patients with cancer of the prostate using a resistive 0.15-T imager and compared their results with MR scans of 22 normal and seven BPH patients. They were unable to determine differential zones in the prostate, nor were signal intensity changes between any of the groups noted.

The reason for the lack of agreement between our studies and those of Poon et al. is not entirely known. The difference might be related to an increased signal-to-noise ratio and less contrast resolution in their low magnetic force instrument (0.15-T) as compared with the 0.3- to 0.8-T machines used by ourselves and others.

Based on our experience and that of most other investigators, intraprostatic cancer can be detected by MRI. Because other prostatic lesions such as chronic prostatitis may reveal similar MRI findings, the specificity of MRI for prostatic cancer is low. Specific figures for the sensitivity and specificity for the diagnosis of prostatic cancer are unavailable because large studies with pathologic confirmation of the MRI results have not been reported. Until such studies are documented, the accuracy of MRI for screening for prostatic cancer will remain undetermined. Based on the studies to date, it is unlikely that MRI will be a satisfactory screening modality.

The use of MRI for staging prostatic cancer appears much more promising. The anatomic boundaries of the prostate are more readily appreciated with MRI than with CT, particularly in regard to levator ani muscles, seminal vesicles, and the bladder neck (Bryan et al. 1984; Buonocore et al. 1984; Demas et al. 1985). Pelvic lymph nodes have been assessed by MRI, and in a few patients, accurate detection of enlarged nodes has been accomplished. Dooms et al. (1984) compared CT and MRI to evaluate lymph nodes in a variety of anatomic sites, including 14 patients with pelvic pathology. Normal nodes (7–11 mm) were only occasionally seen by MRI but pathologic nodes (15–50 mm) were imaged by both MRI and CT. They concluded that: (a) the relationship of nodes to surrounding tissues was better seen on MRI; (b) lymph nodes have an intermediate intensity between that of fat and muscle; and (c) MRI can differentiate abnormal lymph nodes from other pelvic pathology, such as lymphoceles, aneurysms, and fibrosis.

Lee et al. (1984) reported an MRI study of surgically confined abdominal and pelvic lymph nodes in 20 patients with lymphadenopathy initially detected by CT in 19 patients and by ultrasound in one. MRI was performed using a 0.35-T imager. Only two patients with a prostatic primary were studied. In general lymph nodes as small as 8 mm were identified on MRI, but intranodal architecture was not identified even in larger nodes. The enlarged nodes were best seen on transaxial MRI. Similar information was obtained by both MRI and CT in 13 patients. In five patients nodes were more easily differentiated from pelvic or abdominal vessels with MRI than with CT. MRI was unable to differentiate tumor types or to detect microscopic metastases. We recently studied eight patients with prostatic cancer who had MRI prior to radical prostatectomy and pelvic lymph node dissection (complete pathologic staging) and found that the accuracy of MRI with respect to the pathologic stage of prostatic cancer was 78% (Williams et al. 1986). MRI was capable of detecting local spread to periprostatic tissues and seminal vesicles but in comparison to CT, MRI had improved accuracy in detecting enlarged lymph nodes, particularly using coronal scans (Fig. 5.13). Microscopic metastases were not detected by MRI. In addition, MRI detected pelvic bone metastases in one patient with a negative radioisotope bone scan.

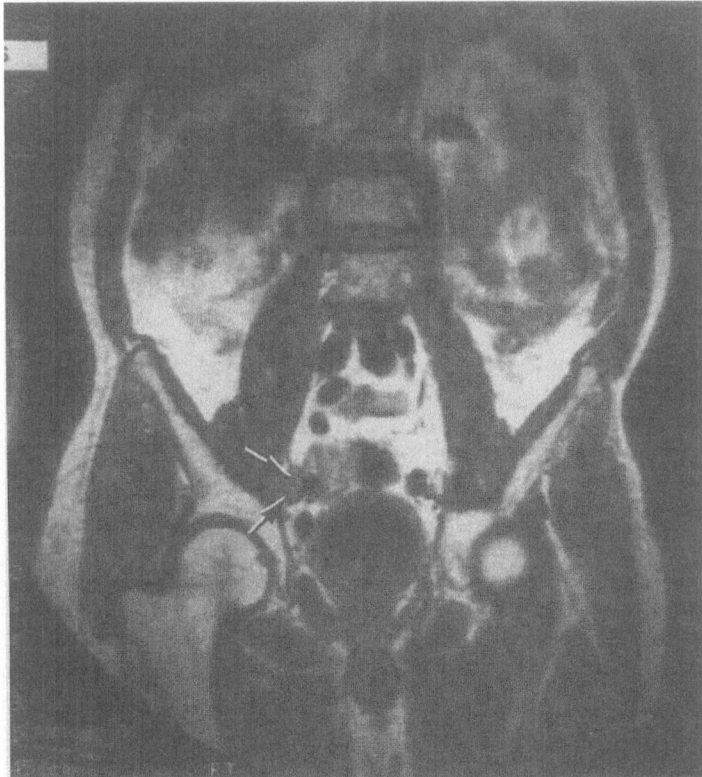

Fig. 5.13. T_1-weighted MRI—coronal image of tumorous pelvic lymph node (*arrows*).

In summary, MRI appears very promising for clinical staging of prostatic cancer due to its ability to depict clearly the anatomic boundaries of the prostate and the pelvic vessels and their surrounding lymph nodes. Comparisons of a large group of pathologically staged patients with those clinically staged by both MRI and CT will be required before MRI can be recommended as the definitive study.

Perhaps the most promising adjunct to MRI is the use of paramagnetic contrast materials to enhance spatial and contrast resolution. There are a variety of materials currently under study which fall into two categories, i.e., nitroxide-stable free radicals and metal ion chelates (Runge et al. 1984). These contrast materials increase MRI signal intensity by indirectly enhancing relaxation of protons surrounding the contrast material. Use of these materials has shown renal enhancement and intravenous urogram-like studies in animals (Brasch et al. 1983; Ehman et al. 1985). We have also shown that nitroxide-stable free radicals are capable of enhancing experimental human renal tumors in nude mice (Brasch et al. 1984). Although contrast materials have not yet been used to study human prostatic tissue or tumors, it is very likely that contrast enhancement may improve the ability to image prostatic abnormalities more definitively in the future. It is also possible that these contrast materials might be attached to prostatic monoclonal antibodies, thus providing an even more specific scanning modality.

MRI is an evolving modality which will require further study to determine the optimal imaging techniques for diagnosis and staging of prostatic cancer. Currently MRI has advantages over CT, particularly in local staging; however, the definitive studies have yet to be reported. The addition of paramagnetic contrast materials, and/or prostate-specific monoclonal antibodies attached to such materials, has the potential to improve prostatic MRI in the future.

Magnetic Resonance Spectroscopy

Magnetic resonance spectroscopy (MRS) is an analytic method which has only recently been extended to in vivo studies of humans. The basic principles are similar to MRI except that while MRI uses encoded magnetic resonance signals to produce a visual image directly related to the number and position of susceptible nuclei (primarily protons), MRS uses the same information to provide the identity and relative amounts of specific chemical groups within the tissue examined, i.e., a chemical shift spectrum (Bottomley 1983).

A chemical shift is produced by slight changes in the element's resonance frequency that reflect the structure of the chemical compound into which the element is incorporated (Fig. 5.14) (Morgan and Hendee 1984). MRS is available with some modification on current clinical MR imagers using magnetic field strengths of 1.5 T and above. With MRS techniques not only can ^{1}H in tissues be analyzed, but other less abundant nuclei, such as ^{31}P, ^{13}C, ^{19}F, and ^{21}Na, can be precisely identified and measured. MRS thus enables a noninvasive, nondestructive, and instantaneous means of monitoring intracellular metabolism.

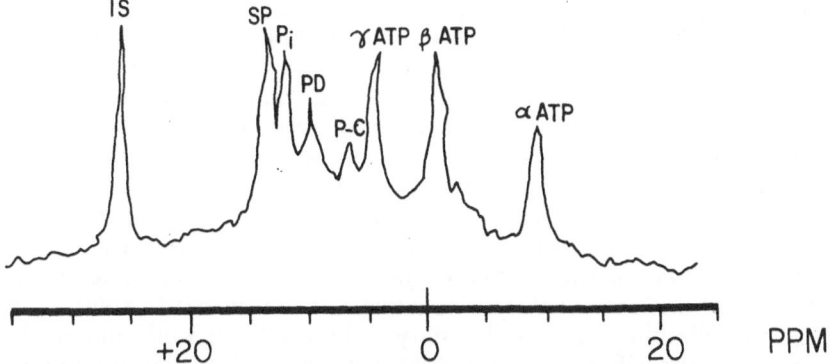

Fig. 5.14. ^{31}P chemical shift (MRS) of an in vivo rat kidney. Chemical shifts measured in parts per million (ppm) from the internal standard. Peak assignments used were β-ATP, α-ATP, and γ-ATP. *IS*, internal standard; *P-C*, phosphocreatine; *PD*, phosphodiester; *P$_i$*, inorganic phosphate; *SP*, sugar phosphate.

Extensive studies of in vitro and in vivo ^{31}P-MRS have indicated that this technique may be more specific than either MRI or proton MRS in differentiating between inflammation, infection, neoplasia, and ischemia. The analytic superiority of ^{31}P-MRS is based on the following: the signal intensity per nucleus is large even compared to hydrogen; all phosphorus atoms in the body are ^{31}P and thus are magnetically susceptible; and ^{31}P-MRS spectra are simple to interpret. Because ^{31}P-MRS measures intracellular ATP and pH, changes in cellular metabolism should be detectable before alterations appear in MRI and long before abnormalities are detected by either ultrasound or computed tomography. Thus, significant information about the normal function of organs and the metabolic response of these organs to injury and disease can be assessed.

Although specific ^{31}P-MRS studies in patients with prostatic cancer have not as yet been reported, MRS may be capable of detecting neoplasia at an early stage. Indeed, studies on human neuroblastoma and renal cancer have shown spectral differences between benign and malignant tissues and have accurately predicted therapeutic responses from chemotherapy and radiation therapy (Ross et al. 1984; Moris et al. 1985).

Lymphangiography

Lymphangiography has been used widely for staging pelvic and retroperitoneal malignancies for the past 20 years. The accuracy of lymphangiography is reportedly high in patients with seminoma, lymphoma, or prostatic cancer. The reports of lymphangiographic staging in prostatic cancer patients for the most part do not provide confirmatory surgical staging data. The recent addition of fine needle aspiration biopsy of abnormal nodes observed on lymphangiography has provided confirmation of positive lymphangiographic diagnoses; however, few studies have surgically confirmed negative fine needle aspiration biopsy.

Lymphangiography, to be useful, requires strict adherence to interpretive criteria. Prando et al. (1979) have stated that specific criteria for positive lymphangiography include a sharply defined concave filling defect at the periphery of a node not traversed by lymphatics (Fig. 5.15), and/or a crescent-shaped (rim sign) area at the edge of a node representing the residual functioning portion of the node. Nonspecific but suspicious criteria include central defects in a node less than 8 mm in diameter and nonopacification of a group of nodes. The limitations of lymphangiography include: (a) the studies are frequently equivocal; (b) the studies are optimally performed only by experienced clinicians who do them often; (c) false-positives occur from nonmalignant diagnoses in up to 30% of cases; (d) false-negatives range from 33% to 66%; and (e) lower limb thrombophlebitis or pulmonary emboli, although infrequent, do occur. Previously nonopacification of the "obturator nodes" was considered an important limitation of lymphangiography; however, Merrin et al. (1977) have shown them to be readily visualized.

Review of reported lymphangiography studies in prostatic cancer patients reveals a wide range of accuracy (48%–83%), sensitivity (33%–88%), and specificity (63%–95%) for lymphangiography alone, emphasizing a high false-

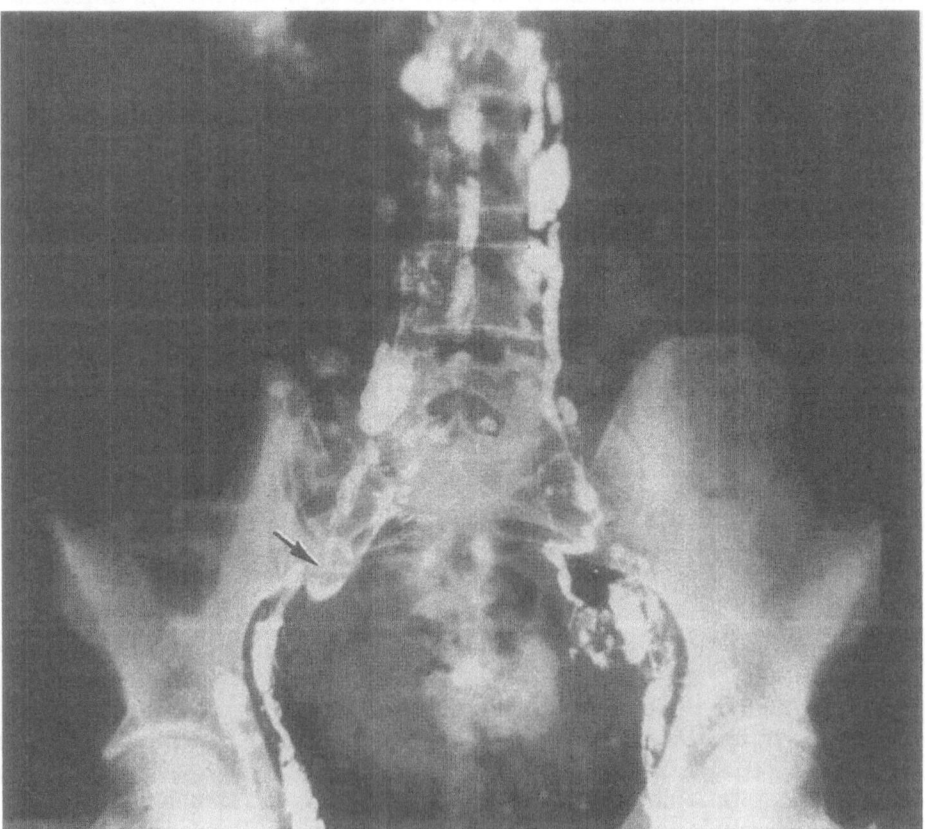

Fig. 5.15. Lymphangiography in patient with prostatic cancer. Tumorous node noted by *arrow*.

negative rate and the need for standardization of criteria for positivity (Loening et al. 1977; Merrin et al. 1977; Prando et al. 1979; Levine et al. 1981; Shankagiri et al. 1982). Lymphangiography is not particularly helpful in low-stage, low-grade prostatic cancer because the majority of patients will have a normal lymphangiogram that would not exclude micrometastases. Lymphangiography is most useful for patients with locally extensive or high-grade tumors. In these patients lymphangiography may well obviate surgical staging.

Fine needle aspiration biopsy of opacified nodes has added a significant dimension to the applicability of lymphangiography. Although there are very few studies of patients with positive lymphangiography and subsequent confirming fine needle aspiration biopsy, with or without surgical corroboration, the results are encouraging (78%–89% accuracy) (Correa et al. 1981; Efrimidis et al. 1981; Kidd et al. 1984). Gothlin and Hoien (1980) have even described finding positive nodal aspirates in 6 of 24 patients with normal lymphangiography, suggesting that lymphangiography may be best used to localize nodes for aspiration rather than for its intrinsic diagnostic utility. Unfortunately only 60%–75% of aspiration attempts were successful, but the accuracy increased with the number of nodes aspirated. The morbidity of fine needle aspiration biopsy is negligible and thus the approach seems very reasonable in patients with a high probability of nodal metastases.

Lymphangiography is not recommended for pelvic staging in patients with low-stage/grade cancer because the probability of nodal metastases is low. Patients with higher stage (A_2, B_2, C) and/or grade (Gleason sum greater than 5) lesions have a higher probability of having tumorous nodes and thus may benefit from either lymphangiography or pelvic CT with associated fine needle aspiration biopsy.

Monoclonal Antibodies and Immunodiagnostic Scanning

The recent development of techniques to mass produce monoclonal antibodies (MABs) to tissue- or tumor-associated antigens is truly one of the most outstanding discoveries in the last decade (Kohler and Milstein 1975). The previous problems with polyclonal antisera have largely been overcome by MABs and thus have allowed the development of many innovative applications in urologic oncology.

Prostatic cancer-related MABs have been developed from prostatic cancer tissue, prostatic tumor markers, and the human prostatic cancer cell lines PC-3, DU-145, and TURP-27 (Vessella et al. 1985). The majority of these MABs are not specific to prostatic cancer but cross-react with normal prostatic tissues or other urologic cancer cells.

Recently an MAB to a unique human prostatic antigen (PA) was developed (Pontes et al. 1982). Evidence is accumulating that PA may be a very useful marker of prostatic cancer and may be helpful in immunodiagnostic imaging. PA serum levels have been found to be elevated in 10% of patients with BPH, in 58% with prostatic cancer stages A and B, in 68% with stage C, and 92% with stage D (Pontes et al. 1982; Che et al. 1984). These levels were found to be completely independent of serum acid phosphatase levels. Recently clinical studies have been initiated to correlate PA serum levels with response to therapy and subsequent prognosis.

A human immunoglobulin M-MAB (MHG7) has been isolated and found to be reactive against human prostatic cells (both benign and malignant) on frozen and paraffin-embedded tissue sections (Lowe et al. 1984). Further work will be needed to establish how well MHG7 discriminates malignant from benign cell types. Indeed, one interesting possibility is that MHG7 may identify an antigen associated with prostatic cancer which is also found in "premalignant" cells.

Because prostatic tumor antigens should react with prostate-specific MABs, it follows that conjugation of radioisotopes to prostatic MABs should allow prostatic tumor imaging (Kohler and Milstein 1975; Sobol et al. 1983; Strand and Scheinberg 1983). Using this technology, MABs tagged to ^{131}I or ^{111}I can be infused into patients harboring tumors and then be scanned by scintigraphic imagers. There are currently studies underway to use these techniques in patients with renal and prostatic cancer, but no significant results have as yet been reported. Animal studies using human renal cancer MABs have shown the ability to identify tumors 10 mg or larger (Vessella et al. 1985). In addition, efforts to use paramagnetic agents for coupling with MABs for MRI are in progress. Both of these approaches are quite promising, although their actual ability to diagnose (screen) or stage prostatic cancer is only speculative at present.

Positron Emission Tomography

Positron emission tomography (PET) scanning is a relatively recent innovation in tissue and organ imaging that promises to provide information concerning regional tissue physiology (Phelps and Mazziatta 1985). The basis of PET scanning is the exogenous administration of a positron-emitting radionuclide in the form of a biologic tracer. The radionuclides used commonly are short-lived isotopes of common biologic elements such as ^{11}C, ^{15}O, and ^{13}N. ^{18}F behaves similarly to ^{1}H (which does not emit positrons) and is thus used as a proton substitute. These isotopic radionuclides decay rapidly while emitting positrons (positive electrons). Positrons move a few millimeters in soft tissue, then interact with a negative electron, emitting two 511-KeV gamma rays which move 180° apart and can easily penetrate tissues. These paired rays are coincidentally detected externally by specially constructed gamma detectors (Beaney 1984).

The fundamental enthusiasm surrounding PET scanning is related to the facts that: (a) the substrates which can be radiolabeled are nearly limitless; (b) the method will provide high spatial resolution and detection efficiency; (c) the regional concentration of radioisotopes can be measured; and (d) minute amounts of tracer can be used to provide accurate measurements. Current resolution appears to be in the range of 6–8 mm, but 2 mm resolution scanners are expected within the near future. The primary disadvantage of the method is that the radioisotopes have extremely short physical half-lives (^{15}O, 2 min; ^{11}C, 20 min; ^{13}N, 10 min; ^{18}F, 110 min), necessitating close proximity to a cyclotron where the isotopes are produced.

To date the majority of laboratory studies have focused on brain metabolism and physiologic function, although a few studies have determined that neoplasms (primary brain and breast, and colon metastatic to liver) can be detected using ^{18}F-deoxyglucose as a tracer.

There are as yet no reports on human urologic tumors, although recent studies by Fair and Kadmon suggest that polyamines labeled with positron-emitting radionuclides, such as ^{11}C-putrescine, may be useful for prostatic imaging (Miller et al. 1978; Fair and Kadmon 1983; Kadmon et al. 1985). Their early work has shown that the polyamines, which are known to be in high concentration in the prostate, can be selectively taken up by normal dog prostate and rat prostatic tumors by manipulating the polyamine metabolic enzymes. PET scanning of the normal dog prostate and spontaneous dog tumors using these methods has been successful. Current research relating to development of appropriate radiolabeled putrescine analogues for human PET scanning is underway but no human studies have been completed.

Conclusion

There are a variety of imaging modalities available for prostatic cancer screening but at the present time TRU and MRI are the most promising. The use of MRS, or paramagnetic contrast materials attached to prostatic MABs with MRI, may provide significant advances. It is doubtful whether PET scanning will become universally useful due to its limited availability. Despite these advances, routine annual rectal examination of patients at risk will probably make a greater impact on prostatic cancer survival statistics than any other screening modality.

Local pelvic staging of prostatic cancer is entirely different. CT and lymphangiography are nearly equivalent in their ability to define pelvic lymph nodes, yet neither is helpful in low-stage, low-grade disease and thus they are recommended only in patients with locally extensive or high-grade (Gleason sum 5 or greater) lesions. Fine needle aspiration biopsy of suspicious nodes seen on CT or lymphangiography is a proven modality which should be encouraged. Local extension can be determined by CT, but at present rectal examination is still superior. MRI has great promise, but studies using improved pulse sequences and enhanced spatial resolution, correlated with precise surgical pathologic staging, will be required prior to recommending its routine use.

Finally the development of MABs specific to prostatic antigens and their subsequent use in imaging is expected to improve the diagnosis and staging of prostatic cancer.

References

Bartsch G, Egender G, Hubscher H et al. (1982) Sonometrics of the prostate. J Urol 127:1119–1121
Beaney RP (1984) Positron emission tomography in the study of human tumors. Semin Nucl Med 14:324–341
Bottomley PA (1983) Nuclear magnetic resonance: beyond physical imaging. IEEE Spectrum 20(2):32–38

Brasch RC, London DA, Wesbey GE et al. (1983) Work in progress: nuclear magnetic resonance study of a paramagnetic nitroxide contrast agent for enhancement of renal structures in experimental animals. Radiology 147:773–779

Brasch RC, Weinemann HJ, Wesbey GE (1984) Contrast-enhanced NMR imaging: animal studies using gadolinium–DTPA complex. AJR 142:625–630

Brooman PJC, Griffiths GJ, Roberts E (1981) Per rectal ultrasound in the investigation of prostatic disease. Clin Radiol 32:669–676

Bryan PJ, Butler HE, Lipuma JP (1983) NMR scanning of the pelvis: initial experience with a 0.3T system. AJR 141:1111–1118

Bryan PH, Butler HE, Lipuma JP (1984) Magnetic resonance imaging of the pelvis. Radiol Clin North Am 22:897–915

Budinger TF, Lauterbur PC (1984) Nuclear magnetic resonance technology for medical studies. Science 226:288–298

Buonocore E, Hesemann C, Pavlicek W, Montie (1984) Clinical and in vitro magnetic resonance imaging of prostatic carcinoma. AJR 143:1267–1272

Burks DD, Drolshogen LF, Fleischer AC et al. (1986) Transrectal sonography of benign and malignant prostatic lesions. AJR 146:1187–1191

Carpenter PJ, Schroder FH (1984) Transrectal ultrasonography in the followup of prostatic carcinoma patients: a new prognostic parameter. J Urol 131:903–905

Che TM, Kuriyama M, Johnson E et al. (1984) Circulating antibody to prostate antigen in patients with prostate cancer. Transplant Proc 16:481–485

Chodak GW, Schoenberg HW (1984) Early detection of prostate cancer by routine screening. JAMA 252:3261–3264

Correa RJ, Kidd CR, Burnett L et al. (1981) Percutaneous pelvic lymph node aspiration in carcinoma of the prostate. J Urol 126:190–191

Dähnert WF, Hamper UM, Eggleston JC et al. (1986) Prostatic evolution by transrectal sonography with histopathologic correlation: the echopenic appearance of early carcinoma. Radiology 158:97–102

Demas BE, Hricak HH, Williams RD (1985) Magnetic resonance imaging in the evaluation of urologic malignancies. Semin Urol 3:27–33

Denkhaus H, Dierkopf W, Grabbe E (1983) Comparative study of suprapubic sonography and computed tomography for staging of prostatic carcinoma. Urol Rad. 5:1–9

Dooms GC, Hricak HH, Crooks LE et al. (1984) Magnetic resonance imaging of the lymph nodes: comparison with CT. Radiology 153:181–188

Efrimidis SC, Dan SJ, Nieburgs H et al. (1981) Carcinoma of the prostate: lymph node aspiration for staging. AJR 136:489–492

Egender G, Rapf C, Feichtenger I et al. (1984) Comparative histopathologic and sonomorphological prostate studies. ROFO 140:60–66

Ehman RL, Wesbey GE, Moon KL et al. (1985) Enhanced MRI of tumors utilizing a new nitroxyl spin label contrast agent. J MRI 3:89–97

Emory TH, Reinke DB, Hill AL et al. (1983) Use of CT to reduce understaging in prostatic cancer: comparison with conventional staging techniques. AJR 141:351–354

Fair WR, Kadmon D (1983) Carcinoma of the prostate: diagnosis and staging. World J Urol 1:3–11

Fornage BD, Touche DH, Deglaire M et al. (1983) Real-time ultrasound-guided prostatic biopsy using a new transrectal linear-array probe. Radiology 146:547–550

Fritzsche PJ, Axford PD, Ching VC, et al. (1983) Correlation of transrectal sonographic findings in patients with suspected and unsuspected prostatic disease. J Urol 130:272–274

Gammelguard J, Holm HH (1980) Transurethral and transrectal ultrasonic scanning in urology. J Urol 124:863–868

Golimbu M, Morales P, Al-Askori S et al. (1981) CAT scanning in staging of prostate cancer. Urology 18:305–308

Gothlin JH, Hoien L (1980) Percutaneous fine-needle biopsy of radiographically normal lymph nodes in the staging of prostatic carcinoma. Radiology 141:351–354

Guinan P, Bush I, Ray V et al. (1980) The accuracy of rectal examination in the diagnosis of prostate carcinoma. N Engl J Med 303:499–503

Harada K, Tanahashi Y, Igari D et al. (1980) Clinical evaluation of inside echo patterns in gray scale prostatic echography. J Urol 124:216–220

Holm HH, Juul N, Pederson JF (1983) Transperineal [125]iodine seed implantation in prostatic cancer guided by transrectal ultrasonography. J Urol 130:283–286

Kadmon D, Mahle D, Heston WDW et al. (1985) Effect of estrogen and androgen administration on alpha DCMO-enhanced putrescine uptake by the rat prostate. Prostate 6:343–349

Kidd R, Crane RD, Doil DH (1984) Lymphangiography and fine-needle aspiration biopsy: ineffective for staging early prostate cancer. AJR 142:1007–1112

Kohler G, Milstein C (1975) Continuous cultures of fused cells secreting antibody of predefined specificity. Nature 256:495–497

Lee JKT, Heiken JP, Ling D et al. (1984) Magnetic resonance imaging of abdominal and pelvic lymphadenopathy. Radiology 153:181–188

Lee F, Gray JM, McCleary RD et al. (1986) Prostatic evolution by transrectal sonography: criteria of early diagnosis. Radiology 158:91–95

Levine MS, Arger PH, Coleman BG et al. (1981) Detecting lymphatic metastases from prostatic carcinoma: superiority of CT. AJR 137:207–211

Loening SA, Schmidt JD, Brown RC et al. (1977) A comparison between lymphangiography and pelvic node dissection in the staging of prostatic cancer. J Urol 117:752–756

Lowe DH, Handley HH, Schmidt J et al. (1984) A human monoclonal antibody reactive with human prostate. J Urol 132:780–785

McNeal JE (1968) Regional morphology and pathology of the prostate. Am J Clin Pathol 49:347–357

Merrin C, Wajsman Z, Baumgartner G et al. (1977) The clinical value of lymphangiography: Are the nodes surrounding the obturator nodes visualized? J Urol 117:742–744

Miller TR, Siegel BA, Fair WR et al. (1978) Imaging of canine tumors with ^{11}C-methyl-putrescine. Radiology 129:221–223

Morgan CJ, Hendee WR (1984) Magnetic resonsance spectroscopy. In: Morgan CJ, Hendee WR (eds) Introduction to magnetic resonance 9. Multi-media Publishing, Denver, p 125

Morgan CL, Calkins RF, Cavalcanti EJ (1981) Computed tomography in the evaluation, staging and therapy of carcinoma of the bladder and prostate. Radiology 140:751–761

Moris JM, Evans AE, McLaughlin AC et al. (1985) ^{31}P nuclear magnetic resonance spectroscopic investigation of human neuroblastoma in situ. N Engl J Med 312:1500–1505

Phelps ME, Mazziatta JC (1985) Positron emission tomography: human brain function and biochemistry. Science 228:799–809

Pontes JE, Chu TM, Slack N et al. (1982) Serum prostatic antigen measurement in localized prostatic cancer: correlation with clinical course. J Urol 128:1216–1218

Poon PY, McCollum RW, Henkelman MM (1985) Magnetic resonance imaging of the prostate. Radiology 154:143–149

Prando A, Wallace S, Van Eschenbach AC et al. (1979) Lymphangiography in staging carcinoma of the prostate. Radiology 131:641–645

Pykett IL (1982) NMR imaging in medicine. Sci Am 246:78–88

Rifkin MD, Kurtz AB, Goldberg BB (1983) Sonographically guided transperineal prostatic biopsy: preliminary experience with a longitudinal linear array transducer. AJR 140:745–748

Rifkin MD, Friedland GW, Shortliffe L (1986) Prostatic evaluation by transrectal endosonography: detection of carcinoma. Radiology 158:85–90

Ross B, Smith M, Marshall V et al. (1984) Monitoring responses to chemotherapy of intact human tumors by ^{31}P nuclear magnetic resonance. Lancet I:641–646

Runge VM, Clanton JA, Herzer WA et al. (1984) Intravascular contrast agents suitable for magnetic resonance imaging. Radiology 153:171–176

Sawczuk IS, deVere White R, Gold R et al. (1983) Sensitivity of computed tomography in evaluation of pelvic lymph node metastases from carcinoma of bladder and prostate. Urology 21:81–84

Shankagiri PG, Walsh JW, Hazra TA (1982) Role of computed tomography in the evaluation and management of carcinoma of the prostate. Int J Radiat Oncol Biol Phys 8:283–287

Smith FW (1985) Nuclear magnetic resonance proton imaging in cancer. Eur J Clin Oncol 21:379–387

Sobol RE, Dillman RO, Halpern S et al. (1983) Sero therapy and radio immunodetection of tumors with monoclonal antibodies. In: Molog PJ, Nicolson GL (eds) Cellular oncology—new approaches in biology, diagnosis and treatment. Praeger, New York

Spirnak JP, Resnick MI (1984) Transrectal ultrasonography. Urology 23:461–467

Steyn JH, Smith FW (1982) Nuclear magnetic resonance imaging of the prostate. Br J Urol 54:726–728

Strand M, Scheinberg DA (1983) Monoclonal antibody conjugates for diagnostic imaging and therapy. In: Boss BD, Langman R, Towbridge I, Dulbecco R (eds) Monoclonal antibodies and cancer. Academic Press, New York

Velthoven RV, Vandewalle JC, Lavieter-Nobre et al. (1984) Early diagnosis of prostatic carcinoma: advantages and limits of transrectal ultrasonic examinations. Abstract from 6th EAU Congress, Copenhagen

Vessella RL, Chiou RK, Lange PH (1985) Monoclonal antibodies in urology: review of reactivities and applications in diagnosis, staging, and therapy. Semin Urol 3:158–167

Walsh JW, Amendola MA, Konerding KF et al. (1980) Computed tomographic detection of pelvic and inguinal lymph-node metastases from primary and recurrent pelvic malignant disease. Radiology 137:157–166

Watanabe H et al. (1968) Diagnostic application of the ultrasonotomography for the prostate. Jpn J Urol 59:273–279

Watanabe H, Saitoh M, Mishina T (1977) Mass screening program for prostatic disease with transrectal ultrasonotomography. J Urol 117:746–748

Weinerman PM, Arger PH, Pollack HM (1982) CT evaluation of bladder and prostate neoplasms. Urol Radiol 4:105–114

Weinerman PM, Arger PH, Coleman BG et al. (1983) Pelvic adenopathy from bladder and prostate carcinoma: detection by rapid sequence computed tomography. AJR 140:95–99

Williams RD, Hricak HH (1984) Magnetic resonance imaging in urology. J Urol 132:641–649

Williams RD, Dunn V, Yousef MA, Brown RC (1986) Staging of pelvic malignancies by MRI. J Urol 135:244A

Chapter 6

Update in Staging Systems

P.C. Sogani and W.F. Whitmore, Jr.

Introduction

Aside from purely taxonomic purposes, the staging of prostatic cancer is important to planning mangement, estimating prognosis, characterizing individual patients or groups of patients, and comparing results of various treatments. There is as yet no universally accepted clinical staging classification for prostatic cancer but two systems, the American and the TNM, with various modifications, are widely used (Whitmore 1984).

The American system, proposed in 1956, grouped patients with prostatic cancer into one of four categories: A, B, C, or D (Whitmore 1956). In 1959 the American Joint Committee for Cancer Staging and End Results Reporting recommended the use of Roman numerals I, II, III, and IV, respectively, in place of A, B, C and D, and such was used by the Veterans Administration Cooperative Urological Research Group (1967).

Stage A (I)

Stage A carcinoma of the prostate is clinically unsuspected on digital rectal examination and is identified upon pathologic examination of prostatic tissue either at autopsy or after transurethral resection or enucleation of the prostate for clinically benign prostatic hyperplasia. It has been variably referred to as incidental, occult, clinically unrecognized, or latent. These tumors are clinically inapparent and unexpected and the most appropriate designations may be "incidental" or "clinically unrecognized." An occult tumor is one that manifests itself by metastatic spread and/or paraneoplastic syndromes with the actual site of the primary lesion clinically inapparent. The term "latent" is presumptive since it infers a lack of biologic potential, an implication which may or may not be true.

About 10% of patients undergoing prostatectomy for clinically benign prostatic enlargements are found to have cancer on examination of routine sections of the resected tissue (Sheldon et al. 1980). Examination of step sections may increase this incidence to 20%. Denton et al. (1965) reviewed 500 specimens from transurethral resections of the prostate for clinically benign disease. Among 100 prostates in which both techniques were used, six incidental carcinomas were found on routine sectioning and 15 additional carcinomas on step sectioning, giving a total incidence of 21%. Bauer et al. (1960), in a series of 847 consecutive suprapubic prostatectomies, reported a 6.5% incidence of stage A carcinoma. Bergman et al. (1955), Smith and Woodruff (1950), and Varkarakis et al. (1970) reported 3.5%, 9.5%, and 4.9% incidences, respectively, among patients treated surgically for clinically benign prostatic obstruction.

The incidence of unsuspected prostatic cancer in autopsy series is even higher (Rich 1935; Hirst and Bergman 1954). Approximately two-thirds of patients over the age of 80 and most patients over the age of 90 are found to have prostatic cancer at the time of autopsy (Whitmore 1956; Sheldon et al. 1980).

In early reports by the Veterans Administration Cooperative Urological Research Group (1967), stage A cancer accounted for only about 6% of clinically identified prostatic cancers; more recent reports suggest that as many as 26%–53% of prostatic cancers are diagnosed in clinical stage A (McMillen and Wettlaufer 1976; Murphy et al. 1982; Donohue et al. 1982).

Based on the volume and the grade of stage A tumors, Jewett (1975) suggested that stage A be further subdivided into two categories: stage A_1 and stage A_2. Subsequently, this subdivision of stage A disease has been used widely despite the fact that quantitative criteria distinguishing stage A_1 from stage A_2 have not been well established (Table 6.1). Stage A_1 is generally defined as a low-grade, focal lesion and A_2 as a high-grade, diffuse lesion. The distinction between a focal and a diffuse lesion varies: a focal lesion has been described as being less than three chips (Boxer 1977; Whitmore 1980), less than five chips (Golimbu et al. 1978), less than five microscopic foci (Parfitt et al. 1983), less than 5% of the prostatic specimen (Cantrell et al. 1981), and less than 50% of the resected specimen (Donohue et al. 1977). A subdivision with stage A_f (focal), A_1 (one lobe only), and A_2 (multifocal or diffuse) has also been proposed (Catalona and Scott 1978). Focal disease alternatively has been called stage O and more diffuse disease simply stage A (deVere White et al. 1977). Sheldon et al. (1980) divided the prostate into four quadrants and proposed a subdivision of stage A tumors into three categories: stage A_f—less than three chips with carcinoma; stage A_1—more than three chips with carcinoma, but restricted to one quadrant or to two contiguous quadrants; and stage A_2—more than three chips with carcinoma but involving two noncontiguous quadrants or more. Each of these categories is then further subdivided according to histologic grade.

Stage A_2 lesions have been shown to have a prognosis clearly worse than stage A_1 and possibly worse than stage B_1 lesions. Approximately 75% of stage A_2 tumors are moderately or poorly differentiated, in contrast to about 15% of stage B_1 tumors (Golimbu et al. 1978). For this reason A_2 lesions have been

Table 6.1.   Subdivisions of stage A prostatic carcinoma

Author	Subdivisions	
Jewett (1975)	A_1	Focal
	A_2	Diffuse, high grade
Boxer (1977)	A_1	Well differentiated cancer involving 3 chips or less
	A_2	Cancer involving more than 3 chips or poorly differentiated
Donohue et al. (1977)	A_1	Cancer involving less than 50% of specimen, well differentiated
	A_2	Cancer involving more than 50% of specimen, poorly differentiated
deVere White et al. (1977)	0	Focal
	A	Diffuse, high grade
Catalona and Scott (1978)	A_f	Focal
	A_1	Only one lobe involved
	A_2	Both lobes involved
Golimbu et al. (1978)	A_1	Cancer involving 5 chips or less
	A_2	Cancer involving more than 5 chips, poorly differentiated
Whitmore (1980)	A_1	Cancer involving less than 3 chips
	A_2	Cancer involving 3 chips or more
Sheldon et al. (1980)	A_f	Cancer involving 3 chips or less
	A_1	More than 3 chips of carcinoma, restricted to one quadrant or two contiguous quadrants
	A_2	More than 3 chips of carcinoma involving two noncontiguous quadrants.
Cantrell et al. (1981)	A_1	Cancer involving less than 5% of specimen, low grade
	A_2	Cancer involving more than 5% of specimen or high grade
Parfitt et al. (1983)	A_1	Cancer seen in 5 microscopic foci or less
	A_2	Cancer seen in more than 5 microscopic foci
Golimbu and Morales (1979)	A	Cancer involving 5 chips or less or less than 3 foci in enucleated gland
	B_2	Cancer involving more than 5 chips or 3 foci in enucleated gland or poorly differentiated
McCullough (1980)	A	Cancer seen in 3 microscopic foci or less, well differentiated
	B_2	Cancer involving more than 3 microscopic foci, poorly differentiated

classified by some as stage B_2 (Golimbu and Morales 1979; McCullough 1980).

Subdivision of stage A is justified by evidence of the roles of both mass and grade in tumor natural history; undifferentiated and diffuse stage A prostatic cancers behave more aggressively than focal and well differentiated ones. Cantrell et al. (1981) proposed that low-grade lesions and lesions constituting less than 5% of the resected prostate be considered A_1, whereas those of higher grade or greater bulk be considered A_2. With such a division, among 117 patients followed for 2–15 years, no patient with low-grade lesion had demonstrable progression and only 2% of patients with less than 5% cancer had progression within 4 years. In contrast, of the patients with more than 5% cancer, 32% had progression, and of the patients with high-grade lesions, 17% had progression.

Donohue et al. (1977) reported 23 patients with stage A disease (5 stage A_1 and 18 stage A_2) who had pelvic lymphadenectomy; none of the patients with stage A_1 disease but four (22%) of the patients with stage A_2 cancer had positive nodes. All of the four patients with positive nodes had high-grade primary tumors compared to half of the remaining 14 stage A_2 lesions. Similar experiences were reported by Golimbu et al. (1978): none of four patients with A_1 cancer had positive lymph nodes on lymphadenectomy whereas 6 of 16 patients (37.5%) with A_2 disease had positive pelvic lymph nodes.

Stage B (II)

Stage B carcinoma is clinically evident on digital rectal examination but apparently confined within the limits of the prostatic capsule. In the Veterans Administration Cooperative Urological Research Group studies (1967), stage B lesions accounted for only 8% of prostatic cancers; however, in more recent series stage B lesions have accounted for 22%–29% of patients (McMillen and Wettlaufer 1976; Murphy et al. 1982; Donohue et al. 1982).

Stage B has been variously subclassified (Table 6.2). In 1975 Jewett subdivided stage B cancer into B_1 and B_2 based on a retrospective analysis of 182 traced patients with clinical stage B cancer who underwent radical perineal prostatectomy at the Johns Hopkins Hospital before 1951. Stage B_1 is defined as tumor occupying less than one lobe of the prostate. Included in this category is the "B_1 nodule," the "discrete palpable nodule of firm or stony consistency limited to a part of one lateral lobe, averaging 1 cm or a little more in diameter, with compressible prostate tissue always on 2 and sometimes on 3 sides" (Jewett et al. 1968). Stage B_2 includes tumors larger than B_1 but still clinically confined to the prostate. Of the 103 patients with clinical stage B_1 lesions in Jewett's series, 16% had microscopic evidence of invasion of the seminal vesicles and 27% survived 15 years or more without evidence of cancer. In contrast, of the 79 patients with clinical stage B_2 lesions, 49% had histologic evidence of seminal vesicle invasion and 18% survived 15 years or more without evidence of cancer (Jewett 1975). Thus, this subdivision of stage B patients appears to have clinical significance.

Table 6.2. Subdivisions of stage B prostatic carcinoma

Author	Subdivisions	
Jewett (1975)	B_1	Tumor involving less than one lobe (including Jewett's nodule)
	B_2	Tumor involving one lobe or more
Catalona and Scott (1978)	B_{1n}	Solitary nodule no more than 1.5 cm surrounded by normal prostatic tissue on all sides
	B_1	Tumor involving one lobe of prostate
	B_2	Tumor involving both lobes of prostate
McCullough (1980)	B_1	Nodule 2 cm or less with normal prostate surrounding the tumor
	B_2	Diffuse carcinoma more than B_1
Whitmore (1980)	B_1	Prostatic nodule 2 cm or less confined to one lobe
	B_2	Prostatic nodule larger than 2 cm but confined to one lobe
	B_3	Prostatic nodule involving both lobes

Catalona and Scott (1978) divided stage B into three subgroups: (1) a solitary nodule no more than 1.5 cm in diameter and surrounded by apparently normal prostatic tissue on all sides (B_{1n}); (2) involvement of an entire lobe of the prostate (B_1); and (3) diffuse involvement of both lobes of the prostate (B_2). Generally, the prognosis worsens as the extent of prostatic involvement by tumor increases. McCullough (1980) defined the B_1 tumor as 2 cm or less in diameter with normal prostate surrounding the tumor, and the B_2 tumor as larger than 2 cm in diameter but clinically confined within the prostatic capsule. At the Memorial Sloan-Kettering Cancer Center (MSKCC), B_1 is a prostatic nodule 2 cm or less in diameter confined to one lobe; B_2 is larger than 2 cm in diameter but confined to one lobe; and B_3 is bilobar but within the prostate (Whitmore 1980). There is clearly no unanimity on the subdivision of stage B tumors.

The incidence of lymph node metastases is reported as 8%–21% for stage B_1 (McLaughlin et al. 1976; Wilson et al. 1977; Nicholson and Richie 1977; Catalona and Scott 1978) and 14%–45% for stage B_2 tumors (McLaughlin et al. 1976; Bruce et al. 1977; Golimbu et al. 1978; Catalona and Scott 1978; Fowler and Whitmore 1981).

Stage C (III)

Stage C prostatic cancer includes tumors that extend beyond the prostatic capsule but without evident metastasis. In the Veterans Administration Cooperative Urological Research Group series (1967), 48% of patients presented in clinical stage C, whereas in more recent series, 9%–15% have presented in stage C (McMillen and Wettlaufer 1976; Donohue et al. 1982; Murphy et al. 1982). Stage C tumors have been subdivided into C_1 and C_2 (Carlton et al. 1976): C_1 includes tumors less than 6 cm in diameter and stage C_2 tumors more than 6 cm in diameter. At MSKCC stage C has been subdivided into C_1, C_2, and C_3 (Whitmore 1980). C_1 is an extraprostatic lesion involving one or both lateral sulci only; C_2 an extraprostatic lesion involving the base of either or both seminal vesicles with or without involvement of the lateral sulci; and C_3 an extraprostatic lesion other than C_1 or C_2. These subdivisions were created to better characterize and evaluate local tumor suitability for iodine 125 implantation.

The incidence of pelvic lymph node metastases in patients with stage C tumors ranges between 50% and 80% (McLaughlin et al. 1976; Wilson et al. 1977; Barzell et al. 1977; Bruce et al. 1977; Donohue et al. 1979; Fowler and Whitmore 1981).

Stage D (IV)

Stage D prostatic cancer includes any tumor with evidence of metastasis. In recent series, 10%–28% of patients have presented with stage D disease (McMillen and Wettlaufer 1976; Donohue et al. 1982; Murphy et al. 1982).

Stage D has been subdivided into: (1) D_1, patients with metastasis apparently limited to the pelvic lymph nodes; (2) D_2, patients with metastases beyond the pelvic lymph nodes. Whitesel and associates (1984) have suggested a stage designation of D_0 for patients with persistently elevated serum acid phosphatase but without other evidence of metastatic disease since 17 of 19 patients (89%) with persistently elevated acid phosphatase who were followed for a minimum of 2 years developed clinical evidence of lymph node or osseous metastases. The latter results suggest that the majority of patients who have persistently elevated serum acid phosphatase levels have occult metastases. It has also been suggested that patients with stage D_2 prostatic cancer who relapse following endocrine therapy should be classified as stage D_3 (Catalona 1984). These patients generally have highly malignant tumors, and the majority die of prostatic cancer within 1 year.

TNM System

The tumor, node, metastasis (TNM) system of staging prostatic cancer was originally devised by the International Union Against Cancer and subsequently adopted by the American Joint Committee for Cancer Staging and End Results Reporting (1978; Wallace et al. 1975). In this system the extent of the primary tumor is indicated by T category, lymph node involvement by N category, and other metastatic involvement by M category.

T categories are defined as follows:

T_x: requirements for assessment of the extent of the primary tumor have not been met.

T_0: includes tumors that are not suspected on digital rectal examination but are detected on histologic examination of prostatic specimens. This is subdivided into T_{0a} and T_{0b} (Prout et al. 1980; Catalona 1984). T_{0a} represents clinically inapparent tumor occupying no more than three high power fields or a positive needle biopsy from only one lobe of the prostate. This corresponds roughly to the stage A_1 lesion in the American system. T_{0b} includes clinically unrecognized tumors with more than three high power fields of tumor and/or positive needle biopsies from both lobes of the prostate. This corresponds roughly to stage A_2 lesions in the American system.

T_1: includes tumors evident on digital rectal examination and apparently confined to the prostate. This category is subdivided into: T_{1a}, a 1-cm nodule confined to the prostate and surrounded by apparently normal prostate (the classic Jewett nodule); T_{1b}, a tumor palpably larger than 1 cm but confined to one lobe of the prostate; and T_{1c}, a tumor with induration involving both lobes of the prostate but apparently confined within the prostatic capsule (Catalona 1984; Prout et al. 1980). T_{1b} includes Jewett's B_1 and some of Jewett's B_2 tumors. T_{1c} includes Jewett's B_2 lesions.

T_2: includes intraprostatic lesions that deform the contour of the gland.

T_3: includes tumors extending beyond the prostatic capsule with or without involvement of the lateral sulci and/or seminal vesicles. This corresponds to stage C_1 of the American system.

T_4: includes tumors extending beyond prostatic capsule and fixed to the paraprostatic tissues or invading neighboring viscera. This corresponds to stage C_2 of the American system.

N categories are defined as follows:

N_x: requirements for assessment of the regional lymph nodes have not been met.

N_0: no involvement of the regional lymph nodes.

N_1: denotes a single, homolateral regional lymph node metastasis.

N_2: denotes multiple unilateral or bilateral regional lymph node metastases.

N_3: denotes bulky, fixed regional lymph node metastases.

N_4: denotes juxtaregional lymph node metastases.

M categories are defined as follows:

M_x: requirements for assessment of distant metastasis have not been met.

M_0: no recognized distant metastasis.

M_1: distant metastasis present (site or sites are specified).

In 1983 the American Joint Committee on Cancer proposed the following changes in "T" categorization (Beahrs and Myers 1983):

T_x: minimum requirements to assess the primary tumor cannot be met.

T_0: no tumor present.

T_{1a}: no palpable tumor; on histologic sections no more than three high power fields of carcinoma found.

T_{1b}: no palpable tumor; histologic sections revealing more than three high-power fields of prostatic carcinoma.

T_{2a}: palpable nodule less than 1.5 cm in diameter with compressible, normal feeling tissue on at least three sides.

T_{2b}: palpable nodule more than 1.5 cm in diameter or nodule or induration in both lobes.

T_3: palpable tumor extending into or beyond the prostatic capsule.

T_{3a}: palpable tumor extending into the periprostatic tissues or involving seminal vesicle.

T_{3b}: palpable tumor extending into the periprostatic tissues, involving one or both seminal vesicles: tumor size more than 6 cm in diameter.

T_4: tumor fixed or involving neighboring structures.

Comment

Regardless of the system used, characterization of the local lesion has been and appears destined to remain, at least for the immediate future, largely subjective, variably arbitrary, and often unsupported by meaningful clinical correlations. The use of pelvic CT scan, ultrasound, and magnetic resonance imaging (MRI) promises to improve objective definition of tumor size, location, and extent. Although primary tumor grade and volume each has prognostic relevance, tumor volume–prostatic volume relationships to prognosis remain to be better examined.

The TNM system seems destined for ultimate widespread adoption not only because it permits an abbreviated but definitive characterization of the tumor relative to local extent (T category), regional spread (N category), and distant dissemination (M category), but because specification of the minimal requirements for these various categorizations reduces one potentially significant variable. The latter feature is often either lacking or unaddressed in alternative staging systems. Dissatisfaction with definitions of T categories and with the obligatory requirements for the various T, N, and M categorizations have been limiting factors in acceptance of the TNM system. The A, B, C, D system has received widespread use because its stage stratifications are relatively gross, simple, and noncontroversial and because there are no obligatory evaluation requirements for the various stage classifications. Both systems will continue to suffer from the uncertainties created by continuously evolving changes in clinical staging techniques and criteria and by technical and interpretational differences with the same clinical staging techniques performed at different institutions.

In a disease where end results are so dependent upon case selection, uniformity in classification and in clinical staging characterizations is especially critical.

References

American Joint Committee for Cancer Staging and End Results Reporting (1978) Manual for staging of cancer. Whiting Press, New Jersey, pp 119–124

Barzell W, Bean MA, Hilaris BS, Whitmore WF Jr (1977) Prostatic adenocarcinoma: relationship of grade and local extent to the pattern of metastases. J Urol 118:278–282

Bauer WC, McGavran MH, Carlin MR (1960) Unsuspected carcinoma of the prostate in suprapubic prostatectomy specimens. Cancer 13:370–378

Beahrs OH, Myers MH (eds) (1983) Manual for staging of cancer. JB Lippincott, Philadelphia, pp 159–163

Bergman RT, Turner R, Barnes RW, Hadley HL (1955) Comparative analysis of one thousand consecutive cases of transurethral prostatic resection. J Urol 74:533–548

Boxer RJ (1977) Adenocarcinoma of the prostate gland. Urol Survey 27:75–82

Bruce AW, O'Clevieachain F, Morales A, Awad SA (1977) Carcinoma of the prostate: a critical look at staging. J Urol 117:319–322

Cantrell BB, Deklerk DP, Eggleston JC, Boitnott JK, Walsh PC (1981) Pathological factors that influence prognosis in stage A prostatic cancer: the influence of extent versus grade. J Urol 125:516–520

Carlton CE Jr, Hudgins PT, Guerriero WG, Scott R Jr (1976) Radiotherapy in the management of stage C carcinoma of the prostate. J Urol 116:206–210

Catalona WJ (1984) Prostate cancer. Grune & Stratton, Orlando, pp 57–83

Catalona WJ, Scott WW (1978) Carcinoma of the prostate: a review. J Urol 119:1–8

Denton SE, Choy SH, Valk WL (1965) Occult prostatic carcinoma diagnosed by the step section technique of the surgical specimen. J Urol 93:296–298

deVere White R, Paulson DF, Glenn JF (1977) The clinical spectrum of prostate cancer. J Urol 117:323–327

Donohue RE, Pfister RR, Weigel JW, Stonington OG (1977) Pelvic lymphadenectomy in stage A prostatic cancer. Urology 9:273–275

Donohue RE, Fauver HE, Whitesel JA, Pfister RR (1979) Staging prostatic cancer: a different distribution. J Urol 122:327–329

Donohue RE, Mani JH, Whitesel JA et al. (1982) Pelvic lymph node dissection. Guide to patient management in clinically locally confined adenocarcinoma of prostate. Urology 20:559–565

Fowler JE, Whitmore WF Jr (1981) The incidence and extent of pelvic lymph node metastases in apparently localized prostatic cancer. Cancer 47:2941–2945

Golimbu M, Morales P (1979) Stage A2 prostatic carcinoma. Should staging systems be reclassified? Urology 13:592–596

Golimbu M, Schinella R, Morales P, Kurusu S (1978) Differences in pathological characteristics and prognosis of clinical A2 prostatic cancer from A1 and B disease. J Urol 119:618–622

Hirst AE Jr, Bergman RT (1954) Carcinoma of the prostate in men 80 or more years old. Cancer 7:136–141

Jewett HJ (1975) The present status of radical prostatectomy for stages A and B prostatic cancer. Urol Clin North Am 2:105–124

Jewett HJ, Bridge RW, Gray GF Jr, Shelley WM (1968) The palpable nodule of prostatic cancer: results 15 years after radical excision. JAMA 203:403–406

McCullough DL (1980) Surgical staging of carcinoma of the prostate. Cancer 45:1902–1905

McLaughlin A, Saltzstein SL, McCullough DL, Gittes RF (1976) Prostatic carcinoma: incidence and location of unsuspected lymphatic metastases. J Urol 115:89–94

McMillen SM, Wettlaufer JN (1976) The role of repeat transurethral biopsy in stage A carcinoma of the prostate. J Urol 116:759–760

Murphy GP. Natrajan N, Pontes JE, Schmitz RL, Smart CR, Schmidt JD, Mettlin C (1982) The natural survey of prostate cancer in the United States by the American College of Surgeons. J Urol 127:928–934

Nicholson TC, Richie JP (1977) Pelvic lymphadenectomy for stage B1 adenocarcinoma of the prostate: justified or not? J Urol 117:199–201

Parfitt HE Jr, Smith JA Jr, Seaman JP, Middleton RG (1983) Surgical treatment of stage A2 prostatic carcinoma: significance of tumor grade and extent. J Urol 129:763–765

Prout GR Jr, Heaney JA, Griffin PP, Daly JJ, Shipley WU (1980) Nodal involvement: a prognostic indicator in patients with prostatic carcinoma. J Urol 124:226–231

Rich AR (1935) On the frequency of occurrence of occult carcinoma of the prostate. J Urol 33:215–223

Sheldon CA, Williams RD, Fraley EE (1980) Incidental carcinoma of the prostate: a review of the literature and critical reappraisal of classification. J Urol 124:626–631

Smith GG, Woodruff LM (1950) The development of cancer of the prostate after subtotal prostatectomy. J Urol 63:1077–1080

Varkarakis M, Casto JE, Azzopardi JG (1970) Prognosis of stage I carcinoma of the prostate. Proc R Soc Med 63:91–95

Veterans Administration Cooperative Urological Research Group (1967) Treatment and survival of patients with cancer of the prostate. Surg Gynecol Obstet 124:1011–1017

Wallace DM, Chisholm GD, Hendry WF (1975) TNM classification for urological tumors – 1974. Br J Urol 47:1–12

Whitesel JA, Donohue RE, Mani JH et al. (1984) Acid phosphatase: its influence in the management of carcinoma of the prostate. J Urol 131:70–72

Whitmore WF Jr (1956) Hormone therapy in prostatic cancer. Am J Med 21:697–713

Whitmore WF Jr (1984) Natural history and staging of prostate cancer. Urol Clin North Am 11:205–220

Whitmore WF Jr (1980) Interstitial radiation therapy for carcinoma of the prostate. Prostate 1:157–168

Wilson CA, Dahl DS, Middleton G (1977) Pelvic lymphadenectomy for staging of apparently localized prostatic cancer. J Urol 117:197–198

Chapter 7

Pelvic Lymph Nodes: Diagnosis and Significance

J.I. Harty and W.J. Catalona

Introduction

For more than 50 years, it has been common knowledge that pelvic and abdominal lymph nodes are frequently found to be involved with metastatic spread from carcinoma of the prostate at the time of autopsy (Bumpus 1926). Since the report by Flocks et al. (1959) that lymph nodes with metastatic deposits are frequently found in early prostatic cancer, that is in prostate glands felt clinically to be surgically removable, there has been intense interest in this field. Controversy has arisen concerning the presence or absence of lymph channels in the prostate itself, the exact location of the regional lymph nodes, the incidence of lymph node involvement with metastatic disease in clinically localized prostatic cancer, the need and accuracy of pelvic lymph node dissection, especially when performed with frozen section examination, the extent of pelvic node dissection, and, finally, whether lymph node dissection in prostatic carcinoma is simply an improved staging procedure that produces additional prognostic information or a therapeutic procedure in addition.

This chapter presents evidence in each of these controversial areas and attempts to answer these questions.

Does the Prostate Contain Lymphatic Channels?

In view of our present knowledge of the frequency of lymphatic metastases from prostatic carcinoma, this question may seem strange. However, the presence of intraprostatic lymphatics was a subject of controversy in the mid-1970s.

Classic anatomic studies by Rouviere (1938) of the lymphatic system of the prostate describe a delicate network of lymph capillaries around each acinus that unite to form larger trunks, which run in the interacinar connective tissues to the capsule of the gland. There they form the periprostatic plexus, which drains to the lymph nodes in the pelvis. The clinical observation by Flocks et al. (1959) that pelvic lymph node metastases were frequently found in clinically localized carcinoma raised new interest in the lymphatic drainage of the prostate. Blennerhassett and Vickery (1966) described perineural lymph channels and suggested that these channels were the route of dissemination of neoplastic cells to the periprostatic lymph channels. In a study of lingual nerves, Rodin et al. (1967) disproved Blennerhassett's description of perineural spaces being lymphatic channels as there were no endothelial cells lining these spaces on electron microscopy. Smith (1966) failed to demonstrate intraprostatic lymphatics in animals or humans when he injected a vital dye directly into the prostate through the capsule. On gross section of the prostate, he found that the dye had tracked along tissue planes and reached the capsule and periprostatic lymph channels. No histologic sections were studied as the dye was soluble in the agent used for tissue fixation. He claimed that in the absence of lymphatics, the tumor cells traveled along planes of least resistance, through the capsule, and into the periprostatic lymph channels. Using India ink particles, Connolly et al. (1968) injected small amounts transurethrally in multiple sites into a canine prostate. They demonstrated a functioning prostatic lymphatic system lined with endothelial cells and showed that perineural spaces were not lymphatics. This finding was later confirmed in a human by Peters (cited by Jewett 1975) and in the dog by Shridhar (1979).

Despite these findings and continuing clinical experience with pelvic lymph node dissection, McCullough (1975) and Gittes and McCullough (1974), using iodinated oils and India ink injected into the prostate of rats, dogs, and humans, failed to demonstrate intraprostatic lymphatics or particles in the extraprostatic lymphatics or pelvic lymph nodes. Therefore, they suggested that the prostate was an immunologically privileged site. These findings could not explain the presence of pelvic lymph node metastases in patients with carcinoma pathologically confined to the prostate without penetration through the prostatic capsule at the time of radical prostatectomy unless the cancer had spread initially by hematogenous routes and then infiltrated the pelvic lymph nodes. It seems unlikely, however, that pelvic lymph nodes would be the only sites of metastatic deposits.

Menon et al. (1977) injected [198]Au colloid into the prostate of dogs through an open cystostomy. They found that the isotope left the prostate and was taken up by the regional nodes. There was no significant uptake in other organs or distant lymph nodes, indicating direct spread of the isotope to the pelvic lymph nodes. These findings have been confirmed by Kaplan et al. (1980).

Raghavaiah and Jordan (1979) injected ethiodol into the prostate in ten patients. The ethiodol was distributed in the prostatic lobe, giving rise to an uneven opacification with a fine particular pattern. Later the contrast medium was picked up by the extraprostatic lymphatics. Raghavaiah and Jordan assumed that because of the immediate and uniform distribution of the contrast material in the prostate and the subsequent drainage to the extraprostatic lymphatics, the opacification of the prostate was due to pick up of the ethiodol by the intraprostatic lymphatics. However, there was no histologic confirmation of ethiodol within the lymph channels. With ultrastructural studies using electron microscopy, Furusato and Mostofi (1980) have demonstrated unequivocal evidence that lymphatic channels exist between the muscle cells and fibrous stroma of the prostate.

Commentary

It appears clear that the prostate does have an intraprostatic arrangement of lymphatic channels, which unite to form larger channels of the periprostatic plexus, and that invasion of cancer cells into these lymphatics is responsible for the high incidence of lymph node metastases in patients with prostatic cancer. It is also apparent that invasion of perineural spaces does not represent lymphatic channel invasion and is not a poor prognostic sign. And finally, the prostate is no longer considered an immunologically privileged site.

What Is the Lymphatic Drainage of the Prostate?

Anatomy textbook descriptions of the lymphatic drainage of the prostate describe lymph channels that accompany the blood vessels of the prostate and drain to the lymph nodes along the external iliac and internal iliac nodes (Last 1973). Rouviere (1938) summarized his own findings and those of others by describing four separate pedicles—external iliac, hypogastric (internal iliac), posterior, and inferior—going to three groups of nodes: external iliac, hypogastric, and sacral. However, Raghavaiah and Jordan (1979) have shown that on prostatic lymphography the external iliac nodes are not areas of primary prostatic drainage and also state that the obturator node was not demonstrated in their study. However, the obturator node that they describe as not being demonstrated is located in the obturator foramen and is not the group of nodes that most urologists refer to as obturator nodes. These are generally considered to be the nodes along the proximal portion of the obturator nerve.

Clinically, the hypogastric nodes, especially those along the obturator nerve (obturator nodes), are the most frequently involved in clinically localized disease (Flocks et al. 1959; McLaughlin et al. 1977). These nodes must be considered to be the primary area of spread. The presacral nodes are also commonly involved—usually in association with the hypogastric nodes, although occasionally they are the only nodes involved (Golimbu et al. 1979). The external iliac nodes generally are not involved unless the hypogastric nodes are positive. There is general agreement that from the hypogastric and obturator nodes, spread is to the common iliac and para-aortic nodes.

Commentary

While it seems clear that the anatomic pathways and clinical findings do not concur exactly, from a urologist's viewpoint the main nodes providing drainage of the prostate are those that lie in the triangular space medial to the external iliac vein, along the obturator nerve and vessels, and along the hypogastric artery. From here, spread may go to the external iliac or presacral nodes and finally to the common iliac and para-aortic nodes. However, it must be realized that in isolated cases the external iliac or sacral nodes may be the only nodes involved. This finding has obvious implications which will be discussed in the section on extent of lymph node dissection.

What Is the Incidence of Positive Nodes in Patients with Carcinoma of the Prostate and Which Factors Influence It?

While it is still uncertain whether lymphatic or skeletal spread is the first mode of dissemination (Varkarakis et al. 1975), it has been known for some time that even clinically localized prostatic carcinoma has a high incidence of pelvic lymph node metastases (Ardiuno and Glucksman 1962). Whitmore (1973) was one of the first to emphasize that prostatic carcinoma frequently fails to develop in an orderly fashion from a subclinical disease through various stages of local growth to local invasion, to regional lymph nodes, and then distant metastases.

The development of lymph node metastases depends on many factors, the most important of which appear to be stage of the tumor, grade of the tumor, size of the tumor, extent of prostatic involvement, and seminal vesicle involvement.

Donohue et al. (1982) found positive nodes in 23% of stage A_2 disease, 18% in stage B_1 disease, 35% in stage B_2 disease, and 46% in stage C. Reviewing a collective series, Lieskovsky (1983) reported similar figures.

Smith et al. (1983) studied the influence of grade as well as stage in patients undergoing pelvic lymphadenectomy. They showed a close relationship between the grade of the tumor and the finding of positive nodes; for example, only 4% of well differentiated B_1 patients had positive nodes compared with 33% when the tumor was poorly differentiated (Table 7.1).

Flocks et al. (1959) showed that the size of the gland containing carcinoma was related to the chance of finding positive nodes. When the gland weighed 35 g, 18% of patients had positive nodes; when it weighed 45–80 g, 44% had positive

Table 7.1. Incidence of pelvic node metastasis by histologic grade and clinical stage (Smith et al. 1983)

| Stage | Grade | | | |
	Well differentiated No./total (%)	Moderately differentiated No./total (%)	Poorly differentiated No./total (%)	Totals (%)
A_1	0/28	0/12	0/1	0/41
A_2	0/7	5/19 (26)	3/7 (43)	8/33 (24)
B_1	2/53 (4)	13/94 (14)	3/9 (33)	18/156 (12)
B_2	5/27 (18)	29/106 (27)	9/21 (43)	43/154 (28)
C	5/10 (50)	18/44 (41)	13/14 (93)	36/68 (53)
	12/125 (10)	65/275 (24)	28/52 (54)	105/452 (23)

nodes; when it weighed 80–150 g, 51% had positive nodes; and if it weighed more than 150 g, then 92% of the patients had positive nodes.

Saltzstein and McLaughlin (1977) have shown that when 65% of the gland showed carcinoma on permanent sections, the nodes were found to be positive, while if there was less than 40% involved, the nodes were negative.

Ardiuno and Glucksman (1962) showed that 80% of patients having seminal vesicle invasion also had lymph node metastases. Catalona and Stein (1982b) found a 68% incidence of positive nodes when the seminal vesicle was invaded. Clinically, however, it is often very difficult if not impossible to detect seminal vesicle invasion, and this finding is most frequently made at pathologic examination.

Commentary

It is clear that the overall incidence of positive nodes even in clinically localized disease is high at the time of initial diagnosis. Because the chance of cure by surgery or radiation therapy is low in patients with positive nodes, every attempt should be made to identify those patients by noninvasive methods prior to surgery. Should noninvasive methods prove negative, then pelvic lymphadenectomy should be performed prior to radical surgery.

Which Patients with Prostatic Cancer Need Lymph Node Dissection?

Since the presence of positive lymph nodes is associated with a poor prognosis regardless of treatment, every effort should be made to diagnose positive nodes prior to definitive therapy (Paulson et al. 1982). The high incidence of false-positive and false-negative results associated with noninvasive techniques for assessing pelvic nodes makes pelvic lymph node dissection the most accurate staging procedure in cancer patients. However, it is associated with some complications (Herr 1979; Lieskovsky et al. 1980) and should only be performed in selected patients.

First of all, the patient should have a clinically localized prostatic carcinoma (stage A_2, B_1, B_2, or small C) and should be medically fit to undergo either radical prostatectomy or interstitial radiation if the nodes are negative.

Kramer et al. (1980) have further attempted to select patients for pelvic node dissection based on the Gleason score of the prostatic biopsy. They reported that no patient with a Gleason score of 2–4 had positive nodes, while 93% of those with a Gleason score of 8–10 had positive nodes. Therefore, lymph node dissection was reserved for those with a Gleason score of 5–7. However, others have not found similar results. Sagalowsky et al. (1982), while agreeing that patients with low Gleason scores had negative nodes, found that only 44%, 60%, and 44% of patients with Gleason scores of 7, 8, and 9, respectively, had positive nodes. Zincke et al. (1982) likewise found that the Gleason scoring system, as an indicator for pelvic node status, did not have suitable predictive value. Olsson (1985) found that 20% of patients with a Gleason score of 2–4 had node metastases while 38% of patients with a Gleason score of 8–10 had negative nodes. However, low grade A lesions had only 8% positive nodes and high grade C lesions had 100% positive nodes. Smith et al. (1983) did not find the Gleason score alone to be accurate enough to preclude a lymph node dissection. However, like Olsson, when they combined stage with Gleason score, they found that the incidence of positive nodes was low enough to preclude lymphadenectomy in patients with stage A_1 disease as well as low Gleason score (2–4) stage B_1 tumors and high enough (93%) to avoid lymphadenectomy in patients with poorly differentiated stage C tumors.

The apparent discrepancies between Kramer et al. and others may be due to the limited reproducibility of the Gleason system when interpreted by different individuals (Harada et al. 1977). Another explanation would be that the histology of a needle biopsy is not truly representative of all the disease in the prostate (Lange and Narayan 1983).

Commentary

At the present time, pelvic node dissection should be reserved for those patients who have localized prostatic carcinoma on clinical examination, who have a negative noninvasive evaluation, in whom a therapeutic decision would be based on the findings of node dissection, and who would be medically fit to undergo definitive therapy. Improved standardization of the Gleason scoring system and its universal use by pathologists and urologists may lead to agreement with Kramer et al.'s findings and reduce the number of positive lymph node dissections. The studies by Diamond et al. (1982) and Tannenbaum et al. (1982) of relative nuclear roundness and nuclear surface area may have greater predictability for malignant potential than grade alone. However, these are not currently in general use.

How Extensive Should the Pelvic Lymph Node Dissection Be?

Based on some of the surgical anatomic descriptions of the lymph node drainage of the prostate, the original lymph node dissection encompassed the external iliac nodes, the hypogastric nodes, and the obturator nodes along the proximal portion of the obturator nerve (Whitmore and Mackenzie 1959). This has come to be known as the *standard lymph node dissection*. Some also included the common iliac nodes and even the para-aortic nodes (McCullough et al. 1974; Gill et al. 1974). The dissection is generally carried out extraperitoneally but occasionally transperitoneally (Freiha and Salzman 1977).

More recently, several reports have demonstrated a more limited node dissection, preserving the lymphatics surrounding the external iliac artery and removing the hypogastric and obturator nodes (Paulson 1980; Whitmore et al. 1985). The advantages of this type of dissection, known as a *limited or modified node dissection*, is that it reduces the incidence of lower extremity and genital edema (especially if postoperative external beam radiation therapy is planned), reduces the operating time, and presents a smaller package of nodes to the pathologist for frozen section, reducing the chances for a false-negative result. The limited dissection yielded the same incidence of positive nodes as the standard node dissection (Paulson 1980).

Conversely, Golimbu et al. (1979), based on the original observation reported by Rouviere that the prostate drains to the presacral nodes, found that these nodes and the presciatic nodes were involved in 53% and 47% of patients, respectively, and that in 7% of cases these were the only groups of nodes involved. This finding led them to recommend *extended lymph node dissection*, which encompasses the common iliac, external iliac, hypogastric (obturator), presacral, and presciatic nodes. They noted no additional complications over the standard node dissection and found it added only 30 min to the procedure.

Commentary

Our current policy is to perform staging pelvic lymphadenectomy only in patients who are deemed to be suitable candidates for radical prostatectomy. Our practice is to perform a limited pelvic lymph node dissection with the lateral margin of the dissection being the external iliac vein, the medial margin being the hypogastric artery, the proximal margin being the bifurcation of the external iliac vein, and the distal margin being the femoral canal. This lymph node dissection includes the lymph nodes surrounding the obturator nerves. The available data in the literature and our own experience suggest that this node dissection is approximately 85% accurate as a staging procedure, i.e., approximately 15% of patients with lymph node metastases have metastases in nodes other than the nodes encompassed by this dissection.

It is clear that the procedure should be performed extraperitoneally to reduce the complication rate and that a random "berry picking" node dissection should not be performed, especially in high-stage, high-grade lesions.

What Is the Accuracy of Frozen Section Examination of Pelvic Nodes?

When radical perineal prostatectomy was the common procedure for localized prostatic carcinoma, the lymph nodes were not routinely examined. This lack of examination probably accounts for the disappointing 15-year disease-free survival rate for patients who had greater than a B_1 lesion (Jewett 1975). However, now that radical retropubic prostatectomy had largely replaced the perineal approach, lymph node dissection is routinely carried out.

Initially, because the implications of positive nodes were unknown, it seemed unreasonable to subject the patient to a node dissection and await the results of permanent sectioning before performing a radical retropubic prostatectomy or ^{125}I implantation if the nodes were negative. Consequently, frozen section examination of the nodes became an important part of the management of patients who were candidates for potentially curative therapy with surgery or radiation.

Table 7.2. Incidence of false-negative frozen sections

	No. of cases	Positive FS	Negative FS	PS	False-negative	Sensitivity
Fowler et al. (1981)	42	10 (25%)	32 (75%)	13 (33%)	3 (9%)	10/13 (76%)
Catalona and Stein (1982a)	75	16 (21%)	59 (79%)	27 (36%)	11 (19%)	16/27 (59%)
Sadlowski et al. (1983)	40	5 (13%)	35 (87%)	8 (20%)	3 (9%)	5/8 (62%)
Kramolowsky et al. (1984)	100	43 (43%)	57 (57%)	59 (59%)	16 (28%)	43/59 (73%)

FS, frozen section; PS, permanent section

McLaughlin et al. (1977) and Saltzstein and McLaughlin (1977) were first to report on the accuracy of frozen section of pelvic lymph nodes as part of a broader study. Over the past 5 years several papers have addressed this question more specifically (Fowler et al. 1981; Catalona and Stein 1982a; Sadlowski et al. 1983; Kramolowsky et al. 1984). The results are listed in Table 7.2. All of these series are comparable in the number of patients in each stage and grade. A standard lymph node dissection was carried out in each case, and if palpably enlarged nodes were found, these were submitted first for frozen section and the procedure terminated if the nodes were positive.

The false-negative frozen section rate ranged between 9% and 28%. Catalona and Stein (1982a) noted that the false-negative rate paralleled the incidence of positive nodes in the patient group. For example, in series comprised largely of patients with small, well differentiated clinical stage B_1 lesions in which the overall incidence of positive nodes was low, the incidence of false-negative frozen sections was correspondingly low. On the other hand, in series that had a large proportion of patients with moderately or poorly differentiated clinical stage B_2 lesions in which the overall incidence of positive nodes was high, the corresponding incidence of false-negative frozen sections also was high. Catalona and Stein suggested that a more reliable index of the accuracy of frozen section examination is the *sensitivity* of frozen section, i.e., the percentage of patients with positive nodes that were detected on frozen section. The sensitivity of frozen section in the literature varied between 59% and 76%. Therefore between 24% and 41% of frozen sections were inaccurate.

Analysis of the reasons for false-negative results revealed that they were due either to the surgeon not submitting the positive nodes to the pathologist for frozen section or the pathologist not sectioning and examining the positive nodes. Misinterpretation of the frozen section was rare.

Commentary

If one agrees that pelvic lymph node dissection is only a staging procedure and unlikely to be therapeutic and that patients with positive nodes (even microscopic) have a uniformly poor prognosis, then subjecting a patient to a radical prostatectomy based on a false-negative frozen section will lead to a disappointing result. Based on the findings in the aforementioned studies, certain recommendations can be made to reduce the incidence of false-negative results. First, all nodal tissue should be submitted for frozen section, especially in cases that have a high risk of positive nodes. Secondly, the pathologist should carefully examine the nodes grossly and examine all nodes at 2–3 mm intervals with frozen section. This examination may be time consuming if there are a lot of nodes. If adequate frozen section facilities are not available, then consideration must be given to performing the pelvic node dissection alone initially and verifying the results of permanent sectioning of the nodes before proceeding with a radical prostatectomy.

Is Pelvic Lymph Node Dissection Only a Staging Procedure or Is It Therapeutic?

Flocks (1973) reported a 13% tumor-free survival in patients who had positive nodes, although these also had radioactive gold implantation at the time of surgery. At Memorial Sloan Kettering Cancer Center, Barzell et al. (1977) initially suggested that if the tumor volume and lymph nodes were less than 3 cc, then the patient could be expected to remain disease-free for 5 years. Prout et al. (1980) showed that only 18% of patients with solitary lymph node metastases developed metastatic disease; however, the median follow-up was short—43 months. These reports led Golimbu et al. (1979) to extend the lymph node dissection to include the presacral and presciatic nodes.

However, in a later report from the Memorial Sloan Kettering Cancer Center, Grossman et al. (1982) showed that individuals with only one positive node fared no better than those with multiple nodal metastases in terms of developing distant metastases, although patients with less nodal involvement had a longer interval before exhibiting evidence of metastases. In a subsequent study from the Memorial Sloan Kettering Cancer Center, Fischer et al. (1983) found that 48% of patients with one positive node, 67% of patients with two or three positive nodes, 68% of patients with more than three positive nodes, and 93% of patients with positive common iliac nodes or positive para-aortic nodes manifested distant metastases at an average of 27, 27, 22, and 25 months postimplantation of ^{125}I, respectively. All of these reports are from series where patients underwent ^{125}I interstitial radiation therapy. In a series of patients who underwent radical prostatectomy in conjunction with the pelvic node dissection, Cline et al. (1981) reported that the median time to failure with patients with positive pelvic lymph nodes following radical prostatectomy and pelvic node dissection was less than 2 years. There was no significant difference in the length of time to failure between patients with a solitary node and those with multiple nodes.

Smith and Middleton (1984) confirmed that patients with minimal nodal metastases do not have a prognosis equivalent to those with negative nodes but did find that of those with only one microscopic positive lymph node, 44% were alive and free of disease at 5 years, while only 15% of those with gross nodal disease were alive and free of cancer over a similar period.

Commentary

The finding of positive nodes—even if microscopic—at pelvic node dissection indicates systemic disease which cannot be detected by the usual means, i.e., acid phosphatase elevation or positive bone scan. Although it is conceivable that a rare patient with microscopic disease might be cured with pelvic node dissection, the evidence is becoming clearer with longer follow-up that almost all of these patients will succumb to distant metastases sooner (those with gross nodal involvement) or later (those with microscopic nodal disease).

Summary

In conclusion, the prostate has a well defined system of lymphatic channels, which drain in a fairly predictable fashion to the hypogastric nodes first and then to the external iliac, common iliac, and presacral nodes. Spread of prostatic carcinoma, even clinically localized disease, frequently occurs through these lymphatic channels to these nodes. Pelvic lymphadenectomy remains the most accurate staging technique, although it is associated with complications. These complications can be reduced by performing a more limited node dissection, and node dissection should be reserved for a select patient group. Thorough examination of nodal tissue with frozen sections is important to avoid unnecessary local therapy in the face of systemic disease since it is becoming increasingly clear that pelvic node dissection is not therapeutic in the vast majority of patients.

References

Ardiuno LJ, Glucksman MA (1962) Lymph node metastases in early cancer of the prostate. J Urol 88:91–93

Barzell W, Bean MA, Hilaris BS, Whitmore WF Jr (1977) Prostatic adenocarcinoma: relationship of grade and local extent to the pattern of metastases. J Urol 118:278–282

Blennerhassett JB, Vickery AI Jr (1966) Carcinoma of the prostate: an anatomical study of tumor location. Cancer 19:980–984

Bumpus HC (1926) Carcinoma of the prostate. Surg Gynecol Obstet 43:150–155

Catalona WJ, Stein AJ (1982a) Accuracy of frozen section detection of lymph node metastases in prostatic carcinoma. J Urol 127:460–461

Catalona WJ, Stein AJ (1982b) Staging errors in clinically localized prostatic cancer. J Urol 127:452–456

Cline WA, Kramer SA, Farnham R, Cox EB, Glenn JF, Hinshaw W, Paulson DF (1981) Impact of pelvic lymphadenectomy in patients with prostatic adenocarcinoma. Urology 17:129–131

Connolly JG, Thompson A, Jewett MAS, Hartman N, Weber M (1968) Intraprostatic lymphatics. Invest Urol 5:371–378

Diamond DA, Berry SJ, Jewett HJ, Eggleston JC, Coffey DS (1982) A new method to assess metastatic potentially human prostatic cancer: relative nuclear roundness. J Urol 128:729–734

Donohue RE, Mani JH, Whitesel JA, Mohr S, Scanavino D, Augspurger RR, Biber RJ, Fanver HE, Wehlaufer JN, Pfister RR (1982) Pelvic node dissection: guide to patient management in clinically locally confined adenocarcinoma of the prostate. Urology 20:559–565

Fischer H, Kleinert H, Whitmore WR Jr (1983) Stratification of node positive patients undergoing I-125 implantation: effect of these to distant metastases. Abstract 302, American Urological Association Meeting, Las Vegas, 1983

Flocks RH (1973) The treatment of stage C prostatic cancer with special reference to combined surgical and radiation therapy. J Urol 109:461–463

Flocks RH, Culp D, Porto R (1959) Lymphatic spread from prostatic carcinoma. J Urol 81:194–196

Fowler JE, Torgerson L, McLeod DG, Stutzman RE (1981) Radical prostatectomy with pelvic lymphadenectomy: observations on the accuracy of staging with lymph node frozen sections. J Urol 126:618–619

Freiha FS, Salzman J (1977) Surgical staging of prostatic cancer: transperitoneal versus extraperitoneal lymphadenectomy. J Urol 118:616–617

Furusato M, Mostofi FK (1980) Intraprostatic lymphatics in man: light and ultrastructural observations. Prostate 1:15–23

Gill WB, Marks JE, Strans FH, Sylora HO, Diamond HM (1974) Radical retropubic prostatectomy and retroperitoneal lymphadenectomy following radiotherapy conversion of stage C to stage B carcinoma of the prostate. J Urol 111:656–661

Gittes RF, McCullough DL (1974) Occult carcinoma of the prostate: an oversight of immune surveillance—a working hypothesis. J Urol 112:241–244

Golimbu M, Morales P, Al-Askari S, Brown J (1979) Extended pelvic lymphadenectomy for prostatic cancer. J Urol 121:617–620

Grossman HB, Batata M, Hilaris B, Whitmore WF Jr (1982) [125]I implantation for carcinoma of the prostate. Further followup of the first 100 cases. Urology 20:591–598

Harada M, Mostofi FK, Corle DK, Byer DP, Trump BF (1977) Preliminary studies of histologic prognosis in cancer of the prostate. Cancer Treat Rep 61:223–225

Herr HW (1979) Complications of pelvic lymphadenectomy and retropubic prostatic ^{125}I implantation. Urology 14:226–229

Jewett HJ (1975) The present status of radical prostatectomy for stages A and B prostatic cancer. Urol Clin North Am 2:105–124

Kaplan WK, Whitmore WF III, Gittes RF (1980) Visualization of canine and human prostatic lymph nodes following intraprostatic injection of technetium-99m-antimony sulfide colloid. Invest Radiol 15:34–38

Kramer SA, Spahr J, Brendler CB, Glenn JF, Paulson DF (1980) Experience with Gleason's histopathologic grading in prostatic cancer. J Urol 124:223–225

Kramolowsky EV, Narayana AS, Platz CE, Loening SA (1984) The frozen section in lymphadenectomy for carcinoma of the prostate. J Urol 131:899–900

Lange PH, Narayan P (1983) Understaging and undergrading of prostatic cancer. Argument for postoperative radiation as adjuvant therapy. Urology 21:113–118

Last RJ (1973) Anatomy, regional and applied, 5th edn. Chruchill Livingstone, Edinburgh, p 29

Lieskovsky G (1983) Pelvic lymphadenectomy. In: Glenn's Urologic Surgery, Philadelphia, JB Lippincott, pp 939–947

Lieskovsky G, Skinner DG, Weisenburger T (1980) Pelvic lymphadenectomy in the management of carcinoma of the prostate. J Urol 124:635–638

McCullough DL (1975) Experimental lymphangiography. Experiences with direct medium injection into the parenchyma of the rat testis and prostate. Invest Urol 13:211–219

McCullough DL, Prout GR Jr, Daly JJ (1974) Carcinoma of the prostate and lymphatic metastases. J Urol 111:65–71

McLaughlin AP, Saltzstein SL, McCullough DL, Gittes RF (1977) Prostatic carcinoma: incidence and location of unsuspected lymphatic metastases. J Urol 115:89–94

Menon M, Menon S, Strauss W, Catalona WJ (1977) Demonstration of the existence of canine prostatic lymphatics by radioisotope techniques. J Urol 118:274–277

Olsson CA (1985) Staging lymphadenectomy should be antecedent to treatment in localized prostatic carcinoma. Urology 25:4–6

Paulson DF (1980) The prognostic role of lymphadenectomy in adenoma of the prostate. Urol Clin North Am 7:615–622

Paulson DF, Ling H, Hinshaw W, Stephani S (1982) The Uro-Oncology Research Group. Radical surgery and radiotherapy for adenocarcinoma of the prostate. J Urol 128:502–504

Prout GR Jr, Heaney JA, Griffin PP, Daly JJ, Shipley WV (1980) Nodal involvement as a prognostic indicator in patients with prostatic carcinoma. J Urol 124:226–231

Raghavaiah NV, Jordan WP Jr (1979) Prostatography. J Urol 121:174–177

Rodin AE, Larson DL, Roberts DK (1967) Nature of the perineural space invaded by prostatic carcinoma. Cancer 20:1772–1779

Rouviere H (1938) Anatomy of the human lymphatic system (translated by MJ Tobias). Edward Brothers, Ann Arbor

Sadlowski RW, Donohue DJ, Richman AV, Sharpe JR, Finney RP (1983) Accuracy of frozen section diagnosis in pelvic lymph node staging biopsies for adenocarcinoma of the prostate. J Urol 129:324–326

Sagalowsky AI, Milam H, Reveley LR, Silva FG (1982) Prediction of lymphatic metastases by Gleason histologic grading in prostatic cancer. J Urol 128:951–952

Saltzstein SL, McLaughlin AP (1977) Clinicopathologic features of unsuspected regional lymph node metastases in prostatic adenocarcinoma. Cancer 40:1212–1221

Shridhar P (1979) The lymphatics of the prostate gland and their role in the spread of prostatic carcinoma. Ann R Coll Surg Engl 61:114–122

Smith JA, Middleton RG (1984) Pelvic lymph node metastasis from prostatic cancer: significance of disease extent. Abstract 228, American Urological Association Meeting, New Orleans

Smith JA Jr, Seaman JP, Gleidman JB, Middleton RG (1983) Pelvic lymph node metastases from prostatic cancer. Influence of tumor grade and stage in 452 consecutive patients. J Urol 130:290–292

Smith MJ (1966) The lymphatics of the prostate. Invest Urol 3:439–444

Tannenbaum M, Tannenbaum S, DeSanctis PN, Olsson CA (1982) Prognostic significance of nuclear surface area in prostate cancer. Urology 19:546–551

Varkarakis MJ, Murphy GP, Nelson GMK, Chehval M, Moore RJ, Flocks RH (1975) Lymph node involvement in prostatic carcinoma. Urol Clin North Am 2:197–212

Whitmore WF Jr (1973) The natural history of prostatic cancer. Cancer 32:1104–1112

Whitmore WF Jr, Mackenzie AR (1959) Experiences with various operative procedures for total excision of prostatic cancer. Cancer 12:396–405

Whitmore WF Jr, Hilaris B, Batata M, Sogani P, Herr H, Morse M (1985) Interstitial reduction: short term palliation of curative therapy? Urology [Suppl] 25:24–98

Zincke H, Farrow GM, Myers RP, Benson RC Jr, Furlow WL, Utz DC (1982) Relationship between stage and grade of adenocarcinoma of the prostate and regional pelvic lymph node metastases. J Urol 128:498–501

Chapter 8

Management of Localized Adenocarcinoma of the Prostate

C.A. Olsson

Introduction

Appropriate management of the patient with localized adenocarcinoma of the prostate remains a controversial topic for various reasons. First, prostatic cancer occurs in an age group in which many other diseases affect the health of the host. Second, the biologic hazard presented by adenocarcinoma of the prostate can be exceedingly variable. This variability is dependent not simply on host factors, such as age and state of health, but also on factors indigenous to the tumor, such as degree of differentiation and metastatic potential. Finally, the majority of studies of the efficacy of one treatment modality versus another have consisted of uncontrolled analyses of patient survival comparative to historical controls alone; few randomized studies of treatment efficacy have been conducted.

This chapter will reflect the prejudice of its author in assuming a surgical approach to the patient with localized adenocarcinoma of the prostate. The premises upon which this prejudice is based will be thoroughly studied by presenting a historical perspective of the diagnosis, staging, and management of localized prostatic cancer over the last 20 years.

Radiation Therapy

Until the late 1960s, the appropriate management of the patient with localized adenocarcinoma of the prostate was traditionally thought to be radical prostatectomy. A series of articles published around this time suggested that 5-, 10-, and 15-year survivals approximating 75%, 50%, and 30%, respectively, could be achieved with this form of management (Jewett et al. 1968; Belt and Shroeder 1972; Culp and Meyer 1973). The premises upon which any continuing enthusiasm for radical prostactectomy was based included the concept that, if the disease were confined to the prostate, excision of that structure should render the patient free of his disease. Up until that time, no other treatment modality had demonstrated similar efficacy with as little, or less morbidity.

Initial reports of the efficacy of radiation therapy in these patients were received by urologists with little enthusiasm, as these reports predominantly consisted of 5-year analyses of treatment outcome in a disease which, because of its slowly progressive characteristics, required longer term studies (Bagshaw 1969). However, by the early 1970s, the pioneering work of Bagshaw and Ray demonstrated that a 10-year survival expectancy of 48% could be achieved by means of regional irradiation of the prostate and surrounding pelvic structures (Ray and Bagshaw 1975). Some of the patients enjoying this 10-year survival had been subjected to endocrine manipulation as well; nevertheless, the fact that equal treatment efficacy had been demonstrated by means other than surgery constituted a compelling reason for the urologist to re-evaluate his thoughts when counselling the patient regarding treatment options.

At that time considerable morbidity was associated with radical prostatectomy. Although surgical mortality was quite modest, sexual impotence could be anticipated in the vast majority of patients undergoing radical prostatectomy. Urinary incontinence was reported to occur in as many as 25% of cases (6). The rectum could be anticipated to be injured in perhaps 3% of cases; this injury would potentially require additional surgery to correct it. Finally, minor complications such as urethral stricture might necessitate bothersome urethral dilation at intervals for life.

Few if any of the complications resulting from radiation therapy of similar patients were fully understood at that time. The apparently equal treatment efficacy offered by an apparently less morbid, noninvasive form of therapy became an attractive prospect for both the patient and his physician alike. In this manner, the popularity of a radiation treatment option became well established.

A variety of innovative radiation therapy approaches had been developed during this interval for patients with localized prostatic cancer, in attempts to improve upon the efficacy (or reduce the morbidity) of curative regional external radiotherapy techniques. Interstitial irradiation with implantation of iodine 125 was promoted predominantly at New York Memorial Hospital; simultaneously a combined approach utilizing interstitial implantation of gold 198 along with adjunctive external radiation therapy was promoted by the group at Baylor University (Whitmore et al. 1972; Carlton et al. 1975).

During the subsequent decade (extending from the early 1970s to the early 1980s) those urologists who maintained their prejudice favoring extirpative approaches faced not only an ethical dilemma in continuing this prejudice, but also a decidedly difficult task in advising patients, many of whom were already aware of the apparently equal treatment efficacy offered by radiation therapy approaches. Maintenance of erectile potency was often cited by the patient as a major reason for his selecting a radiation therapy approach. Less often (but with more emphasis) the sophisticated patient would base his treatment decision upon the desire to remain free from any significant urinary symptoms, in particular urinary wetting. Most importantly, though, the majority of patients would select an approach consisting of external radiation therapy, hoping to achieve adequate treatment for their malignancies without any surgical intervention.

Selection Criteria

The past 20 years have brought improved understanding about adequate staging of the patient with clinically localized prostatic cancer. Several institutions have reported upon both the incidence and prognostic impact of pelvic lymphadeno-pathy in the patient presumed to have localized prostatic cancer (Hilaris et al. 1977; Babayan et al. 1980; Kramer et al. 1981). Together, these reports represent some of the most reproducible biologic data ever reported. Regardless of the institution reporting, it is an inescapable conclusion that a certain number of patients clinically thought to have localized prostatic cancer will in fact have already experienced metastatic disease at the time of presentation. Similarly, without question is the negative prognostic impact that pelvic lymph node metastases exert upon the patient's clinical course.

The incidence of pelvic lymph node metastases in clinically staged A_2 prostatic cancer approximates 30%; the incidence for patients with presumed stage B disease is approximately 15%. When there is the clinical presence of extracapsular disease detected by rectal examination, the incidence of lymph node metastases rises to approximately 50% (Donohue et al. 1977; Wilson et al. 1977; Golimbu et al. 1978). These figures assume considerable importance when viewed in terms of the negative prognostic influence conferred by the presence of pelvic lymph node spread from localized prostatic cancer. For example, nearly 50% of men with pelvic lymph node metastases can be expected to develop bony metastases within 2 years (Olsson and deVere White 1982). This figure rises to 90% or more 5 years after discovery of lymphadenopathy (a progression rate 6 times worse than that experienced by a patient with a similarly staged local tumor without adenopathy).

These data present the urologist with two compelling reasons to accurately stage the patient with prostatic cancer presumed to be localized to the gland. First, the physician has an obligation to instruct the inquisitive patient relative to his prognosis following therapy. Second, the presence or absence of pelvic lymph node metastases may have a profound effect upon the selection of treatment options available to the patient. For example, at this time there is little if any evidence that the patient with pelvic lymph node metastases can be cured by lymph node resection along with radical prostatectomy; similarly, there is little evidence to support the premise that pelvic radiation therapy has the ability to significantly alter the adverse prognostic influence of pelvic node metastases. When pelvic lymph node spread has been documented the patient should be considered to have systemic disease.

Noninvasive techniques of pelvic lymph node staging fall far short of clinically acceptable accuracy. A significant number of patients whose pelvic lymph node architecture is studied by either lymphangiography or pelvic CT scanning will manifest lymph node metastases that are undetectable by these diagnostic modalities; a smaller percentage of patients will be incorrectly judged by these studies to have lymph node spread when there is none (Paulson and Uro-

Oncology Research Group 1979). Some have suggested that tumor grade can be utilized to predict the presence or absence of pelvic lymphadenopathy in patients with prostatic cancer, particularly at the extremes of tumor differentiation or dedifferentiation. For example, it was thought that patients with Gleason 2–4 primary tumors would rarely experience metastases and that those individuals whose primary tumors were scored at the Gleason level of 8–10 would always be found to have metastatic disease (Kramer et al. 1980). Our own work, as well as that of others, suggests that one cannot depend upon tumor grade alone to predict the presence or absence of pelvic lymph node metastases. For example, in our own experience, 20% of patients with Gleason 2–4 primary tumors demonstrated lymphadenopathy and nearly 50% of patients with high grade (Gleason 8–10) primary tumors were free from lymph node spread at the time of exploration (Olsson et al. 1982).

Because of the above data, we continue to advise that the patient with adenocarcinoma of the prostate presumed to be localized to the gland after adequate rectal examination, radioisotopic bone scan, and assay of serum prostatic acid phosphatase undergo pelvic exploration in an effort to document freedom from systemic disease with certainty. For two reasons, those patients selecting external radiation therapy do not generally avail themselves of this degree of pretreatment staging accuracy. In the first place, once the physician and patient have decided upon a noninvasive form of therapy, they are hard-pressed to accept pelvic exploration solely as a diagnostic procedure. In the second place, there is substantial fear among some radiation therapists that significant peripheral lymphedema will occur if a pelvic lymph node exploration has been conducted prior to administration of pelvic field radiation therapy. This fear is rather unfounded, provided the surgeon limits his regional lymph node resection to a quadrilateral area bounded inferiorly by the obturator nerve, superiorly by the external iliac vein, posteriorly by the hypogastric artery, and anteriorly by the pelvic side wall. These surgical boundaries interfere little, if at all, with the lymphatic drainage from either lower extremity, so that the combined influence of surgery and radiation therapy should not result in peripheral lymphedema.

Of course, those forms of radiation therapy that utilize the implantation of radioactive materials into the prostate do not suffer from this deficit. Surgical staging is carried out in the process of exposing the prostate for administration of the radioactive material. In a similar vein, surgery for localized prostatic cancer has undergone evolution as well. There has been a significant trend away from a perineal approach to radical prostatectomy and toward the retropubic approach, which allows the surgeon an opportunity to assess the patient fully for the possibility of pelvic lymph node metastases prior to continuing with extirpation of the gland. This latter approach requires the dedicated participation of the surgical pathologist, who must carry out careful intraoperative histologic studies on excised pelvic nodes. This is not an easy task but, at the same time, does not constitute an insurmountable obstacle. With increasing experience, our pathologists are able to detect the vast majority of patients with pelvic node metastases by means of frozen section analysis of excised nodes at the time of surgical exploration. In our own experience, the number of instances in which they are wrong (and a radical prostatectomy is conducted only to find that the patient did have microscopic tumor deposits in one or more pelvic nodes) is acceptably small (3% or less).

Problems with Radiation Therapy

The popularity of radiation treatments for patients with localized prostatic cancer continued to flourish during the 1970s. As experience with these treatment modalities increased, a variety of data became available causing a reconsideration of the potential hazards and benefits of these approaches.

One of the first issues that became apparent to the practicing urologist sending his patient for external beam radiation therapy was that the promised safety of the treatment modality with regard to preservation of erectile potency was not realized in all individuals. Many a disgruntled patient who chose a radiation therapy approach in order to preserve his sexual function was sorely disappointed. Overall, as additional data became available for review, it was realized that 40% of men undergoing curative levels of external beam radiation therapy would lose erectile potency following treatment (Pistenma et al. 1976).

In time, other complications consequent to external radiation therapy of the prostate became apparent both to the patient and his physician. Disabling radiation cystitis occurred in approximately 3%–5% of individuals, some of whom had to undergo urinary diversion for relief of symptomatology (Kurup et al. 1984). A small but significant (5%) number of patients developed permanent radiation proctitis. A larger number of patients experienced the development of urethral stricture disease.

Some of the complications were related to the radiation sources employed. In general, the use of treatment delivery units employing low energy sources such as cobalt 60 resulted in higher doses of radiation being administered to surrounding structures (rectum, bladder, and urethra). It also became apparent to the urologist that there were differential abilities of one radiation therapy group versus another. Suboptimal treatment plans employing inappropriate levels of radiation administered daily or else appropriate dosages administered through suboptimally designed portals can result in a substantial increase in complications.

Complications resulting from the combined use of interstitial gold followed by external radiation therapy generally parallelled the types and incidence of complications experienced with external radiation treatment. Interstitial irradiation with iodine 125, on the other hand, had been shown to be associated with a lower percentage of posttreatment complications (Hilaris et al. 1974). With this treatment technique, the likelihood of erectile impotence fell to 5%. Provided the distribution of the iodine-containing needles was patterned so as to yield even dosimetry, the likelihood of scatter effect resulting in radiation proctitis or cystitis was remarkably low (Hilaris et al. 1974).

Treatment Failures After Radiation Therapy

Of even greater concern than the complications attendant upon radiation treatment techniques was the fact that prostatic biopsies following definitive radiation therapy continued to demonstrate apparently unaltered prostatic cancer cells. Initially, this phenomenon was thought to be related to the timing of the posttreatment biopsy: a slowly replicating tumor such as adenocarcinoma of the prostate could not be expected to show a loss of cellular integrity within a period as short as 6 months following the completion of radiotherapy (Cox and Stoffel 1977). Additional studies addressing this premise were appropriately conducted, demonstrating that while there was a gradual decrease in the percentage of positive biopsies obtained in previously irradiated prostates, approximately one-third of patients continued to manifest a chronically positive prostatic biopsy in excess of 2 years following conclusion of therapy (Kurth et al. 1977; Kiesling et al. 1980; Scardino et al. 1982). This figure was remarkably similar regardless of the technique of radiation therapy employed, although radiation genetic studies suggest that the number of positive biopsies following interstitial iodine 125 therapy could be expected to be somewhat higher than those following definitive external radiotherapy (Cupps et al. 1980).

The proposition provided to explain the persistence of cancer cells in the prostate of a patient presumed to be "cured" by radiation therapy was that they represented a "dormant" pool of cells that were rendered metabolically and reproductively inactive by the radiation therapy (Cox and Stoffel 1977). This proposition continued to imply that these "dormant" cells were of no potential danger to the host. However, by the early 1980s, this proposition had been largely refuted. This population of prostatic cancer cells remaining in the gland following definitive radiation therapy was further investigated in terms of architecture, metabolic activity, and capability of undergoing cellular division. Electron microscopic analysis showed the cells to retain all of the characteristics of nonirradiated prostatic cancer cells: loss of cellular polarity, cytoplasmic granularity, and the same nuclear anatomy, including the prominent nucleoli often associated with cancer (Kiesling et al. 1979). In fact, the only prominent architectural change that could be ascribed to radiation therapy was the degree of fibrosis surrounding each cell. Other workers conducted immunoperoxidase staining of the irradiated prostatic cancer cells in a search for acid phosphatase secretion; the cells stained positively for acid phosphatase, an observation leading to the presumption that the cells retained metabolic activity (Mahan et al. 1980). Finally, these irradiated cells, upon transfer to the nude mouse model, yielded the development of apparently healthy tumor explants, an indication that they had retained their potential to divide.

By the early 1980s, longitudinal analyses of the clinical course of patients whose postradiotherapy biopsies showed the presence or absence of residual prostatic cancer cells were available for review. The majority of these studies indicated that there was a two- to fourfold difference in prognosis depending upon whether the gland had been "sterilized" of all tumor cells or whether there was residual tumor (Kiesling et al. 1980; Scardino et al. 1982). Disease progression could be anticipated in about 50% of patients with a positive posttreatment biopsy, compared with a 15% likelihood in patients whose prostatic biopsies were negative. Only one study, that of Cox, presented conflicting data, suggesting that the presence of residual cancer cells in prostatic biopsies following definitive radiotherapy did not pose a threat for the host (Cox and Stoffel 1977). This latter study, however, could be criticized on many grounds. In the first place, the study was composed largely of stage C patients, in whom treatment failure is such a prominent expectation that differences between groups of patients might be more difficult to recognize. Secondly, many of the patients underwent endocrine therapy (including orchiectomy), and the potentially profound influence of endocrine manipulation upon biopsy findings as well as time of treatment failure was not taken into account.

A good deal of criticism has been registered against some studies relative to the actual frequency with which positive posttreatment biopsies occur. Obviously, if one carries out prostatic biopsy only on those glands that remain hard and nodular following radiation therapy, the percentage of positive versus negative biopsies will be high indeed. A study in which posttreatment biopsies are conducted routinely or in a random fashion would be more likely to reflect the true incidence of radiation treatment failure. These data are now available and suggest that, even when the prostate is palpably normal and the interval from treatment to biopsy is appropriately extended to 1 year following external radiation therapy or 2 years in the case of interstitial radiation, approximately 30% of biopsy specimens will demonstrate residual tumor cells (Freiha and Bagshaw 1984; Scardino et al. 1982; Vernon and Williams 1983). This figure, combined with the observed number of individuals whose glands retain (or redevelop) nodularity, suggests that definitive radiation therapy fails to eradicate localized prostatic cancer in more than one-third of individuals treated.

Survival After Radiotherapy

The traditional aim of cancer treatment has been total eradication or cure of the disease process. In prostatic cancer, we have become used to lesser treatment objectives for a variety of reasons. First, the patient most frequently presents with disease advanced to the point where curative treatments are not possible. Secondly, it is a malignancy characterized by a slow tumor doubling time occurring in an age group in which death from other causes is not unlikely. However, in younger individuals with disease localized to the prostate we must orient ourselves to attempts at cure. This leads the present discussion to one of the greatest concerns with regard to the efficacy of radiation therapy in the management of such patients. Excellent survivals are actually experienced at the 5-year interval, regardless of the form of radiation therapy employed. For example, there is an overall 5-year survival expectancy approximating 90% in patients with stage B disease treated by external radiotherapy sources, by interstitial iodine 125, or by interstitial gold plus adjunctive external radiotherapy. Disease-free survival, on the other hand, is decidedly less optimistic in these patient cohorts. Figures reported from institutions employing these three types of radiation therapy techniques in patients with stage B prostatic adenocarcinoma suggest that only two-thirds of patients are free of disease after the 5-year interval (Ray and Bagshaw 1975; Carlton et al. 1975; Whitmore 1984). The persistence of disease (and, in some cases, the development of metastases) by the 5-year interval is certainly predictive of a less optimistic outlook at the 10- and 15-year follow-up periods, a fact to be regarded with concern in counseling the younger individual about available treatment options.

Of particular interest in this regard is the individual undergoing interstitial radiation therapy wherein patient selection and surgical staging criteria are similar, if not identical, to those employed by individuals favoring a radical prostatectomy approach. When considering similar patient groups, that is to say those individuals with negative lymph nodes, the 5-year disease-free survival achieved with interstitial iodine 125 remains at the 65% level. Thus, it is safe to presume that radiation therapy has failed in approximately one-third of patients treated. The adverse influence of this observation on patient survival is unlikely to be experienced within the first 5 years following therapy. However, this salutary phenomenon may not be the result of any treatment rendered but simply a reflection of the relatively slow progress of the disease. Even those figures reflecting a 10-year experience following radiation therapy of the prostate may not be sufficiently valid to review when considering treatment options for the younger individual with the disease. For example, if a patient has developed metastatic disease by the 5th year, he may remain asymptomatic for a few additional years and then be placed on endocrine therapy which might give him a favorable response so that he will continue to live and be included in 10-year survival statistics.

Few data are available reflecting the long-term efficacy of radiation therapy in altering disease progression. In 1984 Bagshaw reported a 15-year survival expectancy (in actuarial terms) of 37%±8% in patients presumed to have disease localized to the prostate (most patients did not undergo surgical lymph node staging). However, only 22 patients had reached the 15-year observation. Furthermore, an 8% probability of error may reduce the actual observed 15-year survivability to less than 30%.

Survival After Surgery

The above figures reflecting the efficacy of radiotherapy in patients with localized prostatic cancer should be contrasted with the 10- and 15-year survival advantage enjoyed by the patient undergoing radical prostatectomy. In many series, the crude 10- and 15-year survival expectancies after radical prostatectomy for stage B disease are 75% and 50%, respectively. These figures are consistent with actual cure, rather than arrest of the disease process, as in many instances they reflect 100% age-adjusted survivals at those intervals (Jewett et al. 1968; Belt and Shroeder 1972; Culp and Meyer 1973; Walsh and Jewett 1980).

One of the Bellweather radical prostatectomy series against which other forms of therapy have been compared is the original Hopkins series published by Jewett et al. in 1968. This series reviewed 103 patients with stage B_1 adenocarcinoma of the prostate treated by radical perineal prostatectomy. In this series there was a 27% 15-year survival. A careful analysis of the series, however, indicates that this should not serve as a reflection of the potential of radical surgery in curing patients with localized disease by today's standards. For example, a later Hopkins series was published in concert by Walsh and Jewett in 1980. In this latter series the follow-up of 57 patients with stage B_1 disease showed a 51% 15-year survival, a figure identical with what could be anticipated in a group of patients of similar age without the diagnosis of cancer. It is important to analyze the reason for the twofold difference in survivability between the early and later Hopkins series. The patients in the later series were accessed between the years 1951 and 1963, whereas the earlier series reflected a cohort of patients undergoing prostatectomy between 1909 and 1953. It is quite obvious that numerous advances have been made not only in the staging of prostatic cancer but also in the management of operative patients in the 50-year time span separating the earliest and last patients analyzed. None of the patients in the early Hopkins series underwent radioisotopic bone scanning; many of them did not enjoy the benefit of serum acid phosphatase determination prior to their prostatectomy. Even the later Hopkins series may not reflect our present-day capabilities, for none of the latter individuals had undergone surgical lymph node staging.

Thus the urologist suggesting management for the patient with localized adenocarcinoma of the prostate must take into account the long-term potential for cure that may be achieved with radical surgical approaches comparative with the potential for treatment failure in similar individuals treated by radiation techniques. This is all the more essential when counseling the younger individual with this disease. This does not suggest that there are not treatment failures resulting from radical prostatectomy, on the other hand. These will be addressed in later parts of this discussion.

The above data, comparing long-term survival in patients undergoing radical prostatectomy versus radiotherapy, may be brought under critical scrutiny, based upon the possibility that subtle but important differences may characterize patient groups selected for different treatment modalities. Certainly, as mentioned previously, the patient group undergoing external radiotherapy may be significantly disadvantaged by the fact that surgical lymph node staging is not generally achieved, so that at least a small percentage of patients with microscopic lymph node metastases overlooked by noninvasive lymph node staging techniques are included in survival analyses. Furthermore, at least some of the individuals selected for noninvasive external radiotherapy might represent patients who would be denied surgical treatment options because of significant intercurrent coronary artery disease, and the like. In addressing the latter point first, one can simply analyze the 5-year overall survival achieved by external radiotherapy. If large numbers of individuals with marginal life expectancy because of intercurrent illness had been oriented to external radiotherapy rather than to surgery for localized prostatic cancer, one would anticipate a significantly lower 5-year crude survival rate than has been reported with the latter form of therapy.

Neither of the above critiques relative to differences in patient selection for radiation versus surgery can be anticipated in those individuals undergoing interstitial radiation therapy. Since surgical candidacy must be ascertained, patient selection criteria employed by groups conducting interstitial radiotherapy are generally the same as those employed by groups favoring radical prostatectomy approaches. Furthermore, patients undergoing interstitial radiotherapy are generally subjected to the same pelvic lymphadenectomy as is experienced by those undergoing radical prostatectomy, so that at least retrospective analyses of disease-free survival data among similarly stratified patients are possible.

Randomized or concurrently conducted treatment comparisons in patients with localized adenocarcinoma of the prostate are essential but rare. The Uro-Oncology Research Group (UORG) attempted to conduct such a study during the 1970s (Paulson et al. 1982). Patients with localized prostatic cancer, as judged by (a) digital rectal examination demonstrating freedom from capsular penetration or seminal vesicle invasion, (b) normal serum prostatic acid phosphatase determination, and (c) normal radioisotopic bone scan and radiologic bone survey, underwent pelvic lymphadenectomy. Those individuals in whom histologic examination revealed negative lymph nodes were then randomized to receive definitive external beam radiation therapy versus radical prostatectomy. In 1982 the initial report comparing the two treatment modalities was published, demonstrating a statistically significant advantage for those patients undergoing radical prostatectomy. This report has been widely criticized on many grounds, only one of which, in this author's opinion, is possibly justified: There was indeed a smaller number of patients in the radical prostatectomy versus the radiation therapy arm in the final analysis and this discrepancy has never been adequately explained. Another criticism that has been brought against the study is that, as in many multi-institutional trials, there is bound to be differential quality of care rendered the patient from institution to institution. This might assume particular importance when comparing radiation therapy in one institution versus another, as delivery instruments might differ significantly. However, the UORG did avail itself of referee radiation therapists whose quality control responsibility included a review of the dosimetry in each instance. The final criticism registered against the UORG study was the criterion employed in discriminating differences between the two treatment arms. Because of the short duration of the study, patient survival was not considered. Rather, the time to first evidence of treatment failure was registered as an end point. That point was said to be achieved when serum prostatic acid phosphatase was measured to be in the abnormal range on at least two occasions, or else when the patient developed a positive radioisotopic bone scan or soft tissue metastases.

The use of time to first evidence of treatment failure, rather than survival, as an end point in judging therapeutic efficacy in patients with localized adenocarcinoma of the prostate should really not be criticized. In fact, analyses employing treatment failure as an end point are likely to be more rewarding than those analyzing survival for a number of reasons. Firstly, intercurrent illness (and death therefrom) can be removed from consideration, an important point to achieve in slowly progressive lesions occurring in elderly populations. Secondly, the use of patient survival as an end point reflects not only initial therapy but also the potential contributions of additional treatments during the course of disease progression. Such is not the case when employing first evidence of treatment failure in an analysis.

Our own experience with comparison of treatment failures in patients with localized adenocarcinoma of the prostate has been previously reported (Olsson et al. 1985). One hundred and three surgically staged patients underwent treatment by external radiotherapy, interstitial iodine 125 implantation, or radical prostatectomy. Treatment selection was not randomized, but selected by the patient after informed interview. Even after removing the stage C patients from consideration, patients undergoing radical prostatectomy experienced a statistically significant advantage over those treated by external radiation therapy, as judged by time to first evidence of treatment failure, as defined by the UORG study group. Those individuals undergoing interstitial irradiation did not show as many distant metastases as the external radiotherapy group, for reasons which cannot be explained. However, when combining both local and distant failure in all treatment subgroups, patients treated by radical surgery enjoyed a statistically significant advantage over either radiation therapy patient cohort, with actuarial analyses extending to 90 months following treatment.

Complications of Radical Prostatectomy

With the above data suggesting greater efficacy of radical prostatectomy versus radiation therapy, one must readdress the issue of morbidity attendant upon radical prostatectomy. Obviously, life has quality as well as length and many patients would "rather be dead" than suffer the consequences of urinary incontinence. There are other men who would rather trade away a small survival advantage in order to maintain sexual potency. This latter issue is assuming even greater importance in modern society, where examples of late divorce and remarriage are not uncommon. Although the well informed patient may be totally aware of the potential for prosthetic devices to improve both urinary incontinence and loss of sexual potency, there is no question that these two potential complications taken together represent a major hurdle for the individual attempting to decide upon his course of therapy.

Urinary Incontinence

Is urinary incontinence really a major problem in individuals undergoing radical prostatectomy? The answer to this question is clearly "No," provided the surgeon is experienced in the conduct of the procedure. Unfortunately, because of the impressive popularity of radiation therapy over recent years, an entire generation of urologists has gone untrained in the performance of radical prostatectomy. Urologists with a reawakened interest in the operation should avail themselves of the opportunity to work with colleagues who are experienced in the operation before undertaking the procedure alone; if they do not, the untoward consequence of urinary incontinence may assume a very high incidence indeed. In good hands, the incidence of urinary wetting following radical prostatectomy should be approximately 3% (Walsh 1980).

Several features are important to the preservation of urinary control in patients undergoing radical prostatectomy. First, the patient should be instructed in external sphincter exercises prior to surgery so that he may become aware of the necessary muscular structures he may be required to employ during the early postoperative period. The patient may be simply instructed in gluteal contraction exercises, as the perineal body, anal, and external urinary sphincters generally contract with gluteal contraction. Most individuals will simultaneously contract the abdominal musculature as well; a degree of patience on the part of the physician will allow the individual to perceptually recognize his ability to achieve sphincteric contraction while the abdomen is relaxed.

During the course of the procedure, the entire urethra should be thoroughly identified before transecting the prostatic apex. The urethra is best transected in a stepwise fashion, regardless of whether the procedure is carried out perineally or retropubically. The anterior (retropubic approach) or posterior (perineal approach) hemicircumference should be transected first and a tagging suture placed that will keep the urethra from retracting into the perineal body (this traction suture may later be used as one of the anastomotic sutures). After total urethral transection, gentle traction on the previously described suture will cause the entire urethral circumference to reappear. The surgically destroyed bladder neck should be reconstructed to a diameter approximating 28–30 French caliber. The method by which this reconstruction is conducted is not as important as ensuring that the thickest muscular ring possible is provided for the vesicourethral anastomosis. One may close the bladder neck defect from each side, from the front, or from the posterior aspect in order to ensure that a thickened muscular ring is available. Vesicourethral anastomosis is carried out with 6 or 8 interrupted sutures (the author employs 2.0 chromic catgut for this purpose). An indwelling urethral catheter is advanced into the bladder and its retaining bag inflated to 15 cc prior to securing the vesicourethral sutures. Gentle traction on the catheter balloon will ensure that the sutures can be tied without tearing the fragile urethral tissues. The catheter should remain indwelling following surgery for a period of 10–12 days. This length of time is usually sufficient to ensure that the anastomosis is watertight and that the patient can initiate perineal exercises (if necessary) without discomfort.

On the day the catheter is removed, the bladder should be filled with 250 cc saline. With the patient in the upright position, the retaining bag is deflated and the catheter removed. The patient is immediately allowed to void, but is instructed in stopping and starting exercises so that he may gain confidence in his abilities at urinary control. The majority of patients are comfortably continent from the time of catheter removal and may not require any perineal exercise at all, except for moderately severe Valsalva maneuvers. A number of patients will have initial stress urinary incontinence that will require perineal exercise to overcome; a smaller number of patients may experience passive incontinence for a number of weeks before regaining urinary control. By the end of the first postoperative month, nearly all patients will have achieved both passive and stress-resistant urinary control.

Erectile Potency

It has been shown by Donker and Walsh that erectile potency can be predictably preserved during the course of radical prostatectomy, at least when conducted from the retropubic route (Walsh and Donker 1982). Their fine anatomic studies have demonstrated the location of neurovascular bundles extending along the side of the membranous urethra and prostate. Evidently the cavernous nerves contained in these bundles of tissue are essential to the maintenance of erectile potency and may be spared by modifying the radical prostatectomy slightly. After securing the dorsal vein complex, the neurovascular bundles can be separated from each side of the urethra and prostatic apex prior to urethral transection. Thereafter, the prostate may be dissected in a retrograde fashion, taking care to strip the neural tissue from the side of the prostatic capsule as the dissection proceeds. Walsh reports that more than 80% of men are potent within a year following this modified radical retropubic prostatectomy. It is probable that some degree of damage to the cavernous nerves is experienced by the majority of patients, as a much smaller number are potent immediately; nevertheless, it does appear that the nerve damage is reversible. In our own (considerably smaller) experience with this operation, approximately 50% of patients are potent 6 months following surgery and all of the patients who have thus far reached the 1-year observation interval have regained erectile potency.

Positive Tissue Margins

A substantial amount of criticism has been registered against modified radical retropubic prostatectomy since, by setting out to minimize tissue margins, one is contravening a major principle of cancer surgery—that of excising the tumor with a wide margin of normal tissue. Eggleston and Walsh (1985) have analyzed 7 of their first 100 patients, in whom the resection margins were positive for malignant cells. In no instance could they find that the positive tissue margin occurred as a result of the nerve-sparing procedure, as the positive tissue margin was not situated in the region where the neurovascular bundle was situated. On the other hand, others have not agreed with this analysis on the basis of their experience.

We ourselves try to limit the modified radical retropubic prostatectomy to those individuals with stage A_2 or B_1 disease. The best of all candidates is the patient with the B_1 nodule. Because Eggleston and Walsh have shown that preservation of a single neurovascular bundle is apparently sufficient for erectile potency, patients with an entire lobe occupied by cancer may have the neurovascular bundle sacrificed on the side of the tumor and preserved on the contralateral side. Any patient with a higher stage prostatic cancer is probably not a good candidate for nerve-sparing radical prostatectomy. However, when counseling the patient with stage A_2 or B_1 adenocarcinoma of the prostate who voices concern regarding the impact of treatment on sexual function, one can state with reasonable certainty that the potential for impotence is as low with surgery as with any form of radiation therapy.

Tissue margins positive for adenocarcinoma following radical prostatectomy may be, as Bagshaw et al. (1985) have stated, "prima facie evidence of treatment failure." The incidence of this treatment failure probably varies remarkably from institution to institution. The incidence is likely to rise as more urologists injudiciously apply nerve-sparing prostatectomy to individuals whose disease is so extensive that they are not good candidates for the operation. Even in the best of hands, the incidence of positive tissue margins following radical prostatectomy is 7%. Other workers have reported an even higher number of patients with cancer extending to the resected margin following prostatectomy. This single feature may, in the future, confer a pall upon the long-term survivability that is presently achieved with radical prostatectomy comparative to radiation therapy.

The management of these patients with positive margins remains in doubt today. One could well imagine that a few such patients with a single focus of microscopic disease at a resection margin might in fact be cured because of the tissue necrosis of surgical margins attendant upon placement of ligatures and the like. However, many others may in fact have an extensive amount of microscopic permeation of tissues by viable cancer cells.

There is some evidence to suggest that early administration of radiation therapy in such patients may allow for preservation of long-term survival (Ray et al. 1984). However, the number of patients treated thus far is too small to reach a satisfactory conclusion. Certainly those patients with previously unsuspected seminal vesicle invasion following radical prostatectomy are at high risk. Fortunately, because of the strong positive correlation between lymphadeno-pathy and seminal vesicle invasion, this finding should be infrequent. Neverthe-less, it will continue to occur and should probably warrant adjunctive local therapy, perhaps by the application of external radiation.

Summary

This chapter has provided a historical perspective relative to the treatment modalities employed to treat the patient with adenocarcinoma of the prostate. What has been emphasized is that prostatic cancer is a slow-growing tumor occurring in men at an age when intercurrent illness and general infirmity may surpass the biologic potential of the malignancy. Perhaps the single most important consideration to be borne in mind when counseling the patient facing the prospect of treatment for this disease is his estimated life expectancy. The urologist is well advised to work closely with the patient's primary physician and should carefully search the patient's family history in an attempt to predict (as well as possible) the patient's life expectancy. No absolute chronological limits can be set. However, one can attempt to differentiate between the individual whose life expectancy is rather brief (5 years) and that patient who presents with sufficient youth and freedom from disease to project a rather longer life expectancy (10–15 years), were it not for the discovery of the localized prostatic cancer.

There is no question that radiation therapy, in any of its forms, can achieve cure of prostatic cancer in selected cases. The unfortunate problem for the clinician is that there is presently no good test for relative radiosensitivity of one cancer versus another. On the other hand, the selection criteria necessary to ensure an excellent outcome with surgical therapy are now well established. If the individual truly has disease localized to the gland, as evidenced by appropriate findings on digital rectal examination, serum prostatic acid phosphatase, radioisotopic bone scan and surgical lymphadenectomy, he may be reasonably assured, after radical prostatectomy, of a life expectancy close to that anticipated by men of similar age without the disease.

To be sure, this chapter has not answered all of the controversies relating to the management of the patient with localized prostatic cancer. For example, it has not addressed the concept of nihilism proposed by some: Could it be that localized prostatic cancer of low histologic grade warrants no therapy at all and that similar stage disease of high histologic grade is incurable by any treatment technique? In response to the initial part of the question, our own experience has certainly demonstrated that low-grade lesions can metastasize and adversely affect the survival of the patient. The answer to the second part of the question has yet to be determined in clinical trials. For the young man it can be stated with relative certainty that, regardless of its histologic grade, the disease will have a far more morbid effect on the individual than will radical prostatectomy.

Returning to the basic premises described for radical prostatectomy toward the earlier part of this chapter, it can now be restated that radical prostatectomy can be conducted safely and with little morbidity in the appropriately selected patient. If the disease is truly organ contained, this operation should render the patient tumor free. This certainty compared with the potential failure of radiotherapy to sterilize the gland is sufficient to continue to prejudice this author in favor of a surgical approach when counseling healthy individuals with a diagnosis of localized prostatic cancer.

References

Babayan RK, deVere White R, Austen G Jr, Krane RJ, Feldman M, Olsson CA (1980) Benefits and complications of staging pelvic lymph node dissection in prostatic adenocarcinoma. Prostate 1:345–349

Bagshaw MA (1969) Definitive radiotherapy in carcinoma of the prostate. JAMA 210:326–327

Bagshaw MA (1984) Radiotherapy of prostatic cancer: Stanford University experience. In: Kurth KH, Debruyne FMJ, Schroeder FH, Splinter TAM, Wagener TDJ (eds) Progress and controversies in oncological urology. Alan R. Liss, New York, pp 493–512

Bagshaw MA, Ray GR, Cox RS (1985) Radiotherapy of prostatic carcinoma: long or short term efficacy. Urology [Suppl] 25:17–23

Belt F, Shroeder FH (1972) Total perineal prostatectomy for carcinoma of the prostate. J Urol 107:91–96

Carlton CE Jr, Hudgins PT, Guerriero WG, Scott R Jr (1975) Radiotherapy in the management of stage C carcinoma of the prostate. Trans Am Assoc GU Surg 67:70–74

Cox JD, Stoffel TJ (1977) The significance of needle biopsy after irradiation for stage C adenocarcinoma of the prostate. Cancer 40:156–160

Culp DS, Meyer JJ (1973) Radical prostatectomy in the treatment of prostatic cancer. Cancer 32:1113–1118

Cupps RE, Utz DC, Fleming TR, Carson CC, Zincke H, Myers RP (1980) Definitive radiation therapy for prostatic carcinoma: Mayo Clinic experience. J Urol 124:855–859

Donohue RF, Pfister RR, Weigel JW, Stonington OG (1977) Pelvic lymphadenectomy in stage A prostatic cancer. Urology 9:273–275

Eggleston JC, Walsh PC (1985) Nerve sparing radical retropubic prostatectomy. Pathologic findings in the first 100 cases. J Urol 133: abstract 511

Freiha FS, Bagshaw MA (1984) Carcinoma of the prostate: results of post-irradiation biopsy. Prostate 5:19–26

Golimbu M, Schinella R, Morales P, Kurusu S (1978) Stage A-2 prostatic cancer: clinical, pathological and prognostic difference from A1 and B disease. J Urol 119:618–622

Hilaris BS, Whitmore WF Jr, Batata MA, Grabstald H (1974) Radiation therapy and pelvic node dissection in the management of cancer of the prostate. Am J Roentgenol 121:832–838

Hilaris BS, Whitmore WF Jr, Batata MA et al. (1977) Behavioral patterns of prostate adenocarcinoma following an I^{125} implant and pelvic lymph node dissection. Int J Radiat Oncol Biol Phys 2:631–637

Jewett HJ, Bridge RW, Gray GF, Shelley WM (1968) The palpable nodule of prostatic cancer. Results 15 years after radical excision. JAMA 203:403–406

Kiesling VJ, Friedman HI, McAninch JW, Nachtsheim DA, Nemeth TJ (1979) The ultrastructural changes of prostate adenocarcinoma following external beam radiation therapy. J Urol 122:633–636

Kiesling VJ, McAninch JW, Goebel JL, Agee RE (1980) External beam radiotherapy for adenocarcinoma of the prostate. A clinical follow up. J Urol 124:851–854

Kramer SA, Spahr J, Brendler CB, Glenn SF, Paulson DF (1980) Experience with Gleason's histopathologic grading in prostate cancer. J Urol 124:223–225

Kramer SA, Cline WA Jr Farnham R, Carson CG, Cox EB, Hinshaw W, Paulson DF (1981) Prognosis of patients with stage D-1 prostatic adenocarcinoma. J Urol 125:817–819

Kurth KH, Altwein JE, Hohenfellner R (1977) Follow up of irradiated carcinoma by aspiration biopsy. J Urol 117:615–617

Kurup P, Kramer TS, Lee MS, Phillips R (1984) External beam irradiation of prostate cancer. Cancer 53:37–43

Lindner A, deKernion JB, Smith RB, Katske FA (1983) Risk of urinary incontinence following radical prostatectomy. J Urol 129:1007–1008

Mahan DE, Bruce AW, Manley PM, Fanchi L (1980) Immunohistochemical evaluation of prostatic cancer before and after radiotherapy. J Urol 124:488–491

Olsson CA, deVere White R (1982) Health risk and management of prostate cancer. In: Paulson D (ed) Cancer treatment and research (GU cancer 1), vol 6. Martinus Nijhoff, Amsterdam, pp 121–142

Olsson CA, Tannenbaum M, Babayan R, O'Brien M, deVere White R (1982) Prediction of lymph node metastasis in adenocarcinoma of the prostate (abstr). Presented at Annual American Urological Association Annual Meeting, Kansas City

Olsson CA, Babayan R, deVere White R (1985) Surgical management of stage B or C prostatic carcinoma: radical surgery vs radiotherapy. Urology [Suppl] 25:30–38

Paulson DF, Uro-Oncology Research Group (1979). The impact of current staging procedures in assessing disease extent of prostatic adenocarcinoma. J Urol 121:300–302

Paulson DF, Lin GH, Hinshaw W, Stephani S, Uro-Oncology Research Group (1982) Radical surgery versus radiotherapy for adenocarcinoma of the prostate. J Urol 128:502–504

Pistenma DA, Ray GR, Bagshaw MA (1976) The role of megavoltage radiation therapy in the treatment of prostatic carcinoma. Semin Oncol 3:115–122

Ray GR, Bagshaw MA (1975) The role of radiation therapy in the definitive treatment of adenocarcinoma of the prostate. Ann Rev Med 26:567–588

Ray GR, Bagshaw MA, Freiha FS (1984) External beam radiation salvage for residual or recurrent local tumor following radical prostatectomy. J Urol 132:926–930

Scardino PT, Delaune JM, Hoffman GS, Guerriero G, Carlton CE Jr (1982) The results and significance of prostatic biopsy after definitive radiation for carcinoma of the prostate (abstr). Presented at American Urological Association Annual Meeting, Kansas City, pp 194–195

Vernon SE, Williams WD (1983) Pre-treatment and post-treatment evaluation of prostatic adenocarcinoma for prostatic specific antigen by immunohistochemistry. J Urol 130:95–98

Walsh PC (1980) Radical prostatectomy for the treatment of localized prostatic carcinoma. Urol Clin North Am 7:583–591

Walsh PC, Donker PJ (1982) Impotence following radical prostatectomy: insight into etiology and prevention. J Urol 128:492–497

Walsh PC, Jewett JJ (1980) Radical surgery for prostate cancer. Cancer 45:1906–1911

Whitmore WF Jr (1984) Interstitial I-125 implantation in the management of localized prostatic cancer. In: Kurth KH, Debruyne FMJ, Schroeder FH, Splinter TAM, Wagener TDJ (eds) Progress and controversies in oncological urology. Alan R. Liss, New York, pp 513–527

Whitmore WF Jr, Hilaris B, Grabstald H (1972) Retropubic implantation of iodine[125] in the treatment of prostate cancer. J Urol 108:918–920

Wilson CS, Dahl DS, Middleton RG (1977) Pelvic lymphadenectomy for the staging of apparently localized prostatic cancer. J Urol 117:197–198

Chapter 9

Interstitial Radiotherapy

P.T. Scardino and F. Bretas

Introduction

Interstitial radiotherapy has been used for the treatment of prostatic cancer since the early 1900s. In 1917 Hugh Young reported a series of patients treated with radium needles implanted transperineally, transrectally, and transurethrally (Young and Fronz 1917). Even with the primitive techniques available, several long-term disease-free survivors were reported (Barringer 1942). With the advent of megavoltage external beam irradiation techniques in the 1950s, Bagshaw clearly demonstrated that radiotherapy is effective in controlling prostatic cancer, previously considered "radioresistant" (Ray and Bagshaw 1975). But with time it became clear that doses in the upper range of clinical tolerance (7000 rad) were necessary to control the local tumor in most patients and that such doses led to a high complication rate when external beam therapy was used alone. Basing their work upon the experience of Flocks et al. (1959), a new generation of urologists and radiotherapists initiated the contemporary experience with interstitial radiotherapy ("brachytherapy") in an effort to deliver larger doses of irradiation to the prostate with fewer complications. Modern techniques of brachytherapy include implantation of radioactive seeds of gold, iodine, or iridium, with or without external beam irradiation. The major conceptual limitation of brachytherapy, however, remains the problem of a "geographic miss"—failure to irradiate all areas of the tumor sufficiently because of uneven seed placement.

In 1965 Carlton and Hudgins at Baylor College of Medicine developed a technique combining radioactive gold (^{198}Au) implants with external beam therapy, a technique now applied to over 1200 patients (Carlton et al. 1976; Scardino and Carlton 1983). In 1970 Whitmore and Hilaris pioneered interstitial irradiation with iodine (^{125}I) at Memorial Sloan-Kettering Cancer Center (MSKCC) (Whitmore et al. 1972). Radioactive iridium (^{192}Ir) was developed in

France by Court and Chassagne in 1977, and several studies have been published recently describing this form of brachytherapy, although the follow-up is still too limited for an evaluation of its efficacy.

We now have 20 years of experience with modern techniques of brachytherapy. The large number of patients treated in medical centers around the world and the widespread use of this type of radiotherapy have provided us with substantial information about the indications and contraindications, advantages and disadvantages, pitfalls and complications, as well as the results of these techniques. Although the focus of this review is the experience at Baylor using the combined technique of gold seed implantation plus external beam irradiation, the alternative forms of brachytherapy will be described and compared. Our intention is to provide the busy clinician with a succinct and informative review indicating the status of modern interstitial radiotherapy and describing our day-to-day approach and results.

Treatment Techniques

Radioactive Iodine Implantation

Radioactive iodine implantation is performed through a retropubic approach immediately following bilateral pelvic lymph node dissection (Whitmore et al. 1972, 1985; Kwong et al. 1984; Mag 1985; Peschel et al. 1985; Herr 1980, 1982; Grossman et al. 1982; Hilaris et al. 1977, 1978). Low energy ^{125}I seeds are implanted in a rigidly defined pattern using multiple implant needles placed into the prostate at regular intervals. A finger in the rectum is important to guide the needle so that the seeds are not placed too near the rectal wall. A specially designed instrument is employed to deposit 40–70 seeds in vertical rows at regular intervals as the needle is withdrawn. The geometry of the implant is crucial. The distribution of seeds must be homogeneous to avoid "cold spots." Since the half-value layer for ^{125}I in tissue is only 1.7 cm, seeds must be placed in close proximity to each other within the tumor to avoid a geographic miss (Table 9.1).

Table 9.1. Radiobiology of seed implants

	^{125}I	^{198}Au
Energy level	27 keV	410 keV
$T_{\frac{1}{2}}$	60 days	2.7 days
Activity/seed	Low (0.5 mCi)	High (5–8 mCi)
Seeds/implant	40–50	6–10
Half-value layer (lead)	0.025 mm	2.5 mm
Half-value layer (tissue)	1.3 cm	4.5 cm
Duration of radiation	1 year	14 days
Mean peripheral dose	16–18000 rad	3–3500 rad
Biologically equivalent dose	7000 rad	7500 rad[a]

[a]Combined with 4000 rad external beam.

The recommended dose to the periphery of the prostate is 18 000 rad. Since ^{125}I has a half-life of 60 days, this dosage is delivered over 1 year and is biologically equivalent to 7500–8000 rad delivered by external beam or combined gold seed–external beam therapy.

If any tumor cell lies more than a few millimeters from the edge of the implant it will not receive a tumoricidal dose of irradiation. But the high dose must not strike the rectal wall. Tumor within the seminal vesicles, bladder neck, trigone, or membranous urethra will not be sufficiently irradiated. If the tumor itself is asymmetric, the implant is much less effective. Supplemental external beam therapy carries a high risk of rectal complications.

Combined Gold Seed Implantation and External Beam Irradiation

Combined gold seed implantation and external beam irradiation is also performed through a retropubic approach (Carlton et al. 1976; Scardino and Carlton 1983; Rosenberg et al. 1985). Following a limited staging pelvic lymph node dissection, six to ten radioactive gold seeds are implanted for a total dose of 3500 rad, and this is followed by external beam therapy, according to the following protocol:

Pelvic lymph node dissection		
Negative		Positive
3500 rad	^{198}Au seeds	3500 rad
4500 rad (prostate)	External beam	5400 rad (full pelvis)
8000 rad	Total	8900 rad

A simple implant needle is used. Although the seeds are placed throughout the gland, an effort is made to cluster the seeds in the area of the palpable tumor. If the seminal vesicles or bladder neck are involved, these areas are implanted as well. Since ^{198}Au has a high energy and long "half value" layer in tissue (relative to ^{125}I), precise localization of seeds is not as critical (Table 9.1). These properties allow a gold implant to retain its efficacy even in the previously resected or enucleated prostate. A guiding finger in the rectum is not necessary since the seeds need not closely approximate the posterior capsule. The implant takes only 5–10 min, and the entire operating time averages only 45–75 min, minimizing the exposure of personnel to radiation. There is rarely any significant blood loss or need for a transfusion.

Beginning 14–21 days after the implant, when radiation from the gold seeds is exhausted, a course of external beam radiotherapy is given using a linear accelerator. If the pelvic nodes are negative for metastases, 4500 rad are delivered to the prostate alone using lateral arcs, at 225 rad per day, 4 days a week, for 5 weeks. If the nodes are positive, 5000 rad are given through anterior and posterior opposed portals to the full pelvis at 200 rad per day in a split course with a 2-week rest after 3 weeks of therapy, ending with a boost dose of 400 rad to the prostate through a smaller portal. The rest period is extended if side-effects occur since acute toxic reactions to radiation predict severe late complications. The goal is to deliver 8000–8900 rad to the prostate. The large volume of tissue irradiated by the implanted gold seeds, combined with the external therapy, assures a homogeneous field of irradiation with little chance for a "geographic miss."

Combined Iridium Implantation and External Beam Irradiation

Experience with iridium 192 implantation for prostatic cancer is limited (Court and Chassagne 1977; Martinez et al. 1985; Brindle et al. 1985; Clubb and Summers 1984). Most investigators have combined the implantation with pre- and/or postoperative external beam irradiation. An open retropubic exposure of the prostate is performed with the patient in the lithotomy position so that the perineum is accessible. Hollow steel needles with sealed tips are placed through an acrylic template sutured to the perineum. The needles are inserted at 1-cm intervals under direct vision so that the entire tumor volume is encompassed. The number of needles varies according to the size of the tumor and prostate, but the needles must be kept at least 1 cm from the rectum.

Plain films of the pelvis are taken during the operation to confirm the position of the needles. ^{192}Ir seeds in a nylon ribbon are then loaded into the hollow needles once the patient has returned to his shielded room. To achieve a homogeneous dose, sources of different activity and length are used so that a minimum peripheral dose of 3000–3500 rad is given over 36–50 h. The template, needles, and seeds are then removed. ^{192}Ir provides a low dose rate of 70–90 rad per hour. Approximately 3 weeks later, external beam therapy is begun using a linear accelerator to provide an additional 3000–3500 rad. The goal is to deliver 6500–7000 rad total dose to the prostate.

Rationale for the Selection of Patients and Techniques

Although radical prostatectomy has proved to be an excellent form of therapy for prostatic cancers which are confined to the prostate and immediate periprostatic tissue pathologically (Von Eschenbach 1981), radical surgery will not prove curative if the tumor extends to the surgical margins, seminal vesicles, bladder neck, membranous urethra, or pelvic lymph nodes. The morbidity of radical prostatectomy is not inconsequential. The risk of incontinence remains 1%–3% in the hands of the most experienced surgeons, rising to 10%–15% in less experienced hands. Although the nerve-sparing modification described by Walsh (Lepor et al. 1983) reduces the frequency of erectile impotence to 15%–20% in patients with small tumors, impotence occurs in 50%–60% of patients with microscopic extracapsular extension or seminal vesicle invasion. And some patients are simply too old or infirm to tolerate such surgery safely.

Radiotherapy offers an attractive alternative, even for patients with disease confined to the prostate. If any operation is required, it is more limited; the prostate is left in situ, continence is not threatened, and potency is preserved in the short term (although 25%–79% of patients appear to become impotent over several years). Definitive radiotherapy is applicable to the vast majority of patients with localized disease (clinical stages A_2, B, and C_1), since the treated field can include a margin of periprostatic tissue extending even to the full pelvis. But radiotherapy is not appropriate for stage A_1, which can be left untreated under close observation except in the very young patient (<60 years old), or for large stage C_2 tumors (≥6 cm), in which the local failure rate is prohibitively high. In patients with proven positive pelvic nodes, the role of any type of radiotherapy remains palliative at best.

Experience with external beam irradiation clearly demonstrated that prostatic cancer cannot be considered "radioresistant." Yet definitive external beam therapy is associated with serious complications in about 10% of patients when doses are sufficient (≥7000 rad) to achieve a satisfactory rate of local control. The complications with external irradiation and the growing appreciation of the value of pelvic lymphadenectomy led to the development of modern brachytherapy. The rationale for brachytherapy includes the following points: (a) accurate surgical staging with pelvic lymph node dissection and mobilization of the prostate allows more precise tailoring of the treatment to the actual extent of the disease; (b) implantation of a radioactive source into the prostate makes it possible to administer a higher dose of therapy with less irradiation to surrounding normal structures; (c) more accurate direction of therapy to the tumor mass itself is possible.

Radioactive Iodine Implantation

Implantation of radioactive iodine seeds requires careful patient selection. Whitmore and his co-workers have repeatedly emphasized that iodine seeds are only indicated for palpably well defined, small, symmetric stage B or early stage C tumors which do not invade the seminal vesicles, trigone, ureters, bladder neck, or external sphincter, nor extend to the pelvic side walls. The patient is not considered an appropriate candidate if the prostate is irregular and asymmetric, immobile at cystoscopy, or appears obstructive, if the bladder is trabeculated, or if the patient has obstructive voiding symptoms. A prior prostatectomy creates a shell which cannot be effectively implanted. A "channel cut" transurethral resection of the prostate (TURP) is sometimes an acceptable compromise in patients who otherwise are candidates. But if a TURP becomes necessary for relief of urinary retention within 6 months of the implant, the geometry of the prostate and the implant are altered and the efficacy of the therapy severely compromised.

Iodine implantation does offer the advantages that a high dose of irradiation can be delivered to the prostate with few complications, therapy is completed at a single setting, surgical staging is accurate, and the dosimetry and distribution are more precisely calibrated and defined.

But the disadvantages are many, perhaps the major one being that this technique is applicable to just those small stage B tumors most likely to be confined to the prostate pathologically and therefore most suitable to removal with radical prostatectomy. ^{125}I implantation is just as lengthy, requires the same anesthesia, results in just as much blood loss, and requires just as experienced a physician as a radical prostatectomy if a satisfactory result is to be expected. Furthermore, the possibility of a "geographic miss" is a serious concern because of the short depth of penetration of irradiation from ^{125}I seeds. And when ^{125}I implants have been supplemented with external beam therapy, the complication rate has increased dramatically (Ross et al. 1982), so that effective therapy with ^{125}I seeds is strictly limited to the implanted volume. Iodine implants allow little flexibility. Once the seeds have been placed, therapy cannot be adjusted based on postoperative imaging and isodose curves. Finally, salvage therapy for patients whose tumors are not destroyed by the iodine implant is difficult because of the perivesical fibrosis from the pelvic lymph node dissection and the radiation reaction in the membranous urethra and bladder neck.

Combined Gold Seed Implantation and External Beam Irradiation

Radioactive gold seed implantation is considered a supplement or boost to the prostate which allows a high dose of irradiation to the prostate with fewer complications than with external irradiation alone. The combined treatment is applicable to most prostatic tumors similar to those suitable for external beam therapy: clinical stage A_2, B, or C tumors less than 6 cm in diameter. A major operation is required, so the patients should have a life expectancy of 5 years or more, have no serious medical illnesses contraindicating anesthesia or surgery, and have no prior pelvic radiotherapy. Prior prostatectomy does not exclude the patient, since the few seeds required and the effective depth of penetration of gamma irradiation from ^{198}Au allow adequate irradiation to the resulting prostatic shell (Table 9.1). Patients with urinary retention or severe obstructive voiding symptoms may have a TURP followed by the implant in 6 weeks when the prostatic urethra has healed.

Pelvic lymph node dissection and intraoperative mobilization and palpation of the prostate allow for accurate surgical staging and localization of the tumor mass. The gold seeds are concentrated in the tumor mass, but are also placed uniformly throughout the prostate, and thus provide a precise aiming point for the external beam therapy. The implantation itself is brief and technically simple. Precise placement of the seeds is not essential. Yet a broad homogeneous field of irradiation is achieved by combining the properties of ^{198}Au (deep penetration of tissue) with external beam therapy, so that a "geographic miss" is unlikely.

Gold seeds, although they are "hot" sources of radioactivity, are easy to handle, are quickly placed, and offer little exposure to medical personnel (Scardino and Carlton 1983). Operating time and blood loss are minimal. Since the half-life of ^{198}Au is so short, virtually all of the radiation has dissipated within 14 days. Acute radiation reactions can be detected in time to adjust the planned course of external irradiation so that the acute side-effects are minimized. Similar to external irradiation, the combined treatment offers flexible timing and dose of therapy according to the tolerance and needs of each patient.

Nevertheless, this approach does require an operative procedure; the course of treatment is as long as with external beam therapy; familiarity with ^{198}Au seeds is limited; and precise computation of the dosimetry and distribution of irradiation in vivo has not been uniformly performed.

Combined Iridium Implantation and External Beam Irradiation

Experience with ^{192}Ir implantation for prostatic cancer is too limited to determine the place it may assume in the therapy of these patients. To our knowledge ^{192}Ir implants and external beam therapy have been used in only two medical centers in the United States during the past 4 years (Brindle et al. 1985; Clubb and Summers 1984). Only 47 patients have been reported; only 23 are available for follow-up, and the longest follow-up is 3 years. Iridium implants appear suitable for larger tumors and have been used to salvage prior irradiation failures. But the expense, the ease of learning, and the risks and complications have not been sufficiently analyzed. At this point, the role of iridium remains uncertain.

Complications (Table 9.2)

With almost 1000 patients now reported (Whitmore et al. 1985; Fowler et al. 1979), complications of ^{125}I implantation have been mild in the MSKCC experience, but they may not be apparent for several months after the implantation due to the long half-life of the isotope. Approximately 28% of patients experienced delayed irritative voiding symptoms; bowel complications were rare, although rectal prostatic fistulae have been reported (Abadir et al. 1984). Between 2% and 25% of patients have either prolonged distressing proctitis and/or rectal ulceration or fistula, necessitating colostomy. Potency was preserved in 93% of patients potent before therapy (Herr 1980), although others have reported problems with potency in as many as 24% (Schellhammer et al. 1985). Dry ejaculation may occur in 16% when additional external beam radiotherapy is used (Kwong et al. 1984). In one series, chronic urinary voiding disturbances occurred in 12% of cases (Mag 1985). Although there were four hospital deaths in the first 400 patients in the Memorial series, there have been none in the last 500 cases.

Complications of gold seed implantation and external beam irradiation have been few and are similar to those reported for ^{125}I implantation. Among 523 patients treated before 1980 with total doses of 6500–7500 rad, there were three

Table 9.2. Complications of radiotherapy

	Gold seed[a] (523 patients) (%)	Iodine seed[b,c] (415 patients) (%)
Mortality	0.6	0.7
Major complications	10	3–13
Intestinal	2	3–5
Urinary	2	3–7
Lymphocele/hematoma/abscess	4	3–10
Genital/leg edema		
With PLND[d]	1	3
Without PLND	–	–
Impotence[e]	29	25

[a]Scardino (1983).
[b]Fowler et al. (1979).
[c]Schellhammer et al. (1985).
[d]PLND, pelvic lymph node dissection.
[e]Assessed subjectively by questionnaire.

deaths. With the limited area of dissection and the relatively low dosage of external irradiation required by this procedure, we have seen genital edema in only 3% and lower extremity edema in 3%–8% of our patients. Urinary complications have been rare. Rectal complications have occurred in 13.8%, but in only 1% were the symptoms persistent or disabling (colostomy was required in 0.3% of our earlier series). Erectile potency has been preserved in over 70% of patients potent before treatment.

Results

Differences in patient selection, staging studies, concurrent therapy, methods of follow-up, end points, and data analyses make comparisons of results from one series to another imprecise if not impossible. Several criteria must be met if the data from a reported series are to be considered. A clearly defined staging system should be used. No concurrent hormonal therapy should be employed before the time of treatment failure. A follow-up of 15 years is essential if survival is the end point of the analysis. But if time to treatment failure or progression of disease is the end point, results at 5 and 10 years are meaningful if no other therapy is given in the interim and an adequate evaluation is performed to detect local and distant recurrence.

Radioactive Iodine Implantation

Whitmore has recently analyzed and reported his experience at Memorial Sloan-Kettering Cancer Center with 606 patients, including 239 followed for 5 years or more (Whitmore et al. 1985). The 5-year survival rates were 96% for stage B_1, 76% for B_2, and 69% for C_1 (Table 9.3). Disease-free survival rates from the same institution were reported earlier (Grossman et al. 1982) (Table 9.4). Schellhammer et al. (1985) recently reported 5-year disease-free survival rates of 100% for stage A_2, 100% for B_{1N}, 71% for larger stage B (B_1 plus B_2), and 53% for C_1. Surgically staged patients (with negative nodes) showed 5-year disease-free survival rates of 100% for stage A_2, 100% for B_{1N}, 75% for larger stage B, and 66% for C_1. It should be noted that these patients were carefully selected for tumor characteristics favorable to iodine implantation as described above.

Table 9.3. Survival rates after interstitial irradiation (% ± standard errors)

Clinical stage	Iodine[a,b]			Gold + external[c]		
	No.	5 yr	10 yr[d]	No.	5 yr	10 yr
A and B	155	89	–	373	86 ± 4	55 ± 10
C	82	59	–	102	75 ± 9	43 ± 8

[a]Whitmore et al. (1985).
[b]Schellhammer et al. (1985).
[c]Scardino and Carlton (1983).
[d]10-year data not available.

Table 9.4.   Disease-free survival rates of interstitial irradiation (% ± 2 standard errors)

Clinical stage	Iodine[a]			Gold + external[b]		
	No.	5 yr	10 yr	No.	5 yr	10 yr
A and B	52	60	–	353	58 ± 4	35 ± 5
C	38	24	–	99	41 ± 6	–

[a]Grossman et al. (1982).
[b]Scardino and Carlton (1983).

Table 9.5.   Disease-free survival based on surgical stage. All patients had negative nodes by pelvic lymph node dissection (% ± 2 standard errors)

Surgical stage	Iodine[a]			Gold + external[b]		
	No.	5 yr	10 yr	No.	5 yr	10 yr
A and B						
A_2	7	100	–	71	66 ± 18	–
B						
B_{1N}	7	100	–	24	93 ± 6	71 ± 4
B_1	35	75 ± 16	–	91	73 ± 10	–
B_2				102	81 ± 7	–
C_1	15	66	–	103	60 ± 8	53 ± 10
	64	80		391	74 ± 4	53 ± 9

[a]Schellhammer et al. (1985).
[b]Scardino and Carlton (1983).

The results of therapy based on surgical staging (patients with negative nodes) have rarely been reported (Table 9.5).

Combined Gold Seed Implantation and External Beam Irradiation

We have recently reviewed the results of combined gold seed implantation and external beam therapy in 475 patients treated at Baylor College of Medicine. All had clinical stages A_2, B, or C_1 tumors and none received hormonal therapy before proven recurrence of tumor (Scardino and Carlton 1983). Follow-up was 64 months (mean), ranging from 12 to 180 months. The 5-year actuarial survival rates were 83%±7% for clinical stage A_2, 100% for B_{1N}, 89%±6% for B_1, 82%±4% for B_2, and 75%±9% for stage C_1 (Table 9.3). The disease-free survival (Table 9.4) at 5 years was 57%±6% for clinical stage A_2, 81%±8% for B_{1N}, 62%±5% for B_1, 45%±6% for B_2, and 41%±6% for C_1. These results were achieved in unselected patients. Ten-year actuarial survival (Table 9.3) and disease-free survival rates (Table 9.4) are also available.

Perhaps a better index of the efficacy of interstitial irradiation is apparent in Table 9.5, which lists the 5-year disease-free survival rates by stage for patients with negative nodes on pelvic lymph node dissection. These data suggest that for carefully selected patients treated by iodine implantation, the results are comparable to those with gold seed implantation plus external beam therapy for unselected patients.

However, the efficacy of interstitial radiotherapy for prostatic carcinoma should be judged primarily by the eradication of the local tumor and secondarily by the prevention of distant metastases, recognizing that in some instances the appearance of distant metastases after therapy may only reflect the insensitivity of the staging studies employed rather than progressive dissemination from an uncontrolled primary tumor. Both digital rectal examination of the prostate and prostatic biopsy have been used to assess local control after radiotherapy. Controversy continues to surround the meaning of histologic examination of the prostate after radiotherapy. Some investigators have chosen not to biopsy their patients, claiming that the results are uninterpretable and that there is no definitive treatment even if the biopsy is positive. Yet there is ample evidence from the literature and our own experience that a positive biopsy after radiotherapy is a poor prognostic sign indicating that treatment has failed and that local recurrence or distant metastases will almost certainly appear in time (Scardino and Carlton 1983, 1986; Scardino and Wheeler 1985).

Irradiation of Positive Lymph Nodes

Nodal metastases occur in 8%–68% of patients with clinically localized tumors (normal bone scan and acid phosphatase), depending upon the clinical stage. Full pelvic radiotherapy has often been employed when the nodes are positive (Table 9.6), but the effectiveness of this approach is debatable.

In both the external beam (Bagshaw 1982) and the [198]Au series (Scardino and Carlton 1983), full pelvic radiotherapy was used. In the ^{125}I series (Grossman et al. 1982) only a pelvic lymph node dissection was done. No differences are apparent in the results for patients with positive nodes. Although some other investigators have also shown only slight differences in relapse rates when the pelvis was or was not treated, in the series reported by Paulson and associates the time to relapse was less with extended field irradiation than with expectant management (Kramer et al. 1981).

Post-treatment Biopsy Results (Table 9.7)

A positive biopsy $\geq$ 12 months after the completion of external beam therapy or 18 months after ^{125}I implants indicates that the treatment has failed to eradicate the local tumor (Scardino 1983; Bostwick et al. 1982; Herr and Whitmore 1982).

Table 9.6. Biopsy results after interstitial radiotherapy, by surgical stage

Technique	Negative nodes			Positive nodes
	A$_2$	B	C	D$_1$
Gold seeds (Scardino 1986)	4/18 (22%)	16/67 (24%)	12/22 (55%)	24/36 (67%)
Iodine (Lytton et al. 1979; Schellhammer et al. 1980)	1/6	17/36 (47%)	0/5	5/8 (63%)
	5/24 (21%)	33/103 (32%)	12/27 (44%)	29/44 (83%)

Table 9.7. Incidence and prognostic significance of positive prostatic biopsy results obtained 12 months or more after therapy. (In these patients hormonal therapy was not used before proven recurrence of tumor.[a])

Reference	Total	Negative No.	%	Recurrence No.	%	Positive No.	%	Recurrence No.	%	Follow-up
External beam										
Sewell et al. (1975)	6	6	38	1	17	10	62	8	80	>5
Cosgrove and Kaempf (1976)	9	4	44	0	0	5	56	2	40	5
Kurth et al. (1977)	23	9	39	0	0	14	61	2	14	1–4
Nachstsheim et al. (1978)	29	14	48	0	0	15	52	8	53	1.5–3
Kiesling et al. (1980)	68	29	43	4	14	39	57	11	28	5
Jacobi and Hohenfellner (1982)	64	39	61	7	18	25	39	16	64	4
Freiha and Bagshaw (1984)	64	25	39	6	24	39	61	28	72	8
Total	273	126	46	18	14	147	54	75	51	
[198]Au seeds + external beam										
Scardino (1983)	124	81	65	25	31	43	35	28	65	5
[125]I seeds										
Lytton et al. (1979)	22	11	50	1	9	11	50	1	9	2
Schellhammer et al. (1980) and Herr (1982)	87	60	69	14	23	27	31	18	67	<5
Total	109	71	65	15	21	38	35	19	50	
	506	278	55	58	21	228	48	122	54	

[a]Scardino (1986).

Our recent review of the published literature showed that positive biopsies were reported in 45% of 506 patients (Scardino 1986). At an average follow-up of 4 years the recurrence rate was 54% if the biopsy was positive and only 21% if it was negative. The rate of positive biopsies varied with the clinical stage, ranging from 15% in B_{1N} to 79% in the large stage C tumors. There is no established, satisfactory treatment for patients with a positive postirradiation biopsy. Options include observation, hormonal therapy, regional intra-arterial chemotherapy, interstitial seed implantation, salvage radical prostatectomy, and anterior exenteration.

Discussion and Conclusions

Definitive radiotherapy by a variety of available techniques can often control localized prostatic cancer. However, success requires adequate doses. The attraction of the implant techniques was that high local doses could be given with fewer complications than with external beam irradiation alone. Yet recent experience in the best centers indicates a low complication rate for external beam therapy alone, even using 7000 rad, if no pelvic lymph node dissection is performed. However, implants will continue to be attractive until radiotherapists in most communities can achieve this level of safety at the high doses required.

If the biopsy data accurately reflect the ability of radiotherapy to succeed at the only task we can ask of it—eradication of the local tumor within the field of irradiation—then none of the current techniques is optimal. External beam therapy, even at 7000 rad, is particularly worrisome, with a 61% positive biopsy rate (Freiha and Bagshaw 1984). Even among patients with negative nodes, some 20%–30% of tumors confined to the prostate and 50% of extracapsular tumors are not eliminated. These data and recent clinical experience have fueled the interest of urologists in radical prostatectomy.

Whether further increases in radiation dosage can improve the results of radiotherapy without markedly increasing complications remains to be seen. The implant techniques become even more attractive in this setting, since increased dosages can be delivered with a wide margin of safety.

Which implant technique should be used? If the complex technique can be mastered, iodine implants are safe, but the physics of radioactive iodine and the clinical experience today indicate that iodine implantation is best reserved for patients with small, nonobstructing stage B_1 tumors confined to the prostate—a population, it must be noted, which is also ideally suited for radical prostatectomy. Gold implants combined with external beam therapy provide very high doses of irradiation (8000–9000 rad) with a low complication rate, are technically simple, and are applicable to the full range of patients with clinically localized disease.

Nevertheless, our conclusion at this time is that radiotherapy is effective, and the implant techniques especially so when used for the appropriate lesions. But no technique of radiotherapy appears to be as effective as originally hoped. Overall, only 65%–80% of tumors confined to the prostate and some 45%–55% of extracapsular tumors in patients with negative nodes are eradicated, even with the best available techniques.

A flexible approach can be taken which provides the advantages of each technique. Treatment must begin with an open retropubic exploration and pelvic lymph node dissection with frozen section examination of the nodes and intraoperative palpation of the prostate and seminal vesicles. Regardless of the preoperative clinical stage, if the nodes are negative and the tumor does not palpably extend outside the prostate or into the seminal vesicles, a radical prostatectomy is performed. But if the nodes are positive or the tumor extends beyond the prostate, gold seeds are inserted and external beam therapy is given 3 weeks later.

References

Abadir R, Ross Y Jr, Weinstein SH (1984) Carcinoma of the prostate treated by pelvic and node dissection, iodine-125 seed implant and external irradiation: a study of rectal complications. Clin Radiol 35:359–361

Bagshaw MA (1982) Radiation therapy of prostatic carcinoma. In: Crawford ED, Borden TA (eds) Genitourinary cancer surgery. Lea and Febiger, Philadelphia, pp 405–411

Barringer BS (1942) Prostatic carcinoma. J Urol 47:306–308

Bostwick DG, Egbert BM, Fajardo LF (1982) Radiation injury of the normal and neoplastic prostate. Am J Surg Pathol 6:541–551

Brindle JS, Benson RC Jr, Martinez A, Edmundson GK, Zincke H (1985) Acute toxicity and preliminary therapeutic results of pelvic lymphadenectomy combined with transperineal interstitial implantation of ^{192}Ir and external beam radiotherapy for locally advanced prostate cancer. Urology 25:233–238

Carlton CE Jr, Hudgins PT, Guerriero WG, Scott R (1976) Radiotherapy in the management of stage C carcinoma of the prostate: 452 patients over 11 years. J Urol 116:206–210

Clubb BS, Summers JL (1984) Combined iridium 192 interstitial and external beam radiation therapy for the treatment of prostatic cancer. Cancer Treat Rep 68:1027–1028

Cosgrove MD, Kaempf MJ (1976) Prostatic cancer revisited. J Urol 115:79–81

Court B, Chassagne D (1977) Interstitial radiation therapy of cancer of the prostate using iridium 192 wires. Cancer Treat Rep 61:329–330

Flocks RH, Kerr HD, Elkins HB, Culp DA (1959) The treatment of carcinoma of the prostate by interstitial radiation with radioactive gold (^{198}Au): a follow-up report. J Urol 71:628–633

Fowler JE Jr, Barzell WW, Hilaris BS, Whitmore WF (1979) Complications of ^{125}I implantation and pelvic lymphadenectomy in the treatment of prostatic cancer. J Urol 121:447–451

Freiha FS, Bagshaw MA (1984) Carcinoma of the prostate: results of post-irradiation biopsy. Prostate 5:19–25

Grossman HB, Batata M, Hilaris B, Whitmore WF Jr (1982) ^{125}I implantation for carcinoma of the prostate. Urology 20:591–598

Herr HW (1980) Iodine-125 implantation in the management of localized prostatic carcinoma. Urol Clin North Am 7:605–612

Herr HW (1982) Pelvic lymphadenectomy and iodine-125 implantation of the prostate. In: Johnson DE, Boileau MA (eds) Fundamental principles and surgical technique. Grune and Stratton, New York, pp 63–74

Herr HW, Whitmore WF Jr (1982) Significance of prostatic biopsies after irradiation therapy for carcinoma of the prostate. Prostate 3:339–350

Hilaris BS, Whitmore WF Jr, Batata MA, Barzell W (1977) Behavior patterns of prostatic adenocarcinoma following ^{125}I implant and pelvic node dissection. Int J Radiat Oncol Biol Phys 2:631–637

Hilaris BS, Whitmore WF Jr, Batata MA (1978) Iodine-125 implantation of the prostate: dose response consideration. Front Radiat Ther Oncol 12:82–90

Jacobi GH, Hohenfellner R (1982) Staging management and pretreatment reevaluation of prostate cancer. Dogma questioned. In: Jacobi GH, Hohenfellner R (eds) Prostate cancer. Williams & Wilkins, Baltimore, pp 31–56

Kiesling VJ, McAninch JW, Goebel JL, Agee RE (1980) External beam radiotherapy for adenocarcinoma of the prostate: a clinical follow-up. J Urol 124:851–854

Kramer SA, Cline WA Jr, Farnham R, Carson CC, Cox EB, Hinshaw W, Paulson DS (1981) Prognosis of patients with stage D_1 prostatic adenocarcinoma. J Urol 125:817–819

Kurth KH, Altwein JE, Skoluda D (1977) Follow-up of irradiated prostatic carcinoma by aspiration biopsy. J Urol 117:615–617

Kwong EWH, Huh SH, Nobler MP, Smith HS (1984) Intra-operative iodine-125 prostatic implant following bilateral pelvic lymphadenectomy. Int J Radiat Oncol Biol Phys 10:665–670

Lepor H, Eggleston J, Walsh PC (1983) Radical prostatectomy with preservation of sexual function: anatomical and pathological considerations. Prostate 4:473–485

Lytton B, Collins JT, Weiss RM, Schiff M Jr, McGuire EJ, Livolsi V (1979) Results of biopsy after early stage prostatic cancer treatment by implantation of 125-I seeds. J Urol 121:306–309

Mag S (1985) Radioactive iodine-125 implantation for cancer of the prostate. Prostate 6:293–301

Martinez A, Benson RC, Edmundson GK, Brindle J (1985) Pelvic lymphadenectomy combined with transperineal interstitial implantation of iridium-192 and external beam radiotherapy for locally advanced prostatic carcinoma: technical description. Int J Radiat Oncol Biol Phys 11:841–847

Nachtsheim DA Jr, McAninch JW, Stutzman RE, Goebel JL (1978) Latent residual tumor following external radiotherapy for prostate adenocarcinoma. J Urol 120:312–314

Peschel RE, Fogel TD, Kacinski BM, Kelly K, Mate TP (1985) Iodine-125 implants for carcinoma of the prostate. Int J Radiat Oncol Biol Phys 11:1777–1781

Ray GR, Bagshaw MA (1975) The role of radiation therapy in the definitive treatment of adenocarcinoma of the prostate. Ann Rev Med 26:567–568

Rosenberg SA, Loening SA, Hawtrey CE, Narayana AS, Culp DA (1985) Radical prostatectomy with adjuvant radioactive gold for prostatic cancer: a preliminary report. J Urol 133:225–227

Ross G Jr, Borkon WD, Landry LJ, Edwards FM, Weinstein SH, Abadir R (1982) Preliminary observations on results of combined ^{125}iodine seed implantation and external irradiation for carcinoma of the prostate. J Urol 127:699–701

Scardino PT (1983) The prognostic significance of biopsies after radiotherapy for prostatic cancer. Semin Urol 1:243–251

Scardino PT (1986) The treatment of localized prostate cancer. Scand J Urol Nephrol 20:1–8

Scardino PT, Carlton CE Jr (1983) Combined interstitial and external radiation for prostatic cancer. In: Javadpour N (ed) Principles and management of urologic cancer. Williams & Wilkins, Baltimore, pp 392–408

Scardino PT, Wheeler TM (1985) Prostate biopsy after irradiation therapy for prostatic cancer. Urology [Suppl] 25:39–46

Scardino PT, Frankel JM, Wheeler TM, Meacham RB, Hoffman GS, Seale C, Wilbanks JH, Easley J, Carlton CE Jr (1986) The prognostic significance of postirradiation biopsy results in patients with prostatic cancer. J Urol 135:510–516

Schellhammer PF, Ladaga LE, El-Mahdi A (1980) Histological characteristics of prostatic biopsies after 125 iodine implantation. J Urol 123:700–705

Schellhammer PF, El-Mahdi AE, Ladaga LE (1985) 125Iodine implantation for carcinoma of the prostate: 5 year survival free of disease and incidence of local failure. J Urol 134:1140–1145

Sewell RA, Braren V, Wilson SK, Rhamy RK (1975) Extended biopsy follow-up after full-course radiation for resectable prostatic carcinoma. J Urol 113:371–373

Von Eschenbach AC (1981) Cancer of the prostate. Curr Probl Cancer 5:1–54

Whitmore WF Jr, Hilaris BS, Grabstold H (1972) Retropubic implantation of iodine-125 in the treatment of prostatic cancer. J Urol 108:918–920

Whitmore WF Jr, Hilaris BS, Batata M, Sogani P, Herr H, Morse M (1985) Interstitial radiation: short-term palliation or curative therapy? Urology 25 [Suppl]:24–29

Young HH, Fronz W (1917) Some new methods in the treatment of carcinoma of the lower genitourinary tract with radium. J Urol 1:505–536

Chapter 10

The Case for External Beam Radiotherapy of Certain Adenocarcinomas of the Prostate

M. Bagshaw

First Principles

The surgeons tell us that a first principle for the resection of a neoplasm intended to effect a cure is the total excision of all malignant tissue. A corollary would dictate that the burden in morbidity or mortality, or the risk–benefit ratio, should not be excessive. Similarly, a first principle of radiation therapy dictates that the neoplastic cells must be either destroyed or rendered incapable of further replication by adequate irradiation, and damage to normal structure and function must be minimal.

Surgical failure occurs when the neoplasm is not totally resected, and radiation failure occurs when the reproductive capacity of the neoplastic cells has not been destroyed.

Incomplete resection can occur if the primary neoplasm is understaged preoperatively and the tumor has penetrated beyond the plane of surgical cleavage, for example, to involve the seminal vesicles or the periprostatic fat. Similarly, radiation may fail if the neoplasm has extended beyond the volume of tissue to be irradiated, or if all of the cells within the irradiated volume have not been sterilized. The latter is always a possibility because the probability of sterilization of neoplastic cells, as a function of radiation dose, is a logarithmic event which can only be predicted on a statistical basis. Radiation therapy is less likely than surgery to fail in the treatment of prostatic cancer because of an anatomic miss, because the radiation treatment volume is usually substantially larger than the volume of tissue which can be resected. On the other hand, radiation therapy may fail because owing to the geometry of the Poisson distribution, enough cells to commence replication within the target volume may have survived lethal bombardment by the ionizing radiation. Since the response to irradiation is logarithmic and the maximum dose that can be delivered is dictated by the tolerance of the normal tissues, smaller tumors with fewer cells are more likely to be sterilized than larger ones. In prostatic cancer, as with most neoplasms, a systematic relationship exists between stage and the ability to sterilize the primary tumor. Stage embodies the concept of anatomic location as well as mass. Anatomic extent is probably not as important in radiotherapy as in surgery, while mass, or cell number, is probably more important in radiotherapy than in surgery. Thus, surgery and radiation therapy for localized prostatic cancer have similar limitations. For complete surgical resection, perhaps the ability to resect all neoplastic cells is a more rigid requirement than is the ability to encompass all neoplastic cells for radiation therapy.

Survival Patterns for Stage B Tumors

Figure 10.1 shows an advantage in survival after radiation therapy for patients in whom the primary tumor is confined to the prostate as opposed to those with extracapsular extension. Even for those with extracapsular extension, a survival expectation of 18% at 15 years has been achieved (Bagshaw 1985; Bagshaw et al. 1985). Figure 10.2 indicates that there is little difference in survival pattern between irradiated patients with either stage T_1 (B_1) or T_2 (B_2) disease, whereas in the surgical series of Elder and Jewett (Elder et al. 1982) there was a substantially poorer survival in clinical stage B_2 (approximately 26%) vs B_1 (approximately 52%) following radical prostatectomy. This decrease was clearly correlated with the fact that on pathologic examination, 66% of the clinically staged B_2 patients had extracapsular extension. Thus in radiation therapy, it appears to be less important to make a pretherapeutic distinction between B_1 and B_2 lesions than it is in surgery. In fact, the same is true for those with occult carcinoma with multiple chip involvement. Depending upon how one defines the subcategories, the survival pattern after X-irradiation is nearly identical for patients with A_2, B_1, and B_2 lesions, i.e., approximately 40% actuarial survival at 15 years.

In the B_1 tumor, the relative effectiveness of radiation therapy as compared with surgery is more difficult to ascertain. We have adopted as our B_1 (T_{1a}) designation a somewhat more restricted definition than that employed by Elder et al. (1982), and more nearly as originally described by Jewett (Jewett et al. 1968), that is, a palpably discrete nodular lesion averaging 1 cm or a little more in diameter, limited to a part of one lateral lobe. Using this restricted definition, we have achieved an actuarial survival of 62% at 15 years in 40 patients (Fig. 10.3). This seems indistinguishable from the 51% estimated survival after surgery, as reported by Walsh and Jewett (1980). Since there may have been differences in distribution of histopathologic grade, it is not possible to say that the outcome in terms of survival is better or worse for one or the other method. There is no obvious difference. Certainly, if the surgeon could be sure that all of the tumor is confined to a nodule 1 cm or a little more in diameter, the outcome should be perfect, and it would be better than could be achieved by radiation. Even with a nodule as small as 1 cm or a little more, at our present limiting dose

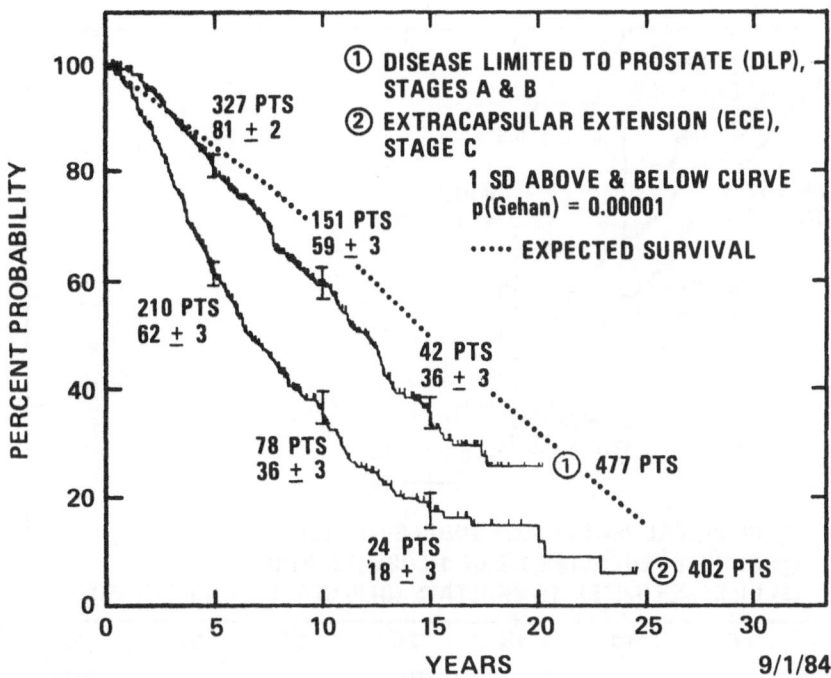

Fig. 10.1. Kaplan and Meier (1958) survival data for patients with prostatic cancer treated by high energy external beam irradiation (4–6 Mv linear accelerator), according to whether or not there was extracapsular extension of the disease.

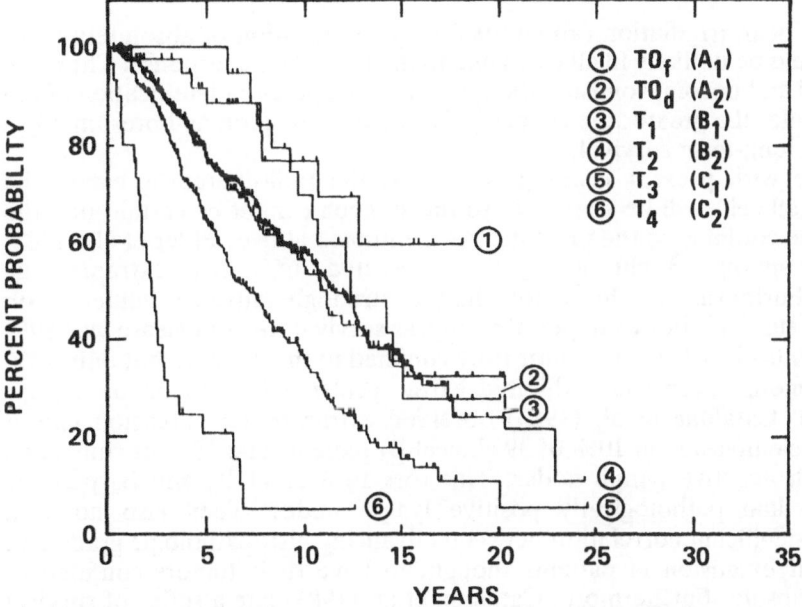

Fig. 10.2. Kaplan and Meier (1958) survival data for patients with prostatic cancer treated by high energy X-irradiation (4–6 Mv linear accelerator), according to a refined TNM staging system.

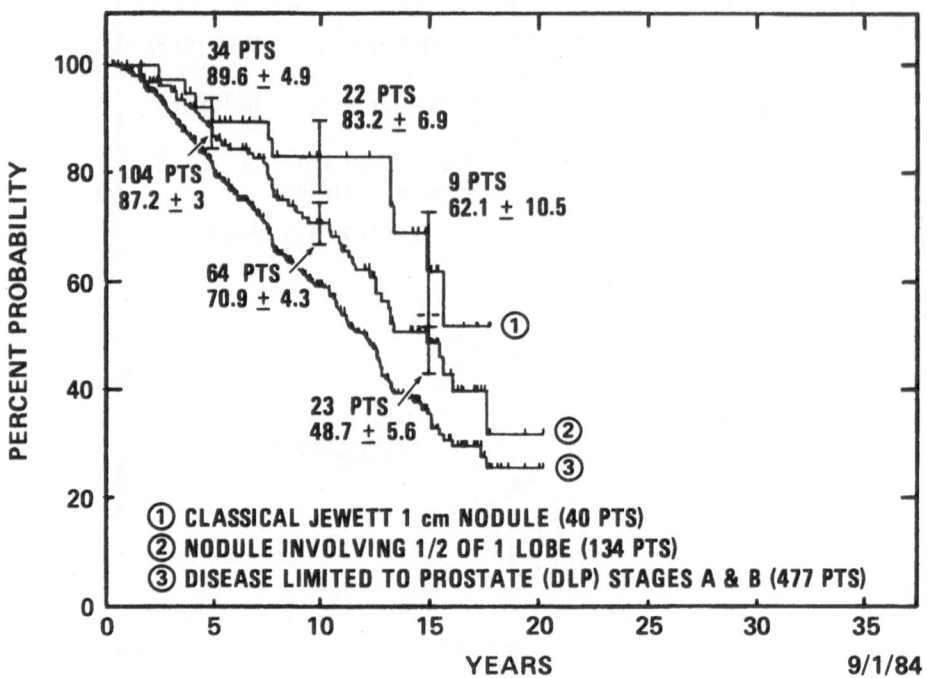

Fig. 10.3. Kaplan and Meier (1958) survival data for patients with nodular carcinoma of the prostate treated by external beam X-irradiation (4–6 Mv linear accelerator).

for external bean irradiation (about 7000 rad), sterilization of absolutely all of the cells would be unlikely in all cases due to the logarithmic response. Thus, the more skilled and uncompromising the surgeon in the precise identification of the solitary nodule, the greater the chances of complete resection and presumably a high rate of long-term survival.

Of course with present techniques, just as the radiotherapists cannot be certain that all cells will be sterilized, so the surgeon cannot be certain that the tumor will be confined to the prostate. As mentioned above, Elder et al. (1982) found that among 53 clinical B_2 cases resected, 66% had extraprostatic extension. Furthermore, this status had a strikingly adverse influence on disease-free survival. For example, the 15-year survival free of disease was 50% among patients (7 of 14) with tumor truly confined to the prostate but only 13% (4 of 32) among those who exhibited extracapsular extension on pathologic examination. Catalona et al. (1983) observed extracapsular extension and/or seminal vesicle invasion in 10% of 39 clinical B_1 patients and 38% of clinical B_2 patients with negative lymph nodes. This rose to 8 of 11 B_1 and B_2 patients (73%) who had pathologically positive lymph nodes. They also noted a statistically significant correlation between advancing histopathologic grade and extracapsular extension in patients thought to have their tumors confined to within the capsule. Furthermore, Catalona et al. (1983) cite a series of surgical reports which demonstrated tumor extension beyond the prostatic capsule in up to 56% of the patients with clinical stage B tumors. In a series of 215 cases carefully selected for radical perineal prostatectomy, Gibbons et al. (1984) found microscopic extracapsular disease in 49 of 195 (25%) clinical stage B patients, even though no extracapsular extension had been detected by two experienced urologists, and no patient with known adenopathy was included. Probably the most rigorous case selection for radical prostatectomy was that reported by Jewett et al. (1968). They reported that 475 patients underwent radical prostatectomy among 3711 patients referred with prostatic cancer. Among these, 292 patients had "a palpably discrete nodule of firm or stony consistency limited to a part of one lateral lobe, averaging 1 cm or a little more in diameter, with compressible prostatic tissue always on two, and sometimes on three sides." One hundred and three of these were evaluable and at risk for at least 15 years. In 17 cases (16.5%), tumor cells were found beyond the prostate, and these patients fared poorly. Only one survived 15 years, and he had cancer. Ten others died with cancer. It is clear that present preoperative staging techniques preclude the ability to select patients in whom all of the malignant tissue can be excised. Current investigation of the use of imaging techniques (ultrasound, CT scanning, and MRI scanning) could improve preoperative staging, but an analysis of this is beyond the scope of this essay.

The presence of prostatic neoplasm in the periphery of the gland and the multicentricity of origin, 97% and 85% respectively according to Byar et al. (1972), at least today provide room for honest error; and it is this honest error on the one hand for surgery, and the inability to sterilize 100% of neoplastic cells on the other hand for radiation therapy, which creates an overlapping margin of uncertainty for each method. Given the above, the decision as to the method of therapy often depends upon other factors. These include the age of the patient and therefore the expected longevity, the health status of the patient, the morbidity of surgery versus the morbidity of radiation treatment, and the emotional ability of the patient to tolerate the lack of certain knowledge of complete sterilization following irradiation.

Treatment Technique

The Stanford technique for prostatic irradiation has been reported in detail elsewhere (Bagshaw 1984). Patients selected for definitive treatment are first surveyed by appropriate studies to rule out distant hematogenous metastases. Lymphangiograms are often performed in patients with intermediate or high-grade neoplasms in order to document adenopathy and assist in the set-up procedures. A preliminary mini CT scan is performed to localize the position of the prostate within the pelvic girdle. The localizing CT is obtained with a flat table top placed upon the CT patient support assembly (therapy tables are usually flat whereas CT tables are usually concave), and with vertical and left and right laser side lights in order to establish index marks on the skin for patient positioning. Next, the patient is placed in the supine position upon a radiation therapy simulator patient support assembly; a Foley catheter is inserted into the rectum, and the balloon distended and then tugged snugly against the internal rectal sphincter. A metallic clamp is slipped over the Foley catheter and locked into position against the anus. Thus, the Foley catheter marks the position of the internal sphincter, and the metallic clamp, the position of the anus. Several milliliters of 2% lidocaine are instilled into the penile urethra for topical anesthesia . Following this, several milliliters of Hypaque-50% are instilled, and a Zipser clamp is placed across the glans penis, entrapping the contrast media within the penile urethra. This demonstrates the position of the external sphincter and the pelvic diaphragm, and hence the distalmost portion of the prostate.

About 100 ml of thin barium contrast is instilled into the rectum through the Foley catheter, and two sets of localization films are obtained, one centered 4 cm superior to the symphysis pubis, the other centered at the symphysis pubis. The table is adjusted so that the isocenter is located about 10 or 11 cm above the table top. Cross-sectional contours are obtained at the central axis planes of the localization films for preparation of the treatment plans. The treatment plans may also be prepared directly from the CT images, providing the proper anatomic level has been established. These localization films are then used to prepare the position and shape of the extended pelvic field and the prostatic boost. At Stanford, both 4 Mv and 6 Mv linear accelerators have been used for this treatment program, and the four-field techniques is recommended for energies up to 10 Mv or 12 Mv.

The anterior and posterior parallel opposed fields are octagonal or "stop-sign" fields which extend inferiorly from L5 to approximately the ischial tuberosities. It is important to be sure that the position of the external sphincter, as indicated by the urethrogram, is positioned within the field perimeter, and that the position of the anus is positioned outside the field perimeter. This is an important point since these two anatomic sites are frequently at nearly the same cross-sectional level. If it is not possible to exclude the anus in the anterior posterior parallel opposed pair, special care must be taken to shield the anus from exposure from the lateral fields. The left and right margins of the field are approximately 1–15 cm lateral to the widest diameter of the true pelvis. The superior and inferior corners of these parallel opposed anterior and posterior radiation fields are trimmed, converting them from rectangular to octagonal fields. The lateral fields have the same isocenter and superior and inferior margins as the anterior and posterior fields. The lateral pelvic field is presently constructed by using the Styrofoam-Cerrobend system for creating individualized outboard collimators. Using the lateral orthogonal companion to the AP extended pelvic localization film, the posterior margin of the lateral field is established by tracing a line that extends from the anus superiorly along the midlumen of the rectum in a curvilinear fashion, and parallel to the hollow of the sacrum. This extends superiorly to the S2 segment, at which point the posterior margin is deviated toward the central plane of the sacrum, and then the margin extends superiorly to intercept the superior border of the field at L5. Inferiorly, the anus is blocked out of the lateral field, and the inferior margin is adjusted to be certain it is external to the external sphincter of the urethra, as demonstrated by the intraurethral contrast. The anterior margin now courses superiorly, following the midplane of the pubic bone up to the superior pubic symphysis. The field then extends directly superiorly to the level of L5. Conceptually, this field is shaped to provide maximum protection to the posterior wall of the rectum and the anus, and to ensure that the lymph nodes of the pelvis, which generally follow a line that extends from the posterior pubic symphysis to the sacral promontory, are well encompassed.

The boost field for the prostate alone is adjusted to encompass the prostate and the seminal vesicles. Usually it extends from the pelvic diaphragm inferiorly to the acetabulum superiorly and is approximately 8 or 9 cm square. The prostatic boost is delivered through left and right moving beam therapy which subtends a lateral arc of 120°. In practice, the extended pelvic fields are started first and the dose is carried to 2600 rad at the isocenter point, taking care to treat every field every day. At this dose level, the patient is usually commencing to experience modest diarrhea and, therefore, the program is switched to the prostatic boost, and an additional 2000 rad is given. At this point, the four-field technique is resumed for an additional 2400 rad. This provides 7000 rad in 7 weeks to the prostate, and 5000 rad in 7 weeks to the first echelon lymphatic drainage. Nearly all patients tolerate this program well. It is rare to require further rest periods for medication other than occasional Lomotil. The key points of the technique include careful trimming of all radiation fields to minimize normal tissue exposure, protection of the posterior wall of the rectum and the anal sphincter, applying treatment to all fields every day, and inserting the prostatic boost during the middle one-third of the therapy rather than at the end.

Treatment Sequelae

In the well selected and carefully followed series of Gibbons et al. (1984), 18% of the patients suffered a stricture postoperatively, and 16 required more than one dilatation. Abnormal urinary control was present in 8% of 213 patients. Twelve incontinent patients wear an appliance for urine collection. Ninety-three per cent of 146 patients had erectile impotence. Adverse sequelae in the Stanford series have not been reported recently. A comprehensive review of side effects and complications in 898 patients is now nearly complete, and inspection of the data suggests a reduction in sequelae as compared to previous reports. A review in 1976 based on 430 patients (stages A, B, and C inclusive), showed urethral stricture in 16, or 3.7% (Pistenma et al. 1976). The incidence of stricture was related to multiple preradiotherapeutic transurethral resection of the prostate. One patient with persistent tumor required a colostomy, and three had fecal stress incontinence and urinary stress incontinence. Erectile potency was maintained in 65 of the evaluable 110 patients (59%). In a study by Pilepich et al. (1981) which detailed adverse sequelae following irradiation, urethral stricture was noted in 5.2% and proctitis in 4.5% of irradiated patients. In the Patterns of Care Outcome Studies drawn from 163 randomly chosen radiation therapy facilities, major complications following radiation therapy requiring admission to the hospital occurred in 28 of 619 (4.5%) patients evaluated (Leibel et al. 1984). These involved the urinary tract in 13, the bowel in 8, and both in 3. Sixteen required surgical intervention, and one was fatal. Again, this represents both stage B and stage C carcinoma, a considerably more advanced group of patients than those of Gibbons et al.

It appears that the risk of incontinence is significantly less following radiotherapy. This is certainly true in the Stanford series. Bowel complications appear somewhat greater after irradiation; however, with current radiation techniques, these are rare and can usually be attributed to persistent tumor. A 60% preservation of erectile potency seems possible after X-irradiation, although this probably applies to the younger patients. In the Stanford series, for example, the mean age of those who reported preservation of potency was 59 years, whereas the mean age for the group as a whole was 63 years.

The nerve-sparing surgical procedure introduced by Walsh and Donker (1982) improves preservation of erectile potency after prostatectomy, but whether this is at the expense of tumor recurrence remains to be seen. Byar et al. (1972) observed perineural invasion in 84% of their step-section specimens; and although they could not correlate this with an adverse outcome, the rationale of preserving nerves with potential perineural involvement is reasonably open to question.

Surgery vs Radiotherapy for Clinically Resectable Tumors

Although Paulson et al. (1982) observed an apparent advantage for patients randomly assigned to radical prostatectomy versus those assigned to radiation therapy, with "time to first evidence of distant metastases" taken as the end point, this observation was not confirmed by a retrospective analysis of 51 patients who were identically surgically staged in the Stanford series. The Stanford patients were treated by external beam irradiation in a similar fashion and at about the same time as those treated in Paulson's study. The Stanford observations suffer from not having been randomized; however, the "time to first evident metastasis" in the Stanford group was nearly identical to that observed for the radical surgery group in the Paulson study, and significantly different from the patients in the Paulson study who were irradiated (Fig. 10.4). Also, there is a substantially longer follow-up of the Stanford patients and, at the time of the last analysis, over 80% were surviving at 10 years by actuarial calculation (Fig. 10.5).

Survival Patterns for Stage C Tumors

Although many studies of external beam irradiation of stage C prostatic cancer could be cited, the Stanford experience as shown in Fig. 4.1, curve 2, may be taken as representative of the experience of X-irradiation of more advanced extracapsular prostatic carcinoma (Bagshaw 1985; Bagshaw et al. 1985). Based on survival alone and staged by noninvasive techniques only, actuarial survivals of 62%, 36%, and 18% may be achieved at 5, 10, and 15 years, respectively, in spite of the fact that the patients in the Stanford series have a 60% probability of lymph node metastases, and probably many have occult metastases to other sites at the time of treatment. Two other series bear special mention because they have been coauthored by urologists from institutions with proclivity for surgical

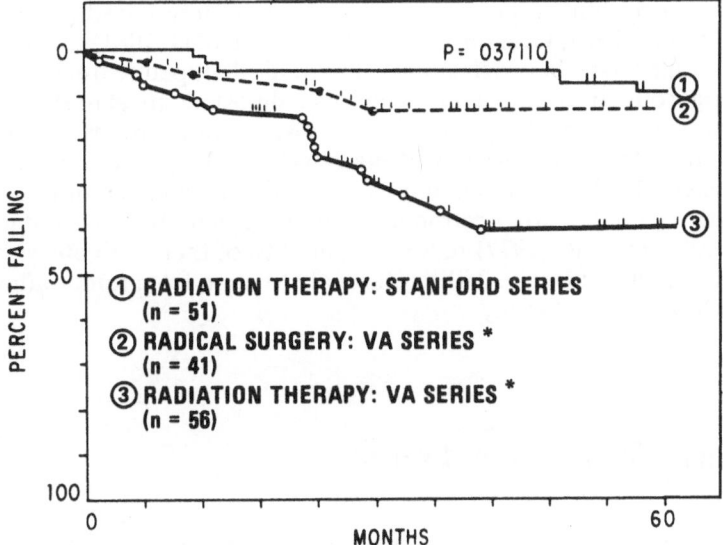

From: Paulson et al, J.Urology, Vol. 128,1982

Fig. 10.4. Time to first evidence of treatment failure (Paulson et al. 1982).

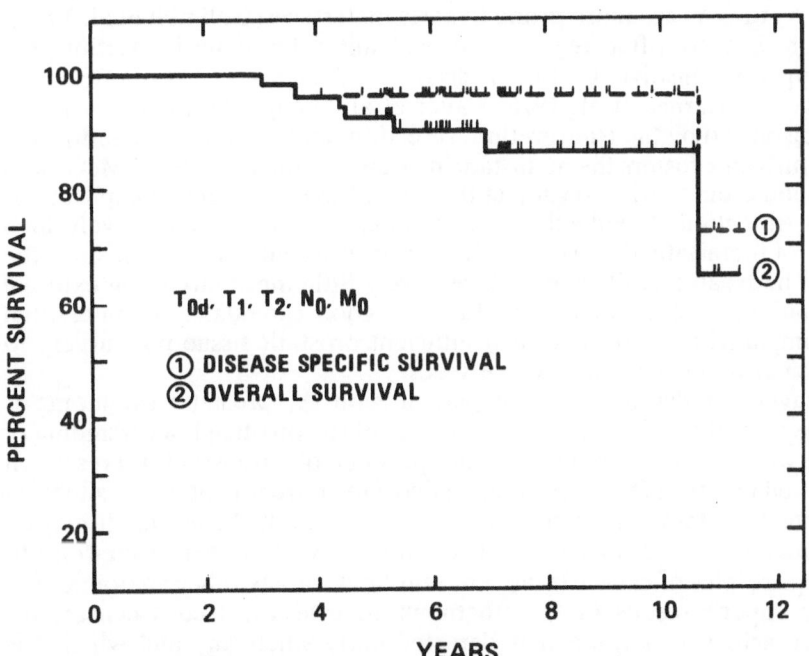

Fig. 10.5. Disease-specific and overall survival in the 51 surgically staged patients with prostatic cancer in the Stanford series. The cohort includes *all patients* with stage A_2 or B disease who had negative adenopathy proven by surgery and were irradiated between 1970 and 1978. An *upward tick* indicates the length of follow-up at the last interrogation for a living patient. A *downward step* indicates death due to tumor (*curve 1*) and death due to any cause (*curve 2*).

treatment from which excellent surgical results also have been reported (Cupps et al. 1980; Gibbons et al. 1979; Gibbons et al. 1984; Zincke et al. 1981). Thus it is fair to assume that the triage between surgical and radiotherapeutic treatment options was fairly rigorous. Both series report survival almost identical to that of the Stanford experience. Even though metastatic disease often occurs, most patients are relieved of local symptoms and many achieve long-term control. Gibbons and associates (1979) noted that only 17 (8%) of 209 patients required a subsequent prostatic operation for obstruction following definitive X-irradiation, whereas Thomlinson et al. (1977) reported that 75% of their patients with stage C disease developed recurrence with urethral obstruction from tumor after resection, even with hormone therapy.

Survival Patterns for Stage A Tumors

Possibly the most difficult stage about which to decide the question of appropriate therapy is stage A or, in our staging system, T_{0f} for focal occult carcinoma (A_1), or T_{0d} for diffuse occult carcinoma (A_2).

Although stage A_2 tumors are thought to behave more aggressively than stage A_1 tumors (Fig. 10.2), the difference in the Stanford series is not statistically significant. A_2 tumors are more prone to early metastasis (Golimbu et al. 1978), and although they are often regarded as well suited for radical resection, the outcome appears sensitive to tumor grade, and survival deteriorates with increasing grade (Barnes et al. 1976; Bauer et al. 1960). The tumor itself will have been disturbed by the transurethral resection, and there is some indication that this disturbance fosters the metastatic process (Leibel et al. 1984; McGowan 1980). It would seem unwise to subject the patient to the possible complications of a radical resection if, indeed, he must look forward to a relatively high expectation of metastatic disease as well. This is especially of concern since the patients can be treated easily and with relatively little morbidity using external beam irradiation. Such patients are often not good candidates for interstitial iodine-125 implants because there is insufficient prostatic tissue postsurgery to hold a sufficient number of radioactive seeds.

The management decision for the patient with A_1 prostatic carcinoma is probably the most difficult. Stage A_1 carcinoma of the prostate is a carcinoma of the prostate which is discovered within the specimen of a transurethral resection and is observed in only a few chips. Many advocate no treatment in this situation because of the long-term nature of prostatic cancer and the belief that it may be treated successfully at a later date. This point of view, however, is contrary to the general principles of cancer treatment that hold for any other anatomic site. Clearly, the superb results in the treatment of true vocal cord cancer, for example, are achieved because it is detected early when tiny and when it is confined to the vocal cord. Either surgical resection or radiation therapy has a greater than 90% chance of achieving a cure in this situation. One may argue that 90% of the patients with occult carcinoma of the prostate will never manifest clinical disease and, therefore, why treat 100% to prevent a more aggressive manifestation of the disease in the other 10%? One might understand this argument if, indeed, the only therapeutic option were radical prostatectomy with its unavoidable morbidity and occasional mortality. Low though they may be, they do exist, and one can understand the reluctance to advise radical surgery for a neoplasm of such low potential for aggressive behavior. On the other hand, radiation therapy, especially if limited to the prostate, is an extremely well tolerated procedure of insignificant morbidity. Irradiation is a small price to pay for the assurance that the A_1 lesion will not resurface in 5 or 10 years as a full-blown symptomatic, or even worse, metastatic, malignancy. We have encountered proven progression from A_1 to advanced B, or even C disease in a few patients, and whenever it occurs one wishes that radiotherapy had been carried out at the time of the initial diagnosis. Here the age of the patient plays an important role. Usually the A_1 lesion is well differentiated. Surely if that is not the case, then radiotherapy should be carried out. Even when the tumor is well differentiated, if the patient is relatively young, say below 65, then irradiation should be considered. If the patient is over 70 years of age or infirm, one could avoid treatment with little chance that the neoplasm would become clinically manifest.

Lymph Node Metastases

It is unknown whether radiation therapy can stop the progression of prostatic carcinoma once lymph node metastasis has occurred; however, when such metastases are *overt*, irradiation interrupts disease progression in only a relatively small number of patients. In our staged patient series, the survival among the 61 patients who had biopsy-proven lymph node metastases diminished to less than 20% at the 10th year (Fig. 10.6) (Bagshaw 1985). By contrast, in the cohort of 85 staged patients who had no demonstrable lymph node metastases, over 70% are surviving at the 10th year. In general, overt lymph node metastases of the more radioresistant neoplasms are difficult to sterilize with tolerable doses of X-irradiation. It is thought, however, that microscopic metastases, e.g., those with relatively small cell numbers, can be sterilized, and indeed this has been well demonstrated in certain other neoplasms, such as carcinomas of the head and neck. It may be that more than is easily apparent is accomplished by treating patients who have microscopic prostatic metastases in lymph nodes. For example, there is a unique cohort of patients in the Stanford series where this appears to be the case. Originally, treatment was being given to the prostate and periprostatic tissue only. In the late 1960s, interest broadened to include investigation of lymphadenopathy (Pistenma et al. 1979); and upon discovering that a substantial number of patients had positive lymph nodes, the treatment program was gradually modified to include not only the prostate, but also the regional lymph nodes. Over a period of several years, some patients received radiation treatment restricted to the prostate, while others received treatment to the prostate plus the pelvic lymph nodes. If one compares the survival within the group of patients with disease limited to the prostate, that is, stage B, between those who received treatment localized to the prostate and those receiving treatment to the prostate plus the pelvic adenopathy, a statistically significant long-term survival advan-

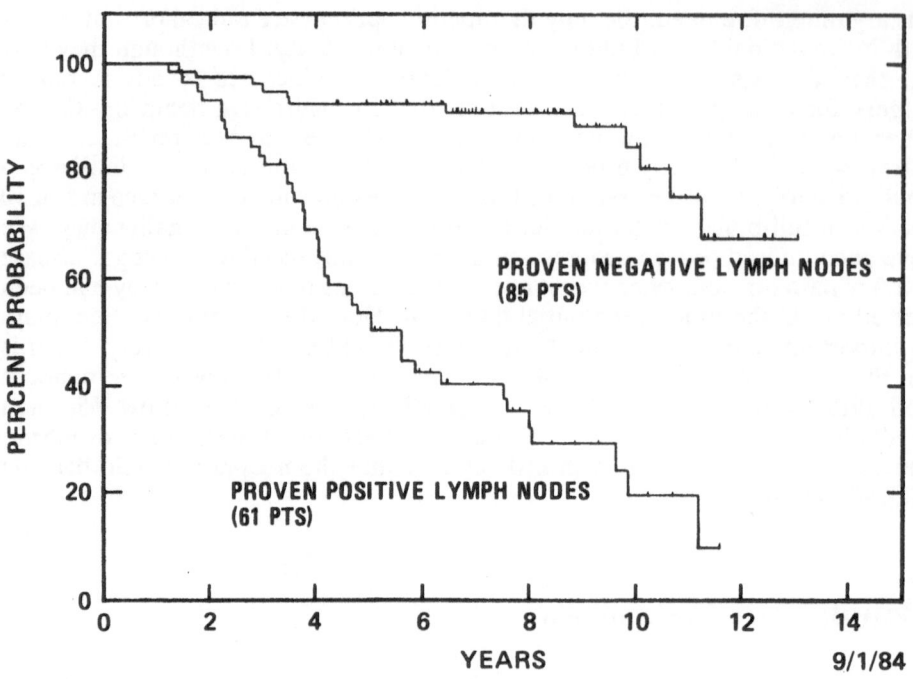

Fig. 10.6. Duration of survival of patients surgically staged for lymphadenopathy (Kaplan–Meier plot) after X-irradiation.

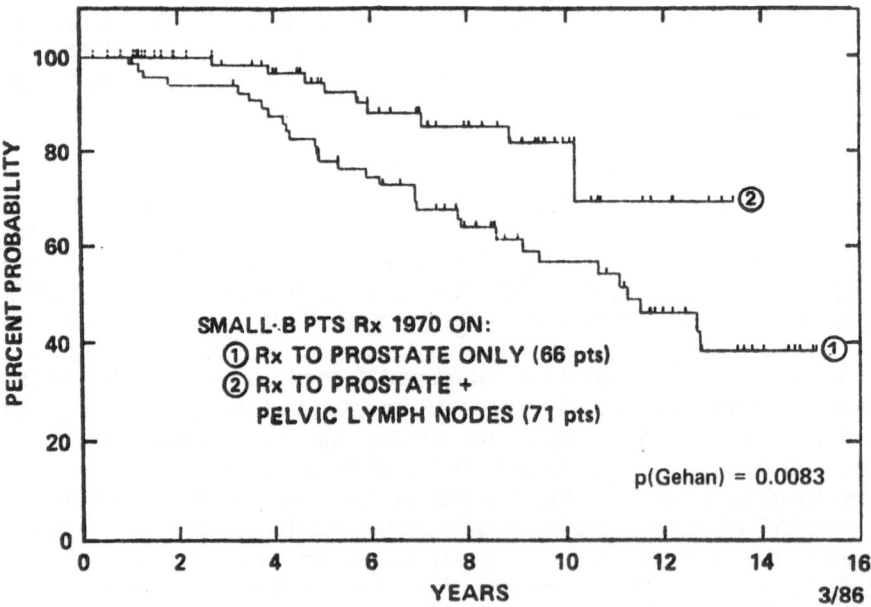

Fig. 10.7. Duration of survival (Kaplan–Meier plot) of stage B patients treated by X-irradiation between 1970 and 1978, according to whether the radiation treatment included the pelvic lymph nodes. Approximately 20% of the patients may have had lymph node metastases.

tage is observed in the patients who received extended-field irradiation (Fig. 10.7) (Bagshaw 1985). This suggests that for some patients there is a window of time when the metastatic process may be arrested in the lymphatic system and, providing there is only microscopic disease, may be sterilized by X-irradiation. Similarly, McGowan (1981) found a survival advantage for patients who received extended-field irradiation. In his series, the survival advantage was observed in patients with stages B_2 and C.

Summary

Radical surgery and definitive X-irradiation have much in common in the treatment of carcinoma of the prostate. They are both local modalities and, therefore, to a certain extent, limited by their ability to encompass the full extent of disease within or in continuity with the target organ. Surgery is advantageous because if the entire neoplasm is resected, then the patient is cured. It is disadvantageous because of the inability to determine in many cases the true extent of the tumor and the significant probability that the surgical excision may transect extracapsular neoplasm. Radiotherapy has the advantage of being able to encompass a more generous target volume than surgery, making it less sensitive as to whether or not the capsule has been penetrated. Radiotherapy is disadvantaged because it is impossible to know, except on a statistical basis, whether or not all of the cells have been truly sterilized. However, as the tumor burden increases, the ability of external beam irradiation alone to sterilize the tumor diminishes. Certain adjunct treatments, such as radioactive implant boost, sensitization by chemotherapeutic agents, radiosensitization by hyperthermia, or boost by neutron therapy may increase the probability of sterilizing the more bulky neoplasms.

Because of the lower morbidity expected from skillfully executed radiotherapy, the treatment may be implemented in situations of relative low- grade malignancy which might not warrant radical surgery. In view of these considerations, recommendations for local external beam radiotherapy are as follows:

Stage A_1: Localized radiation therapy to the prostate only, using a small treatment volume in patients with a long life expectancy.

Stage A_2: External beam irradiation including potential regional adenopathy, except in the very elderly.

Stage B_1: Either external beam irradiation or radical surgery for the truly nodular B_1 lesion: radiation therapy preferred for patients who might be a poor surgical risk, or used as a back-up for patients who have incomplete resection.

Stage B_2: Radiation therapy preferred, with treatment of regional adenopathy. If surgery is used, postoperative radiotherapy may also be used in the event of incomplete resection.

Stage C: Radiation therapy with treatment of both the primary tumor and regional adenopathy.

Stage D: Aggressive palliative irradiation (5000–6000 rad, in 5 or 6 weeks) to relieve overt or impending local symptoms.

References

Bagshaw MA (1984) A technique for external beam irradiation of carcinoma of the prostate. In: Levitt SH, Tapley N (eds) Technological basis of radiation therapy: practical clinical applications. Lea & Febiger, Philadelphia, pp 244–270
Bagshaw MA (1985) Potential for radiotherapy alone in prostatic cancer. Cancer 55:2079–2085
Bagshaw MA, Ray GR, Cox RS (1985) Radiotherapy of prostatic carcinoma: long- or short-term efficacy. Urology 25:17–23
Barnes R, Hirst A, Rosenquist R (1976) Early carcinoma of the prostate: comparison of stages A and B. J Urol 115:404–405
Bauer WC, McGavran HM, Carlin MR (1960) Unsuspected carcinoma of the prostate in suprapubic prostatectomy specimens. Cancer 13:370–378
Byar DP, Mostofi FK, VA Cooperative Urological Research Group (1972) Carcinoma of the prostate: prognostic evaluation of certain pathologic features in 208 radical prostatectomies. Cancer 30:5–13
Catalona WJ, Fleischmann J, Menon M (1983) Pelvic lymph node status as predictor of extracapsular tumor extension in clinical stage B prostatic cancer. J Urol 129:327–329
Cupps RE, Utz DC, Fleming TR, Carson CC, Zincke H, Myers RP (1980) Definitive radiation therapy for prostatic carcinoma: Mayo Clinic experience. J Urol 124:855–859
Elder JS, Jewett HJ, Walsh PC (1982) Radical perineal prostatectomy for clinical stage B2 carcinoma of the prostate. J Urol 127:704–706
Gibbons RP, Mason JT, Correa RJ Jr, Cummings KB, Taylor WJ, Hafermann MD, Richardson RG (1979) Carcinoma of the prostate: local control with external beam radiation therapy. J Urol 121:310–312
Gibbons RP, Correa RJ Jr, Brannen GE, Mason JT (1984) Total prostatectomy for localized prostatic cancer. J Urol 131:73–75
Golimbu M, Schinella R, Morales P, Kurusu S (1978) Differences in pathological characteristics and prognosis of clinical A2 prostatic cancer from A1 and B disease. J Urol 119:618–622
Jewett HJ, Bridge RW, Gray GF Jr, Shelley WM (1968) The palpable nodule of prostatic cancer. JAMA 203:403–406
Kaplan EL, Meier P (1958) Non-parametric estimations from incomplete observations. Am Stat Assoc J 53:457–480
Leibel SA, Hanks GE, Kramer S (1984) Patterns of care outcome studies: results of the national practice in adenocarcinoma of the prostate. Int J Radiat Oncol Biol Phys 10:401–409
McGowan DG (1980) The adverse influence of prior transurethral resection on prognosis in carcinoma of prostate treated by radiation therapy. Int J Radiat Oncol Biol Phys 6:1121–1126
McGowan DG (1981) The value of extended field radiation therapy in carcinoma of the prostate. Int J Radiat Biol Phys 7:1333–1339
Paulson DF, Lin GH, Hinshaw W, Stephani S, Uro-Oncology Research Group (1982) Radical surgery versus radiotherapy for adenocarcinoma of the prostate. J Urol 128:502–504
Pilepich MV, Perez CA, Walz BJ, Zivnuska FR (1981) Complications of definitive radiotherapy for carcinoma of the prostate. Int J Radiat Oncol Biol Phys 7:1341–1348
Pistenma DA, Ray GR, Bagshaw MA (1976) The role of megavoltage radiation therapy in the treatment of prostatic carcinoma. Semin Oncol 3:115–122
Pistenma DA, Bagshaw MA, Freiha FS (1979) Extended-field radiation therapy for prostatic adenocarcinoma: status report of a limited prospective trial. In: Johnson DE, Samuels ML (eds) Cancer of the genitourinary tract. Raven Press, New York, pp 229–247
Thomlinson RL, Currie DP, Boyce WH (1977) Radical prostatectomy: palliation for stage C carcinoma of the prostate. J Urol 117:85–87
Walsh PC, Donker PJ (1982) Impotence following radical prostatectomy: insight into etiology and prevention. J Urol 128:492–497
Walsh PC, Jewett HJ (1980) Radical surgery for prostatic cancer. Cancer 45:1906–1911
Zincke H, Fleming TR, Furlow WL, Myers RP, Utz DC (1981) Radical retropubic prostatectomy and pelvic lymphadenectomy for high-stage cancer of the prostate. Cancer 47:1901–1910

Chapter 11

Hormonal Therapy in Metastatic Prostatic Cancer

J. Trachtenberg

Introduction

The concept of hormonal therapy for prostatic cancer was introduced in 1941 by Huggins and Hodges with the prospect of curing even the most advanced of cases. They reasoned that since normal prostatic epithelium is androgen dependent, prostatic cancer should be similarly dependent. They and others then demonstrated that human prostatic cancer could be made to regress by the administration of pharmacologic doses of estrogens or by castration (Huggins et al. 1941; Spirnak and Resnick 1983). However, after a decade of enthusiastic and optimistic use of these forms of androgen ablation in all stages of prostatic cancer, it became apparent that hormonal therapy was not to be the panacea initially envisaged. Clinical studies conducted from 1942 to 1983 failed to define clearly the indications for this treatment except to demonstrate that hormonal therapy could not cure prostatic cancer. Studies by Vest and Frazier (1946), Nesbit and Plumb (1946), and Nesbit and Baum (1950) all suggested that hormonal therapy prolonged survival of patients with metastatic disease. However, the Veterans Administration Cooperative Urological Research Group (VACURG) (1967) failed to demonstrate any survival benefit of early hormonal therapy in advanced disease. Lepor et al. (1982) compared the survival of patients with metastatic disease treated immediately prior to the introduction of hormonal therapy with that in patients treated immediately after. After accounting for changes in survival in the population as a whole they could not find a statistical difference in survival between these two groups.

In spite of these conflicting and indeed disappointing results, hormonal therapy continues to play an important role in the treatment of prostatic carcinoma. The exact place of androgen ablation in the treatment is still not entirely defined. It seems certain that this form of therapy is not curative but equally clear that hormonal therapy can play an important role in alleviating bony metastatic pain and improving symptoms which are secondary to tumor compression. Virtually all other aspects of the use of this form of therapy in the treatment of prostatic cancer remain controversial. What is the optimal form of this therapy? At what stage of the disease is it best instituted? Finally, and probably of most importance, is there or is there not any advantage to hormonal therapy in terms of survival?

Androgen Action

The exact methods by which androgens promote their characteristic actions on tissue such as the prostate are still being elucidated. Briefly, androgen-dependent tissues derive their sources of androgen from either the testes or the adrenals. Under the influence of pituitary-derived hormones both the testes and the adrenals produce androgens. The testes produce more than 95% of the major circulating powerful androgen, testosterone. The adrenals produce large quantities of the weak androgens, androstenedione and dehydroepiandrosterone, but these steroids are generally not considered to be significantly stimulating to the prostate (Walsh 1975). In the blood, testosterone is bound tightly to TEBG, a specific carrier protein, and albumin. Only the unbound or "free" fraction is available for intracellular use. Testosterone passively diffuses into the prostate, where it is converted by the cytoplasmic membrane bound enzyme 5α-reductase into dihydrotestosterone. It is this molecule that is the active intracellular androgen (Anderson and Liao 1968). It binds specifically and with high affinity to an intracellular receptor protein. This receptor steroid complex then undergoes a transformation which allows it to interact with the genome and then initiates transcription and protein production (Baxter and Funder 1979). The aim of hormonal therapy is to prevent this final step. This can be accomplished by any method that interferes with either androgen production or utilization.

Methods of Androgen Ablation

Orchiectomy

Although many patients and some physicians find castration psychologically unacceptable, this treatment remains the standard to which all other forms of therapy have been compared. Bilateral orchiectomy rapidly and directly removes the source of the majority of the powerful circulating androgen, testosterone. It can be performed with little morbidity and mortality in virtually any patient. It is also associated with few significant side-effects except for loss of libido and impotence. This form of therapy obviates any question of therapeutic compliance.

Estrogen Therapy

The administration of estrogens reduces the pituitary release of luteinizing hormone, thereby removing the central stimulation for the testes to produce androgens. Castrate levels of testosterone are usually achieved by 7–21 days when oral doses of 3 mg and greater of diethylstilbestrol (DES) or its equivalent are delivered (Shearer et al. 1973). Furthermore, the serum carrier protein for androgens, TEBG, is raised by estrogen therapy, thereby decreasing the amount of free or "active" hormone in the serum. Also there is the possibility that estrogens may themselves have cytotoxic effects on prostatic cancer. Although appealing to many, this theory has yet to be substantiated. Low levels of estrogen receptors have been demonstrated in the prostate, which would provide a direct site for action of estrogens, but their significance remains unknown (Ekman et al. 1983). A correlation between prostatic tumor estrogen receptor content and response to estrogen therapy has not been demonstrated.

Estrogen therapy obviates any surgical procedure. Although this mode of treatment is simple, the side-effects of this medical form of castration are numerous. Immediate side-effects consist of nausea, vomiting, headaches, and fluid retention. Long-term side-effects consist of gynecomastia, loss of libido and potency, and an increase in serious cardiovascular events. The latter is of great significance since mortality due to thromboembolic events has been reported to be 300% higher than in age-matched populations not on estrogen therapy (Glashan and Robinson 1981). Indeed, the initial doubts about the benefits of hormonal therapy arose when the first VACURG study (1967) found that stage D patients treated with 5 mg DES daily had similar survival data to those treated with delayed therapy. This observation has been attributed by many to a marked increase in early cardiovascular mortality that perhaps obscured potential later cancer deaths. Three milligrams of DES per day has been shown to be as effective as castration although the incidence of side-effects is higher (Blackard et al. 1970). The second Veterans Administration study demonstrated that a daily dose of 1 mg DES, in spite of not consistently reducing serum androgen levels to the castrate level, led to similar clinical results as were achieved with 5 mg, without the associated side-effects. Other estrogenic agents are available but they offer no advantage over DES (Table 11.1).

Table 11.1. Estrogens used in treating prostatic cancer

Agent	Mechanism of action	Usual dose
Diethylstilbestrol	Pituitary inhibition ?Direct cytotoxic effect	1–5 mg daily (oral)
Ethinylestradiol (Estinyl)	Pituitary inhibition ?Direct cytotoxic effect	0.05 mg once–twice daily
Chlorotrianisene (Tace)	Pituitary inhibition	12 mg twice daily (oral)
Premarin	Pituitary inhibition	5–15 mg daily (oral)
Stilbestrol diphosphate (Honvol)	Pituitary inhibition	100–1000 mg daily (oral) 250–500 mg daily (i.v.)

Estramustine	Pituitary inhibition
	Cytotoxic effect
	  blocks cytoplasmic
	  estramustine receptor
		14 mg/kg/day (oral)

Estramustine has been advocated as an estrogenic agent that has the added benefit of providing a nitrogen mustard moiety to effect a cytotoxic action at the tumor site. More recently estramustine has been demonstrated to bind to protein receptors within the cytoplasm of prostatic cells and to inhibit growth. Nonetheless, an EORTC prospective trial that randomized patients with previously untreated advanced disease to either 3 mg DES daily or 280 mg estramustine per day for 8 weeks followed by 140 mg twice a day failed to show any significant difference between these two treatments (protocol 30762) as regards response of metastases, response of the primary tumor, distant progression, and overall survival and death due to cancer.

Other Drug Therapies

In view of the side-effects of estrogen therapy a variety of drug therapies have been devised that do not rely on these agents.

Luteinizing Hormone Releasing Hormone and Its Analogues

In 1971, Schally and co-workers successfully isolated, and described the molecular structure of native luteinizing hormone releasing hormone (Pyro-Glu-His-Trp-Ser-Tyr-Gly-Leu-Arg-Pro-Gly-NH2) and subsequently synthesized this hormone (Matsuo et al. 1971). Luteinizing hormone releasing hormone (LHRH) is a linear decapeptide with an active center at amino acids 2–3 and important conformational sites at amino acids 1, 6, and 10. Substitution of the sixth amino acid, glycine, by a variety of D amino acids and deletion of the tenth amino-amide group results in a molecule with a substantial increase in affinity and binding characteristics to LHRH receptors in the brain. These analogues are capable of releasing 15–120 times more luteinizing hormone than the native hormone.

While these agents cause an abrupt increase in LH release and subsequent sex steroid release in both males and females after acute administration (termed the flare period), paradoxically during chronic administration sex steroid levels fall to the castrate level. The exact mechanism of this action is not clear but it probably results from alterations in the central feedback control of LH release, desensitization of the gonad to LH by reduction in gonadal LH receptor sites, and direct gonadal steroid enzyme inhibition. These agents have no effect on adrenal androgen production.

In a recent North American trial 199 patients with previously untreated metastatic prostatic cancer were randomly assigned to receive either 1 mg of a six-leucine LHRH analogue (Lupron, TAP pharmaceutical, North Chicago, Ill.) subcutaneously daily or 3 mg DES per day (The Leuprolide Study Group 1984). Time to first evidence of progression was not different between the two groups. At 1 year the number of patients alive in both groups was also similar. Actuarial survival at 1 year was 87% for those patients treated with the LHRH analogue and 78% for those treated with DES. These rates are not significantly different. The LHRH analogues are not free of side-effects but these tend to be of a minor nature. There were fewer serious cardiovascular complications and incidents of gynecomastia in the LHRH analogue-treated group than in the estrogen-treated group. The long-term side-effects of Lupron therapy were remarkably few; however, they did include episodes of profuse flushing, occasional irritation at the injection site, and impotence. The DES-treated group had a significantly greater incidence of pedal edema, deep vein thromboses, myocardial infarctions, and strokes, as well as gynecomastia and impotence. Although several patients reported an initial increase in bone pain corresponding to the physiologic flare period (days 4–10) induced by Lupron, this tended to resolve spontaneously. Because of the possibility of inducing spinal cord injury during the flare period in those patients with vertebral metastases, several strategies, such as the initial use of antiandrogens or estrogens, have been devised to reduce the impact of this period. In spite of these maneuvers the use of LHRH analogues in patients with any form of neurologic deficit suggesting tumor compression is clearly dangerous and unwarranted. European studies using another LHRH analogue (Buserelin) have confirmed these results and demonstrated that these agents are capable of sustaining their physiologic effects on androgen production for periods greater than 2 years (Tolis et al. 1980). These agents represent an advance in the drug-related hormonal treatment of prostatic cancer. This is not because they are any more effective than estrogen therapy but because their toxicity profile is considerably better. All of the presently available LHRH analogues appear clinically equivalent.

Since the LHRH analogues are small proteins they are degraded if taken orally. Thus earlier preparations were given either by daily subcutaneous injection or nasal spray (e.g., Buserelin, Hoechst and Nafarelin, Syntex). Buserelin is poorly absorbed (<5%) by the nasal mucosa and must be administered as many as six times per day to suppress testosterone production adequately. Nevertheless, when taken as directed it is effective. With Nafarelin this absorption problem has been overcome by inclusion of a bile salt in the carrier solution which is mildly irritating to the nasal mucosa. This has raised the degree of absorption to approximately 20% and has decreased the necessity for multiple insufflations to two per day.

Depot injections are now the main alternative method of administering these analogues. Zoladex (ICI) is an LHRH analogue that is embedded in a *d-l* lactide-glycolide co-polymer medium. When the Zoladex pellet is deposited via a 14 gauge needle subcutaneously, 3.60 mg of the analogue is released over approximately 1 month (the average daily release is 125 µg/day). Several trials have now demonstrated that this mode of administration reduces and maintains serum testosterone at the castrate level for at least 1 month, and early results show this treatment to be equivalent to surgical castration. A new preparation promises to prolong the duration of action to 3 months. Another form of administration which seems to be equally useful is the intramuscular injection of a micro-encapsulated form of a *d*-6-tryptophan LHRH analogue. The period between administrations of this compound is 5 weeks.

Antiandrogens

The antiandrogens are a class of compound that peripherally inhibit the action of dihydrotestosterone, usually by interfering with receptor steroid binding or nuclear translocation. They generally fall into two classes of agent: steroidal and nonsteroidal.

Steroidal. The steroidal agents are typified by cyproterone acetate, medroxy-progesterone acetate, and Megace (megestrol)—progestational agents that have both central and peripheral effects. The central effects cause a decrease in luteinizing hormone release, thereby decreasing testosterone production. At the target site these agents are potent competitors with dihydrotestosterone for cytosolic receptor sites. In addition progestational agents are competitors of testosterone for 5α-reductase. These agents thus have the dual potential to eliminate androgen activity from both testicular and nontesticular sources. However, small-scale clinical trials with Megace have demonstrated an escape from the central effects of this agent after several months of use, leaving only the peripheral effects to yield active hormonal therapy. Furthermore, the anti-androgenic qualities of Megace are limited (Geller and Albert 1983). Few significant side-effects are noted with this treatment.

Cyproterone acetate is a significantly more potent antiandrogen than is Megace. It too has been reported to lose some degree of central effectiveness with chronic administration. In clinical use its strong peripheral activity may compensate for this phenomenon. The EORTC has recently conducted a randomized phase III type trial comparing oral cyproterone acetate (CPA), intramuscular medroxyprogesterone acetate (MPA), and DES in patients with advanced prostatic cancer (protocol 30761). The 5-year survival of these groups was 38%, 32%, and 14% for DES, CPA, and MPA respectively. The survival of those patients receiving DES or CPA was significantly better than that of those receiving MPA. At 3 years the rate of progression was 55%, 80%, and 90% for DES, CPA, and MPA respectively. DES was significantly better than either CPA or MPA in retarding progression. However, cardiovascular toxicity was greater in the DES group (35%) as compared with the CPA (10%) and MPA (19%) groups. The risk of severe cardiovascular complications was highest during the first 6 months of treatment. Increasing age, body weight greater than 75 kg, and the presence of preexisting cardiovascular disease represented adverse factors in the development of cardiovascular toxicity.

Nonsteroidal. Nonsteroidal antiandrogens such as flutamide have little central effect but do have potent peripheral effects. They are noted to be effective clinically with minimal side-effects. Since serum testosterone concentrations do not decrease, potency is usually preserved. However, in younger patients in whom maintenance of potency may be deemed more important, serum testosterone has often been noted to increase to levels 1.5–2 times their initial values, thus calling into question the adequacy of the competitive androgen blockade. Furthermore, recent animal studies have suggested that flutamide does not institute complete androgen blockade even in the presence of normal serum testosterone concentrations (Burton and Trachtenberg 1986). The drug does have few side-effects; they are confined to diarrhea (10%–15%), gynecomastia (25%–50%), and flushing (15%–30%) (Burton and Trachtenberg 1986). Several investigators have been impressed by the ability of this agent to induce hormonal remission with only minimal side-effects and feel that these observations justify large-scale trials (Sogani et al. 1983).

A similar and equipotent nonsteroidal antiandrogen, Anandron (RU 23908, Roussel Pharmaceuticals), has proved equally effective. Its toxicity profile is complicated by several additional minor problems (viz. difficulties with dark adaptation, and alcohol intolerance) and several reported cases of severe idiopathic pulmonitis. At this time the nonsteroidal antiandrogens have not been approved for clinical use in the United States.

Inhibitors of Steroidogenesis

Inhibitors of steroidogenesis such as aminoglutethimide, spironolactone, and ketoconazole impair the production of androgen, usually by inhibition of multiple enzymes in the steroid synthetic pathways. Ketoconazole impairs activity of cytochrome P450-dependent enzymes. These include 17-20 desmolase (catalyzes the conversion of 17OH-progesterone to androstenedione) and 17-hydroxylase (catalyzes the conversion of progesterone to 17OH-progesterone). Ketoconazole induces a very rapid and sustained decrease in both testicular and adrenal androgen production. Castrate levels of androgens are usually achieved within 4–8 h after an initial 400 mg oral dose. Ketoconazole has been used alone in the primary treatment of metastatic prostatic cancer and as an adjunct to the LHRH analogues to prevent the physiologic flare and to reduce adrenal androgens. Although apparently effective, these agents have not as yet been subjected to large-scale trials to determine their long-term clinical safety and effectiveness (Trachtenberg and Pont 1984). Ketoconazole is associated with a 1 in 16 000 incidence of severe but reversible hepatotoxicity. In addition its short serum half-life necessitates multiple daily dosing (no less than every 8 h). Its major side-effect is nausea, which can be seen in as many as 20% of patients. Other less common side-effects are asthenia, which may be related to a mild degree of glucocorticoid insufficiency, and dry skin and mucous membranes. Because of its effects on adrenal androgen production, this agent has also been used in the treatment of patients who have already failed conventional testicular hormonal ablation therapy. There have been several independent reports suggesting that there is marked subjective response to this treatment in approximately half of patients, largely in the form of relief of bone pain. The dose administered is usually in the order of 200–300 mg every 8 h. There is mounting evidence that this response is not only mediated by further diminution of androgen levels but also by the effects of ketoconazole on other cytochrome P450-dependent intracellular activities. In vitro work on androgen-independent human prostatic cancer cell lines (PC 3 and DU 145) shows a significant cytostatic effect of ketoconazole in clinical therapeutic concentrations. Newer analogues of ketoconazole with more specific sites of action, minimal side-effects, and much longer duration of action are presently being evaluated.

Success and Failure of Hormonal Therapy

Escape from the effects of hormonal therapy are usually ascribed to the presence of preexisting clones of cells that are not androgen dependent (Isaacs et al. 1978). After the destruction of the hormone-dependent cells by hormonal therapy, the remaining hormone-independent cells continue to grow and eventually overwhelm and kill the host. The proportion and rate of growth of these cells are variable. This observation seems apparent from the survival statistics of patients with stage D disease treated by hormonal therapy. Ten percent survive less than 6 months, 50% survive 3 years, and 10% survive 10 years or more (Scott et al. 1980).

Some investigators have felt that progression is caused by a second class of cells that are not hormone independent but rather dependent on only small amounts of androgen. This amount of androgen might potentially be provided by adrenal androgens. Following this hypothesis Huggins and Scott performed bilateral adrenalectomies in 1945 on four patients who had failed primary hormonal therapy. All four patients died shortly thereafter from adrenal insufficiency. After glucocorticoid replacement became available in 1951, bilateral adrenalectomy or hypophysectomy was performed in several series of patients with failed primary therapy. The results of these studies were inconclusive but in general tended to show a short-term subjective improvement that did not alter survival (Brendler 1973).

In 1982 Labrie reintroduced the concept of total androgen ablation. Furthermore, he suggested that this form of therapy be instituted at the initiation of primary hormonal therapy. He paired an LHRH analogue (Buserelin, t-butyl-6 serine-1-9 nonapeptide LHRH) and an antiandrogen (RU 23908, Anandron). The advantages of this combination rest in the immediate androgen blockade instituted by the antiandrogen. This blocks the physiologic increase in testosterone caused by the LHRH analogue and also blocks any effects of adrenal androgens. In a pilot trial of nine patients with advanced prostatic cancer (stage C or D) on this regime, Labrie noted a remarkably low rate of progression. He has now enlarged his initial series to include 131 patients with previously untreated stage D prostatic cancer (Labrie et al. 1982, 1985). This trial is uncontrolled and not randomized. Nonetheless, using NPCP criteria for response, Labrie claims that only six patients in this group have relapsed at 1 year. This is in marked contrast to quoted historical trials of hormonal therapy in stage D prostatic cancer which have demonstrated 1-year rates of progression of 25%–40%. Labrie has claimed that the excellent results of his ongoing study justify his reluctance to perform a randomized comparative trial of his form of hormonal therapy versus conventional methods of testicular androgen ablation. Since these observations are of paramount importance in substantiating his findings, several collaborative efforts [the Intergroup Study—NIH, comparing leuprolide plus placebo vs leuprolide plus flutamide; the EORTC study, comparing cyproterone acetate plus orchiectomy vs DES vs orchiectomy; the Roussel study group (France North, France South, and Canada), comparing Anandron plus orchiectomy, orchiectomy plus placebo, and Buserelin plus Anandron] are now underway to determine the efficacy of this mode of treatment. Communications from the latter two of these groups have failed to substantiate Labrie's claims of increased 1-year survival or decreased rate of progression at 1 year. Indeed, the findings of these groups indicated no difference in the number of patients with disease progression or in their survival at 1 year, whether patients were treated with conventional or total androgen ablation (Beland et al. 1986; Schroder et al. 1986; Trachtenberg and Zadra 1986).

Summary

At this time no agent has shown superiority over any other in initiating and maintaining remissions. The choice of appropriate treatment must thus rest on the perceived need to initiate therapy and the treatment that will effect a remission with the minimum of side-effects. Bilateral orchiectomy is both clinically effective and associated with minimal long-term side-effects. As such, orchiectomy must remain the hormonal treatment of choice for those patients accepting castration. Furthermore, because of the unsurpassed rapidity of its action it is also the treatment of choice when therapy is acutely needed as an adjunct to other more distinct measures in the treatment of ureteral obstruction or spinal cord compression.

Because of the proven high incidence of cardiovascular complications, chronic use of DES in doses of 3 mg per day or more should be avoided. One milligram of DES per day may, however, be an appropriate compromise between effectiveness and minimal side-effects. Of those new agents currently available, the LHRH analogues have been subjected to the most extensive trials and have clearly shown themselves to be both effective and associated with minimal side-effects. Care must be taken to avoid those patients who might sustain any permanent effects of the flare period. Because of the necessity for daily subcutaneous injections, patient selection for this treatment should be rigorous as compliance may be a significant problem. This problem may cease as newer formulations of this medication become available in either nasal sprays or depot preparations.

The nonsteroidal antiandrogen flutamide may have a place in treating individuals who are unwilling to accept impotence as a consequence of hormonal therapy. Since serum testosterone levels do not decline and may even rise, these patients must be watched closely for escape from the antiandrogen blockade. The use of this drug as a single agent must be tempered with the realization that failure of therapy may be the price paid for continued potency. Only large-scale comparative clinical trials will determine the appropriate use of this agent.

In view of the poor results of hormonal therapy alone, the concept of hormonal therapy coupled to adjunctive chemotherapy has proved appealing to many who treat metastatic prostatic cancer. Theoretically hormonal therapy should eliminate those cells that are androgen dependent while cytotoxic agents should eliminate the hormone-independent cells. The National Prostatic Cancer Group has made an extensive investigation into this possibility. One protocol compared (a) standard hormonal therapy (DES or orchiectomy), (b) standard therapy with cyclophosphamide and 5-fluorouracil, and (c) Emcyt (protocol 1300). No difference was noted in the distribution of objective response at 1 year. Similarly there was no difference in survival. Another procotol (1700) compared two forms of hormonal therapy alone or with methotrexate. Results of this trial are not as yet available but there is no early suggestion that the latter arm is superior. These data suggest that adjunctive therapy is not presently capable of extending the effects of hormonal therapy alone.

Optimal Time for Initiation of Therapy

For those patients who present with severe bone pain or compromised lower urinary tracts due to compression by tumor, hormonal therapy has proven extremely effective. There thus is no controversy in initiating therapy at this stage of the disease. For those patients with metastatic disease who are asymptomatic at presentation, the introduction of hormonal therapy remains controversial. Does the early introduction of hormonal therapy in any way delay progression of the disease or increase survival time? Initial studies of patient survival before and after the introduction of hormonal therapy suggested that this treatment indeed prolonged life. This finding confirmed the intuitive beliefs of the early practitioners of hormonal therapy. Vest and Frazier (1946) compared 74 patients with either localized or metastatic prostatic cancer treated with bilateral orchiectomy with a similar number and type of patients left untreated in a prior decade. They noted a marked increase in the duration of survival of those patients treated with hormone therapy. Nesbit and Plumb (1946) compared 795 patients treated prior to the advent of endocrine treatment with 75 patients treated by bilateral orchiectomy or estrogens. They compared the survival of those patients in these groups who had evidence of metastatic disease. Fifty percent of the untreated patients were dead at 1 year while only 17% of the treated patients fared similarly; at 2 years 82% of the untreated group were dead, as opposed to 50% of the treated patients. Nesbit and Baum (1950) compared the survival of 263 patients treated with hormonal therapy with survival in the untreated group of the Nesbit and Plumb series mentioned above. At 36 months the treated group had a 34% survival rate compared with 11% for the untreated group. At 5 years the treatment group had 17% survival as compared with 6% in the control group. The above investigators therefore concluded that hormonal therapy significantly "prolonged survival" and should be instituted at the time of diagnosis.

Although these studies seemed to support the view that hormonal therapy prolonged life, they suffered from the fact that the groups compared were from different eras of medical treatment and were never randomized. The first serious questioning of the value of hormonal therapy arose with the first VACURG trial of 1967. This study randomized 1903 patients with stage C and D disease to be treated with placebo, orchiectomy, 5 mg DES per day, or orchiectomy and DES. In stage D disease there was no difference in survival. The study design allowed for cross-over of patients from their initial assigned group although the results were reported by the initial group. All of the stage D patients who had been in the control group ultimately were treated by hormonal therapy. Thus this group represented delayed hormonal therapy. In the DES-treated groups there were fewer cancer deaths. There were, however, more cardiovascular-related deaths in the first year of treatment in this group, and such deaths may have masked cancer-related deaths that might have ultimately occurred with time. Although this study has been subject to significant and valid criticisms, two clear conclusions can be drawn from it. Firstly, delayed hormonal therapy does not decrease survival when compared with early introduction of hormonal therapy. Secondly, DES therapy is associated with a significant increase in cardiovascular morbidity and mortality.

Lepor et al. (1982) reviewed the histories of 65 patients at the Johns Hopkins Hospital with advanced prostatic cancer before the introduction of hormonal therapy (1937–1940) and compared their survival with that of 47 similar patients treated hormonally in 1942 and 1943. After accounting for changing patterns of survival from one decade to the next, these authors could not demonstrate any significant survival benefit for hormonal therapy.

These later studies suggest that hormonal therapy should be reserved for those patients who will clearly benefit from it, viz. patients with pain or obstructive conditions. For asymptomatic patients the risk–benefit ratio of hormonal therapy should be carefully examined as the benefits from early initiation of therapy are not clear. The patient who is asymptomatic and sexually potent and desires to maintain his potency should be carefully followed and treated with flutamide (if available) or treatment should be withheld. If the patient is asymptomatic and impotent then hormonal therapy may be started using either an LHRH analogue or orchiectomy.

The preceding discussion has concentrated on the treatment of patients with D_2 disease. As controversial as the choice of appropriate treatment of this disease is, the correct therapy of D_1 is even more difficult. Hormonal therapy has been used as sole therapy, as adjunctive therapy to radical prostatectomy or radiation therapy, or has been delayed until evidence of disease progression. Since no clear conclusions can be drawn from these studies we suggest that the treatment outlined in the preceding paragraph be followed for patients in stage D_1 as well as D_2.

Acknowledgment. The author wishes to thank the EORTC and the NPCP, who kindly provided clinical trials data.

References

Anderson KM, Liao S (1968) Selective retention of dihydrotestosterone by prostatic nuclei. Nature 219:277–279

Baxter JD, Funder JW (1979) Hormone receptors. N Engl J Med 301:1149–1161

Beland J, Elhilali M (1986) A prospective randomized trial of total androgen ablation in metastatic prostatic cancer (abstr). Proceedings of the Second International Conference on Prostate Cancer. Paris

Blackard CE, Doe RP, Mellinger GT et al. (1970) Incidence of cardiovascular disease and death in patients receiving diethylstilbestrol for carcinoma of the prostate. Cancer 26:249–256

Brendler H (1973) Adrenalectomy and hypophysectomy for prostatic cancer. Urology 2:99–102

Burton S, Trachtenberg J (1986) Effectiveness of antiandrogens in the rat. J Urol 136(4):932–935

Ekman P, Greene GL, Jensen EV, Walsh PC (1983) Estrogen receptors in human prostate: evidence for multiple binding sites. J Clin Endocrinol Metab 57:166–176

Geller J, Albert JD (1983) Comparison of various hormonal therapies for prostatic cancer. Semin Oncol 10(4) [Suppl 4] 34–41

Glashan RW, Robinson MRG (1981) Cardiovascular complications in the treatment of prostatic cancer. Br J Urol 53:624–647

Huggins C, Hodges CV (1941) Studies on prostatic cancer: I. The effect of castration, of estrogen and of androgen injection on serum phosphatases in metastatic carcinoma of the prostate. Cancer Res 1:293–297

Huggins C, Stevens RE, Hodges CV (1941) Studies on prostatic cancer: II. The effects of castration on advanced carcinoma of the prostate gland. Arch Surg 43:209–223

Isaacs JT, Heston WDW, Weissman RM, Coffey DS (1978) Animal models of the hormone-sensitive and insensitive prostatic adenocarcinoma, Dunning R-3327-H, R-3327-HI, and R3327-AT. Cancer Res 38:4353–4359

Labrie F, Dupont A, Belanger A et al. (1982) New hormonal therapy in prostatic cancer: combined treatment with an LHRH agonist and an antiandrogen. Clin Invest Med 5:267–275

Labrie F, Dupont A, Belanger A et al. (1985) Antiandrogens and LHRH agonists in the treatment of prostatic cancer. Medicine/Science 1:435

Lepor H, Ross A, Walsh PC (1982) The influence of hormonal therapy on survival of men with advanced prostatic cancer. J Urol 128:335–340

Matsuo H, Baba Y, Nair RMG, Arimura A, Schally AV (1971) Structure of the porcine Lh and FSH releasing hormone 1. The proposed amino acid sequence. Biochem Biophys Res Comm 43:1334–1339

Nesbit RM, Baum WC (1950) Endocrine control of prostatic carcinoma: clinical and statistical survey of 1818 cases. JAMA 143:1317–1320

Nesbit RM, Plumb RT (1946) Prostatic carcinoma: a follow-up of 795 patients treated prior to the endocrine era and a comparison of survival rates between these and patients treated by endocrine therapy. Surgery 20:263–272

Schroder FH, Klijn JG, de Jong FH (1986) Metastatic cancer of the prostate managed by Buserelin acetate versus Buserelin acetate plus cyproterone acetate. Proceedings of the Annual Meeting of the American Urological Association, New York. J Urol 135:202A

Scott WW, Menon M, Walsh PC (1980) Hormonal therapy of prostatic cancer. Cancer 45:1929–1936

Shearer RJ, Hendry WF, Sommerville IF et al. (1973) Plasma testosterone: an accurate monitor of hormone treatment in prostatic cancer. Br J Urol 45:668–677

Sogani PC, Vagawal MR, Whitmore WF Jr (1983) Experience with flutamide in patients with advanced prostatic cancer without prior endocrine therapy. Cancer 54:744–750

Spirnak JP, Resnick MI (1983) Carcinoma of the prostate: early endocrine therapy is best. Semin Urol 1:269–279

The Leuprolide Study Group (1984) Leuprolide vrs DES in the initial therapy of advanced prostatic cancer: a randomized prospective trial. N Engl J Med 311:1281–1286

Tolis G, Menta A, Kinch R, Comaru-Schally AM, Schally AV (1980) Suppression of sex steroids by an LH-Rh analogue in man. Clin Res 28:676A

Trachtenberg J, Pont A (1984) Ketoconazole in the treatment of metastatic prostatic cancer. Lancet II:433–435

Trachtenberg J, Zadra J (1986) Total androgen ablation therapy in the treatment of advanced prostatic cancer. Proceedings of the Annual Meeting of the American Urological Association, New York. J Urol 135:201A

Vest SA, Frazier TH (1946) Survival following castration for prostatic cancer. J Urol 56:97–111

Veterans Administration Cooperative Urological Research Group (1967) Treatment and survival of patients with cancer of the prostate. Surg Gynecol Obstet 124:1011–1017

Walsh PC (1975) Physiologic basis for hormonal therapy in carcinoma of the prostate. Urol Clin North Am 2:125–140

Chapter 12

Chemotherapy of Prostatic Cancer

R.P. Huben and G.P. Murphy

Introduction

Optimal management of patients with hormone-refractory prostatic cancer remains problematic. While there is some acceptance of the results of numerous clinical studies which have reported that chemotherapy is superior to further hormonal approaches or other supportive measures as a treatment option for hormone-refractory prostatic cancer, there persists a "general pessimism" about the use of chemotherapy in this patient population (Scott et al. 1976; Murphy et al. 1977; Logathetis et al. 1983; Torti 1983). This pessimism may be caused in part by the variability in clinical course of metastatic prostatic cancer and the problems in determining response to therapy in a systemic stage of disease which is particularly difficult to quantify. Since there is reason to question the overall impact of hormonal therapy in advanced prostatic cancer, it is not surprising that the impact of chemotherapy, which may cause a far less dramatic response, is all the more controversial.

Some physicians have chosen to dismiss chemotherapy for prostatic cancer from consideration. Patients considering entry into a treatment program will not infrequently state "My doctor said chemotherapy doesn't work for prostatic cancer." This opinion represents one extreme in the spectrum of attitudes and approaches to advanced prostatic cancer once hormone resistance develops, but it illustrates the underlying feelings and beliefs of a number of investigators and practitioners alike. However, it is critical that urologists and others involved in the care of patients with advanced prostatic cancer have an understanding of the disease (Torti and Carter 1980; deKernion and Lindner 1984). Regardless of the form of therapy, median survival from discovery of distant metastases to death is 1–3 years (Torti and Carter 1980). What treatment, if any, is indicated when hormonal therapy no longer controls the disease? Second-line endocrine manipulation is still widely practiced, although it can be expected to offer little to the patient who fails initial hormonal therapy (deKernion and Lindner 1984). There is increasing acceptance of the view that chemotherapy is generally superior to secondary hormonal maneuvers in terms of palliative response as well as survival, and that it should therefore be used next in the sequence of therapy (Torti 1983). Yet chemotherapy, until the last few years, had rarely been studied systematically in prostatic cancer. A number of reasons for this have been suggested (Murphy 1979; Torti and Carter 1980). Because of inherent problems in staging and determining response to treatment in prostatic cancer, this tumor is often excluded from critical early studies of promising agents (Torti and Carter 1980). A dramatic response to hormonal therapy may dampen enthusiasm for further treatment approaches, and such responses may select out relapsing patients with extensive disease and poor performance status (Murphy 1979; Torti and Carter 1980). Another consideration is the fact that prostatic cancer often occurs in older men with other major health problems, and the unfounded fear that treatment may be worse than the disease (Murphy 1979).

Factors involved in patient selection for a particular treatment are obviously critical to the outcome of studies of the agents utilized. Previous treatment and extent of tumor burden are of recognized prognostic significance, as are performance status and the presence or absence of pain at the initiation of therapy (Slack and Murphy 1983; Murphy 1984). Previous treatment may have consisted of pelvic or palliative focal radiation therapy, which may significantly enhance toxicity of myelosuppressive chemotherapeutic agents (Murphy et al. 1977; Ihde et al. 1980). Prior chemotherapy may also affect the likelihood of response, since early cross-over studies of a number of agents suggest that failure to respond to the first agent lessens the probability of response to a second agent (Scott et al. 1976; Slack et al. 1980b). Why does a patient choose to undergo chemotherapy? A study conducted at three cancer centers examined interactions in the consent process for chemotherapy and determined that patients rely heavily on physician's advice in consenting to therapy (Penman et al. 1984). Primary reasons for accepting treatment were trust in the physician, belief that treatment would help, and fear the disease would get worse without it.

Response Criteria in Advanced Prostatic Cancer

Defining response to treatment is perhaps the most difficult issue in systemic prostatic cancer, and a major cause of the high variability in reported response rates to the same or similar chemotherapy regimens (Torti and Carter 1980). Since this topic is the subject of later sections, response criteria will be discussed briefly. The first major problem concerns the role of bone scans in assessing response to therapy. Bone scans are qualitative rather than accurate quantitative methods of following change in metastatic prostatic cancer (Yagoda 1983). Bone scan changes are evaluable but not measurable. While this limits the sensitivity of bone scans in determining response to therapy, serial bone scans have been reported to indicate accurately the course of prostatic cancer (Fitzpatrick et al. 1978; Chisholm et al. 1982). An alternative view is that only patients with bidimensionally measurable soft tissue lesions are appropriate subjects when response to treatment is the end point of study (Yagoda et al. 1979; Citrin et al. 1984). But such selectivity is usually impractical, since only 10% or less of patients may be evaluable by these standards (Yagoda 1983; Citrin et al. 1984).

The potential bias in studying patients with extensive soft tissue lesions, which may be associated with poorer survival and less responsiveness to chemo-therapy, has also been recognized (Yagoda et al. 1979).

The most widely accepted response criteria in the study of advanced prostatic cancer are those of the National Prostatic Cancer Project (NPCP), which have been extensively described (Murphy and Slack 1980). Criticism of NPCP response criteria has centered around the significance of stabilization of disease as a response category. Early NPCP trials demonstrated convincingly that both survival and duration of response in stable patients paralleled those of partial responders, which strengthens the argument that stabilization is a valid measure of tumor response (Torti and Carter 1980; Slack et al. 1980a; Slack et al. 1984). Others contend that stabilization is merely a reflection of an inherently longer survival due to a more slowly growing tumor rather than a response to therapy (Herr 1982; Yagoda 1983; Beynon and Chisholm 1984). Despite this continuing controversy, the NPCP response criteria represent a major contribution in the systematic investigation of chemotherapy for metastatic prostatic cancer in that they allow comparison of treatment results by established parameters.

Chemotherapy

Both in theory and practice, the ideal approach to chemotherapy for a particular tumor is identification of active cytotoxic agents, followed by the combination of agents to produce additive or synergistic responses. While combination chemotherapy generally produces a higher response rate than do single agents in some tumor systems, many authors have noted that this has not been demonstrated convincingly in studies of prostatic cancer (Torti and Carter 1980; Schmidt 1983; deKernion and Lindner 1984). The results of single agent chemotherapy for prostatic cancer have been the subject of several recent reviews (Torti and Carter 1980; Slack and Murphy 1983; Murphy 1984; deKernion and Lindner 1984).

Three conditions are thought to justify a program of adjuvant chemotherapy: (a) the disease, untreated, should carry a poor prognosis; (b) the agents used should have demonstrated antitumor activity; (c) complications from treatment should be low, i.e., there should be an acceptable risk–benefit ratio (deVere White et al. 1983). A partial update of the results of the clinical trials of the National Prostatic Cancer Project (NPCP) and other recent studies of chemotherapy for prostatic cancer will be reviewed in an attempt to address these concerns.

Clinical Trials

NPCTG Trials

Tables 12.1 and 12.2 summarize the results with single agent and combination chemotherapy in the National Prostatic Cancer Treatment Group (NPCTG) trials in patients failing hormonal treatment with or without prior radiation. The reasons for the conduct of these protocols, as initially described, were to

Table 12.1. Summary of results of chemotherapy in NPCP clinical trials in patients with hormone-refractory tumors without prior radiation

Protocol/study period	Agents	Response rate[a]
100	Cyclophosphamide	46%
(7/73–7/75)	5-Fluorouracil	36%
	Standard therapy	19%
300	Cyclophosphamide	26%
(4/75–6/77)	Imidazole–carboxamide (DTIC)	27%
	Procarbazine	14%
700	Cyclophosphamide	35%
(5/77–4/79)	Hydroxyurea	15%
	Methyl-CCNU	30%
1100	Emcyt	34%
(4/79–12/81)	Methotrexate	41%
	Cis-platinum	36%
1600	Streptozotocin	
(1/82–9/85)	Stilphostrol	
	Megace	Evaluation ongoing
	Megace plus 0.1 mg diethylstilbestrol	

[a]As defined by NPCP criteria.

Table 12.2. Summary of results of chemotherapy in NPCP clinical trials in patients with hormone-refractory tumors and prior radiation

Protocol/study period	Agents	Response rate[a]
200	Estramustine (Emcyt)	30%
(7/74–3/76)	Streptozotocin	52%
	Standard therapy	19%
400	Prednimustine	13%
(3/76–5/77)	Prednimustine plus Emcyt	13%
800	Emcyt	26%
(5/77–4/79)	Vincristine	15%
	Emcyt plus vincristine	24%
1200	Emcyt	18%
(4/79–12/82)	Cis-platinum	21%
	Emcyt plus cis-platinum	33%
1500	Methotrexate	
(1/82–11/85)	Adriamycin plus cyclophosphamide	
	Cis-platinum plus cyclophosphamide plus 5-fluorouracil	Evaluation ongoing

[a]As defined by NPCP criteria.

determine the efficacy of single agents and to examine evaluation of responses. In the studies, regardless of the criteria used, activity or evidence for benefit, both subjective and objective, was found principally with cyclophosphamide, 5-fluorouracil, and Emcyt. Some improvement with the combination of Emcyt and platinum was also seen. This was probably the only situation in these trials which suggested that the combination of agents was of benefit when compared with single agents alone. Methotrexate, at a reduced dosage from that conventionally used, also appears to have some activity, and in current trials use of this agent has been extended to patients with newly diagnosed metastatic disease in combination with diethylstilbestrol or orchiectomy (Scott et al. 1976; Murphy et al. 1979, 1983; Schmidt et al. 1979, 1980; Loening et al. 1981, 1983; deVere White et al. 1983; Slack 1983; Soloway et al. 1983; Schmidt 1984).

Trials following surgery or external radiotherapy for B_2 through D_1 lesions with pelvic lymph node staging and with or without adjuvant chemotherapy using either Emcyt or cyclophosphamide are currently being conducted. Disease-free interval or progression-free survival will be the immediate criterion of response, but further follow-up will be necessary before the results of these adjuvant studies become available.

Other Recent Trials

Combination Chemotherapy

An encouraging report of the effects of chemotherapy for advanced prostatic cancer is that of Ihde et al. (1980), in which 32 patients were treated with a combination of doxorubicin and oral cyclophosphamide. The dosage of doxorubicin was 30 mg/m^2 i.v. on days 1 and 8 and that of cyclophosphamide 100 mg/m^2 p.o. on days 1–14 of each 28-day cycle. Seven patients (32%) were documented to have objective partial responses, and four or 18% of patients had stable disease. Similar to the results of the early NPCP studies, patients with a partial response lived significantly longer than those with no response, and survival of patients with stable disease approximated that of partial responders. While the authors found that no single staging test identified all patients with objective tumor response or progression, a worsening bone scan indicated progressive disease in 11 of 12 patients with such a course. This regimen was fairly well tolerated, except in patients with prior radiation therapy, which was associated with more severe hematologic toxicity.

A high objective response rate to combination chemotherapy in patients with hormone-refractory prostatic cancer was also reported by Logothetis et al. (1983). The agents given were doxorubicin 50 mg/m^2 i.v. on day 1, 5-fluorouracil (5-FU) 750 mg/m^2 i.v. on days 1 and 2, and mitomycin-C 10 mg/m^2 i.v. on day 1 (DMF). Courses were given at increasing intervals which were determined by marrow recovery, with a mean interval of 4–5 weeks between the first and second courses. Objective partial responses were reported in 30 of 62 patients (48%). Of patients with osseous metastases, those with axial skeletal involvement only had a higher response rate (52%) than those with axial and appendicular skeletal involvement (33%); in patients with visceral metastases the highest response rate was in patients with pulmonary parenchymal metastases only (88%), while patients with advanced visceral disease had the expected poorer survival and lower response rate (33%). Patients with axial skeletal metastases only survived significantly longer than patients in the remaining three clinical substages. Responding patients in each clinical category survived longer than nonresponding patients, except for patients with advanced visceral metastases. Although the regimen was delivered to most patients on an outpatient basis, three patients suffered fatal complications of chemotherapy. The authors concluded that the combination of doxorubicin, mitomycin-C, and 5-FU is an effective regimen in hormone-refractory prostatic cancer, although the benefits must be weighed against the toxicity encountered.

The results of a prospective randomized trial of combination chemotherapy versus a single agent were reported by Herr (1982). The combination regimen consisted of methotrexate 45 mg/m^2 and 5-FU 500 mg/^{2} i.v. on days 1 and 8, and cyclophosphamide 75 mg/m^2 orally on days 1–14 of each 28-day cycle. Single drug therapy was chloroethyl-cyclohexy-nitrosourea (CCNU) 130 mg/m^2 orally every 6 weeks. Of the 20 patients receiving combination therapy, three or 15% had partial objective response (as defined by NPCP criteria), and four or 20% had stable disease. There were no partial responses to CCNU and six (30%) patients were stable, resulting in similar overall response rates of 35% and 30% for the two treatment arms. Patients with partial regression or stabilization survived longer than patients whose disease progressed (52 weeks vs 24 weeks, respectively). Subjective improvement occurred in all seven patients who responded to the combination regimen and in three of six patients who were stable on CCNU. The author noted a significant different in the lead time (interval between diagnosis and initiation of chemotherapy) in responders and in those who progressed and suggested that these drug regimens may have selected those patients with slower growing tumors and a longer natural history.

Combination chemotherapy employing three of the most active single agents was reported by Straus et al. (1982). Twenty-three patients who had failed previous hormonal therapy were treated with cyclophosphamide 600 mg/m^2 i.v. and 40 mg/m^2 doxorubicin i.v. on day 1, followed by methotrexate 15 mg/m^2 orally, biweekly days 9 through 20. Courses were repeated every 3 weeks. Response parameters which improved in more than 50% of cases included alkaline and acid phosphatase levels, pain level, performance status, and measurable lung and soft tissue lesions. Seven patients had partial response, seven had measurable response (defined as 50% improvement in all objective parameters except bone scan and enlarged prostate), and eight patients had no response. Mean survivals by response category were 106 weeks, 57 weeks, and 26 weeks, respectively. Pretreatment parameters associated with a significantly decreased survival were age greater than 66 years, increased pain, and poor performance status. Four patients had severe leukopenia and one patient died of sepsis. The authors concluded that response rate and survival in this study compared favorably with previous reports of combination chemotherapy in advanced prostatic cancer.

Stephens et al. (1984) recently reported the results of a Southwest Oncology Group (SWOG) study in which patients were randomized to either a combination of doxorubicin and cyclophosphamide or hydroxyurea as a single agent. There were 43 patients with measurable soft tissue lesions. Objective response was reported in 6 of 19 (32%) on the combination regimen and in only 1 of 24 (4%) randomized to hydroxyurea. The low activity of hydroxyurea in this study confirms the results of an early NPCP study (Protocol 700) in which significant toxicity of hydroxyurea was also reported.

A randomized study in 51 patients with advanced hormone-resistant prostatic cancer comparing a combination of doxorubicin and lomustine (DC) with cyclophosphamide and 5-FU (CF) was recently reported by Page et al. (1985). Regimens consisted of doxorubicin 45 mg/m^2 i.v. and lomustine 450 mg/m^2 i.v. every 3 weeks, or cyclophosphamide 500 mg/m^2 i.v. plus 5-FU 500 mg/m^2 i.v. on days 1 and 8 every 4 weeks. Using NPCP response criteria, the objective partial response rate was 57% for DC and 8% for CF. Stabilization occurred in 14% and 44%, respectively. Overall, there was no significant difference in survival between the two arms, which the authors believed reflected the similar total objective response rate (partial response plus stable disease). Both combinations were well tolerated. Subjectively, the doxorubicin–lomustine combination demonstrated better palliation of pain, but without affording a significant survival advantage over the cyclophosphamide–5-FU combination.

Restriction of response determination to the presence of bidimensionally measurable lesions does not necessarily lessen the variability of results in clinical trials of particular chemotherapy agents in prostatic cancer. Citrin et al. (1984) treated 28 patients with doxorubicin 40–60 mg/m^2 i.v. every 3 weeks for a median duration of 67 days and reported that 25% of patients had a significant reduction (greater than 50%) in bidimensionally measured tumor masses. In a similarly defined group of patients, Scher et al. (1984) reported measurable partial remission in only 2 of 41 (5%) patients receiving doxorubicin on a similar dosage schedule to a total of 500 mg/m^2. The authors of the latter study concluded the doxorubicin has only marginal activity in soft tissue lesion in patients with prostatic cancer. Since the same response criteria were applied to similarly measurable, nonosseous metastases following a similar treatment schedule, the cause of the wide variability in results in these two reports is not readily apparent.

Chemohormonal Therapy

Chemohormonal therapy for prostatic cancer after progression on hormonal therapy, other than in the form of estramustine phosphate, has rarely been studied (Citrin et al. 1983). Since reactivation of prostatic cancer is not associated with a secondary evaluation of plasma testosterone levels, there is little evidence to suggest that further hormonal manipulation is worthwhile after progression occurs on conventional hormonal therapy (deKernion and Lindner 1984). This conclusion is supported by the low response rates to "standard" therapy arms of NPCP Protocols 100 and 200, which consisted in many cases of further hormonal approaches (Scott et al. 1976; Murphy et al. 1977). A pilot study of chemohormonal therapy was recently reported by Citrin et al. (1983). Doxorubicin plus high dose diethylstilbestrol diphosphate (Stilphostrol) was used in 19 patients who had failed hormonal therapy, and the majority of whom had also had secondary hormonal manipulation. Clinical improvement was reported in 10 of 16 (63%) evaluable patients, although toxicity was considerable. Severe myelosuppression was seen in one-third of the patients, and the authors also concluded that the risk of cardiac failure and thromboembolism is significant with this regimen. In the absence of appropriate control arms, which the authors plan, the relative contribution of Stilphostrol to the responses reported is indeterminable.

Because of the limited duration of response to hormonal therapy and questions regarding its impact on patient survival, the early use of both hormonal therapy and chemotherapy is an attractive approach to the management of newly diagnosed metastatic prostatic cancer. Consideration of the nature and implications of tumor cell heterogeneity may also support this approach (Isaacs 1984). Early results of NPCP Protocol 500 suggest some improvement in patient survival with early combination therapy (Murphy et al. 1979). Results of early combined hormonal therapy and chemotherapy were also reported by Servadio et al. (1983). Following diagnosis, bilateral orchiectomy was done and patients then received diethylstilbestrol at 3 mg per day, plus cyclophosphamide 10 mg/kg and 5-FU 10 mg/kg i.v. weekly for a period of 2 years. There was relief of bone pain in 75% of patients, and stabilization or improvement on bone scans in 79%. Encouraging cumulative survivals of 64% at 5 years and 51% at 6 years were reported. Chemotherapy was well tolerated. While there was no control group in this study, the results do suggest that early hormonal therapy in addition to chemotherapy may have a positive effect on patient survival.

Eisenkraft et al. (1984) reported the results of orchiectomy and a four-drug chemotherapy regimen. Agents were oral estramustine phosphate 600 mg/m^2 daily plus cis-platinum 50 mg/m^2, 5-FU 500 mg/m^2, and cyclophosphamide 500 mg/m^2, given i.v. at 3-week intervals. The overall response rate to this regimen was 89%, with an average response duration of 25 months. Analysis of follow-up data also suggested that survival in patients receiving chemotherapy was greater than in patients receiving hormonal therapy alone. Larger, randomized studies are obviously necessary to determine the value of early combination therapy.

Adjuvant Chemotherapy

Another clinical situation in which chemotherapy may be of benefit is in patients with a high likelihood of progression, e.g., patients with limited and resected local lymph node metastases. As previously noted, one-half of these patients will show evidence of progression within 3 years, and 85% will have progressed within 5 years (deVere White et al. 1983). deVere White and co-workers reported the results of a clinical trial of adjuvant chemotherapy in a group of 37 patients with pelvic lymph node metastases. Chemotherapy consisted of cyclophosphamide 750 mg/m^2 and doxorubicin 50 mg/m^2 i.v. every 3 weeks for a 6-month period. Of 12 patients receiving chemotherapy, progression occurred in four, with an average time to progression of 15 months, while in 25 control patients, 12 progressed within an average interval of 12 months. No significant toxicity was reported. These results suggest that early chemotherapy following diagnosis of local nodal involvement may delay the emergence of bone metastases. Protocols 900 and 1000 of the NPCP should help to determine the potential benefit of early adjuvant chemotherapy with lymph node metastases.

Future Approaches

Major areas of research in the development of potential treatment approaches to disseminated prostatic cancer are new hormonal agents, new cytotoxic agents, new combinations of agents based on biochemical modulation, and biologic response modifiers (Creaven et al. 1984). Classes of cytotoxic agents which appear worthy of further investigation include the liquid-soluble antifolates, anthracyclines, nitrosoureas, and platinum analogues (Creaven 1984). Advances in cytotoxic therapy will progress in parallel with our understanding of the cellular and subcellular metabolism of prostatic cancer cells. Immunotherapy of prostatic cancer has been a subject of recent review articles and is at a very early stage (Guinan et al. 1984; Droller 1985). Biologic response modifiers such as interferon are another active research area, but relatively little is known about the likely efficacy of interferon in prostatic cancer. An early study conducted by the National Prostatic Cancer Project (Protocol 2100) using interferon-β (human fibroblast interferon) in a group of 16 patients with hormone-refractory prostatic cancer demonstrated limited efficacy and a high rate of progression during the course of treatment (Bulbul et al. 1986).

An attractive research area is that of early combined hormonal therapy and chemotherapy in newly diagnosed prostatic cancer. An appreciation of the limited benefit of hormonal therapy alone on the ultimate course of prostatic cancer warrants such an approach (Torti and Carter 1980; deKernion and Lindner 1984). In the absence of evidence to suggest that hormone responsiveness is lost after cytotoxic chemotherapy, Yagoda (1983) has suggested that it is not unreasonable to offer chemotherapy alone as initial therapy for metastatic prostatic cancer. Schmidt (1983), however, maintains that the high expected response rate to initial endocrine therapy makes it most difficult to consider any alternative such as chemotherapy alone or in combination with hormone therapy.

Summary

As suggested by the results of early randomized NPCP clinical trials, chemotherapy appears to be superior to other palliative measures in the treatment of hormone-refractory prostatic cancer, both in terms of pain relief and improved survival. Patients who respond to chemotherapy do better than patients who fail to respond. While the opinion persists that this consistent observation reflects the natural history of prostatic cancer rather than true therapeutic benefit, there are frequent reports of both subjective and objective improvement in patients receiving chemotherapy, and the view that chemotherapy "doesn't work" in prostatic cancer is no longer justified. It is only within the future setting of large, randomized clinical trials that the real impact of various treatment approaches on the course of disseminated prostatic cancer will be appreciated. Prospective and retrospective analyses of survival data and patient selection factors from these large cooperative studies will also help to resolve some of the controversies concerning response criteria for chemotherapy of prostatic cancer. While combination chemotherapy may prove more effective than single agent results in future clinical trials, toxicity may be greater. Consideration of the reported toxicity of chemotherapy for advanced prostatic cancer suggests that chemotherapy is fairly well tolerated in this patient population, and the rate of complications is acceptably low in the opinion of some.

In addition to the identification of effective combination chemotherapy, other promising clinical research areas include early chemohormonal therapy of metastatic disease and the use of adjuvant chemotherapy in high-risk patients, such as those with limited or resected pelvic nodal involvement. A number of promising classes of agents in the development of new cytotoxic agents have been identified and should be tested. As continuing progress is made in our understanding of the metabolic and ultrastructural characteristics of prostatic cancer cells, more selective and less toxic agents may evolve. The key to progress in treatment of advanced prostatic cancer in general and in the field of chemotherapy in particular is further randomized phase II and phase III clinical trials. Properly conducted clinical trials of promising agents or combinations of agents remain at present the only means of determining the future role of chemotherapy for advanced prostatic cancer.

Acknowledgment. This work was supported in part by PHS Grants CA-14716-10-53 and CA-28794-06 through the National Prostatic Cancer Project, National Cancer Institute, National Institutes of Health, Department of Health, Education and Welfare.

References

Beynon LL, Chisholm GD (1984) The stable state is not an objective response in hormone—escaped carcinoma of prostate. Br J Urol 56:702–705

Bulbul M, Huben RP, Murphy GP (1986) Interferon-β treatment of metastatic prostate cancer. J Surg Oncol 33:231–233

Chisholm GD, Stone AR, Beynon LL, Merrick MV (1982) The bone scan as a tumor marker in prostatic carcinoma. Eur Urol 8:257–260

Citrin DL, Hogan TF, Davis TE (1983) Chemohormonal therapy of metastatic prostate cancer. A pilot study. Cancer 52:410–414

Citrin DL, Elson P, DeWys WD (1984) Treatment of metastatic prostate cancer. An analysis of response criteria in patients with measurable soft tissue disease. Cancer 54:13–17

Creaven PJ (1984) Cytotoxic chemotherapeutic agents under development with a possible future role in prostate cancer. Prostate 5:484–493

Creaven PJ, Madajewicz S, Mittelman A (1984) New potential treatment modalities for disseminated prostatic cancer. Urol Clin North Am 11:343–353

deKernion JB, Lindner A (1984) Chemotherapy of hormonally unresponsive prostatic carcinoma. Urol Clin North Am 11:319–326

deVere White R, Babayan RK, Krikorian J, Krane RJ, Olsson CA (1983) Adjuvant chemotherapy for stage D_1 adenocarcinoma of prostate. Urology 21:270–272

Droller MJ (1985) Immunotherapy in genitourinary neoplasia. J Urol 133:1–5

Eisenkraft S, Huben RP, Pontes JE (1984) Orchiectomy and chemotherapy with estramustine, cis-platinum, cyclophosphamide and 5-fluorouracil in newly diagnosed prostate cancer with bone metastases. Urology [Suppl] 23:51–53

Fitzpatrick JM, Constable AR, Sherwood T, Stephenson JJ, Chisholm GD, O'Donoghue EPN (1978) Serial bone scanning: the assessment of treatment response in carcinoma of the prostate. Br J Urol 50:555–561

Guinan P, Ray P, Shaw M (1984) Immunotherapy of prostate cancer: a review. Prostate 5:221–230

Herr WW (1982) Cyclophosphamide, methotrexate and 5-fluorouracil combination chemotherapy versus chloroethyl-cyclohexynitrosourea in the treatment of metastatic prostatic cancer. J Urol 127:462–465

Ihde DC, Bunn PA, Cohen MH, Dunnick NR, Eddy JL, Minna JD (1980) Effective treatment of hormonally-unresponsive metastatic carcinoma of the prostate with adriamycin and cyclophosphamide. Methods of documenting tumor response and progression. Cancer 45:1300–1310

Isaacs JT (1984) The timing of androgen ablation therapy and/or chemotherapy in the treatment of prostatic cancer. Prostate 5:1–17

Loening S, Narayana A (1980) Adjuvant chemotherapy to definitive treatment of prostate cancer. Prostate 1:321–355

Loening SA, Scott WW, deKernion J et al. (1981) A comparison of hydroxyurea, methyl-chloroethyl-cyclohexy-nitrosourea and cyclophosphamide in patients with advanced carcinoma of the prostate. J Urol 125:812–816

Loening SA, Beckley S, Brady MF et al. (1983) Comparison of estramustine phosphate, methotrexate and cis-platinum in patients with advanced, hormone refractory prostate cancer. J Urol 129:1001–1006

Logothetis CJ, Samuels ML, vonEschenback AC, Trindale A, Ogden S, Grant C, Johnson DE (1983) Doxorubicin, mitomycin-C, and 5-fluorouracil (DMF) in the treatment of metastatic hormonal refractory adenocarcinoma of the prostate, with a note on the staging of metastatic prostate cancer. J Clin Oncol 1:368–379

Murphy GP (1984) Chemotherapy: Is it effective in treatment of prostatic cancer? Urology [Suppl] 24:41–47

Murphy GP (1979) Management of disseminated prostatic carcinoma. In: Murphy GP (ed) Prostate cancer. PSG, Littleton MA Sci Grp. 13:213–233

Murphy GP, Slack NH (1980) Response criteria for the prostate of the USA National Prostatic Cancer Project. Prostate 1:375–382

Murphy GP, Gibbons RP, Johnson DE et al. (1977) A comparison of estramustine phosphate and streptozotocin in patients with advanced prostatic carcinoma who have had extensive irradiation. J Urol 118:288–291

Murphy GP, Gibbons RP, Johnson DE et al. (1979) The use of estramustine and prednimustine versus prednimustine alone in advanced metastatic prostatic cancer patients who have received prior irradiation. Am Assoc Genitourinary Surg 70:69–71

Murphy GP, Beckley S, Brady MF et al. (1983) Treatment of newly diagnosed metastatic prostate cancer patients with chemotherapy agents in combination with hormones versus hormones alone. Cancer 51:1264–1272

Page JP, Levi JA, Woods RL, Tattersall MN, Fox RM, Coates AS (1985) Randomized trial of combination chemotherapy in hormone-resistant metastatic prostate carcinoma. Cancer Treat Rep 69:105–107

Penman DT, Holland JC, Bahna GF et al. (1984) Informed consent for investigational chemotherapy: patients' and physicians' perceptions. J Clin Oncol 2: 849–855

Scher H, Yagoda A, Watson RC, Serber M, Whitmore W (1984) Phase II trial of doxorubicin in bidimensionally measurable prostatic adenocarcinoma. J Urol 131:1099–1102

Schmidt JD (1093) Cytotoxic agents effective in prostate cancer. Semin Urol 1:299–310

Schmidt JD (1984) Cooperative clinical trials of the National Prostate Cancer Project: protocol 900. Prostate 5:387–399

Schmidt JD, Scott WW, Gibbons RP et al. (1979) Comparison of procarbazine, imidazole-carboxamide and cyclophosphamide in relapsing patients with advanced carcinoma of the prostate. J Urol 121:185–189

Schmidt JD, Scott WW, Gibbons R et al. (1980) Chemotherapy programs of the National Prostatic Cancer Project (NPCP). Cancer 45:1937–1946

Scott WW, Gibbons RP, Johnson DE, Prout GR, Schmidt JD, Saroff J, Murphy GP (1976) The continued evaluation of the effects of chemotherapy in patients with advanced carcinoma of the prostate. J Urol 116:211–213

Servadio C, Mukamel E, Lurie H, Nissenkorn I (1983) Early combined hormonal and chemotherapy for metastatic prostatic carcinoma. Urology 21:493–495

Silverberg E (1986) Cancer statistics, 1986. CA 36:9–25

Slack NH (1983) Results of chemotherapy protocols of the USA National Prostatic Cancer Project (NPCP). Clin Oncol 2:441–459

Slack NH, Murphy GP (1983) A decade of experience with chemotherapy of prostate cancer. Urology 22:1–7

Slack NH, Mittelman A, Brady MF, Murphy GP, Investigators in the National Prostatic Cancer Project (1980a) The importance of the stable category for chemotherapy treated patients with advanced and relapsing prostate cancer. Cancer 46:2393–2402

Slack NH, Murphy GP, participants in the National Prostatic Cancer Project (1980b) Overview of chemotherapy programs of the NPCP. Prostate 1:367–373

Slack NH, Brady MF, Murphy GP, Investigators in the National Prostatic Cancer Project (1984) Stable versus partial response in advanced prostate cancer. Prostate 5:401–415

Soloway MS, deKernion JB, Gibbons RP et al. (1981) Comparison of estramustine phosphate and vincristine alone or in combination for patients with advanced hormone refractory, previously irradiated carcinoma of the prostate. J Urol 125:664–667

Soloway MS, Beckley S, Brady MF et al. (1983) estramustine phosphate versus cis-platinum alone versus estramustine phosphate plus cis-platinum in patients with advanced hormone refractory prostate cancer who had had extensive irradiation to the pelvis or lumbosacral area. J Urol 129:56–61

Stephens RL, Vaughn C, Lane M et al. (1984) Adriamycin and cyclophosphamide versus hydroxyurea in advanced prostatic cancer. A randomized Southwest Oncology Group Study. ICRDB Cancergram, Series CT16, No 84/07,5

Straus MJ, Fleit JP, Engelking C (1982) Treatment of advanced prostate cancer with cyclophosphamide, doxorubicin, and methotrexate. Cancer Treat Rep 66:1797–1802

Torti FM (1983) Prostatic cancer chemotherapy. Cancer Res 85:58–69

Torti FM, Carter SK (1980) The chemotherapy of prostatic adenocarcinoma. Ann Intern Med 92:681–689

Yagoda A (1983) Cytotoxic agents in prostate cancer: an enigma. Semin Urol 1:311–322
Yagoda A, Watson RC, Natale RB, Barzell W, Sogani P, Grabstald H, Whitmore WF (1979) A
   critical analysis of response criteria in patients with prostatic cancer treated with cis-
   diamminedichloride platinum II. Cancer 44:1553–1562

Chapter 13

Clinical Trials in Prostatic Cancer: Methodology and Controversies

H.I. Scher* and A. Yagoda

Introduction

Prostatic cancer is a heterogeneous disorder with varying biologic potential. The prevalence of asymptomatic disease in up to 28% of autopsy series has led some to consider this an innocuous disease of the elderly (Breslow et al. 1977; Mettlin 1983). However, despite new biologic markers (Guinan 1981; Pontes 1983; Zweig and Ihde 1985), the proportion of patients with stages C and D at diagnosis has not changed (Slack et al. 1986) and the annual death rate has remained constant (Silverberg 1985). Although new hormonal therapies have recently been introduced (Trachtenberg 1984; Drago et al. 1985; Labrie et al. 1985; Eisenberg et al. 1986), no consistent improvement in response rate, response duration, or survival has been observed. More disturbing is a recent analysis showing an increase in the proportion of deaths attributable to prostatic cancer for patients diagnosed from 1980 to 1983 (Slack et al. 1986). Clearly, new therapeutic modalities are needed.

Classic phase II response criteria require serially evaluable parameters to assess the effect of therapy (Yagoda et al. 1979; Yagoda 1983; Simon et al. 1985; Wittes et al. 1985; Scher et al. 1986). In advanced disease, prostatic cancer often presents with retroperitoneal lymphadenopathy or a local prostatic mass. Objective clinical and subjective response to androgen ablative therapy, albeit incomplete, will occur in 40%–80% of cases for a median of 12–18 months. Twenty percent of patients respond for 5 years or more (Bayard et al. 1974). Improvement in symptomatology, which is often dramatic, correlates with

*Dr Scher is the recipient of an American Cancer Society Clinical Oncology Career Development Award.

regression in both the primary and the metastatic lesions and with a decrease in acid phosphatase (Nesbit and Baum 1950). Thus, to the uninitiated, the evaluation of chemotherapeutic agents in prostatic cancer would seem straight-forward. However, in contrast to the situation at first diagnosis, hormone refractory disease is often restricted to bony sites which are inherently difficult to evaluate. Too often, clinical trials are based solely on (a) evaluation of "tumor specific" parameters such as an elevated acid phosphatase level, (b) secondary manifestations of the tumor on the host such as bone scintigraphy or elevations in alkaline phosphatase, or (c) subjective parameters such as pain and performance status. These are inaccurate and subject to innumerable, and often non-treatment-related, variations (Yagoda et al. 1979; Yagoda 1983). This in part explains why, despite a vast literature suggesting the contrary, few patients with hormone resistant prostatic cancer achieve significant clinical benefit from systemic chemotherapy (Yagoda 1983; Eisenberg et al. 1985; Scher and Sternberg 1985; Tannock 1985). In a recent review only 4.5% of 1464 patients entered on randomized chemotherapy trials had objective tumor regression (Eisenberger et al. 1985). The results of chemotherapy and hormonal manipulation must be evaluated in the context of the recognized response rates to the latter therapy.

Comparison of treatment results is further hampered by the variable natural history of disease, variable response criteria, and inconsistencies in reporting of results (Whitmore 1973; Yagoda et al. 1979; Yagoda 1983; Tannock and Murphy 1983; Glatstein and Makuch 1984; Eisenberger et al. 1985; Scher and Sternberg 1985; Tannock 1985; Torti and Lum 1985). In many studies, statistical significance is mistaken for "clinical" significance (Richards 1984), and the only therapeutic "benefit" is a demonstration of prolonged survival for responders vs nonresponders. Although selected patients do experience subjective improvement, the typical response durations are measured in weeks, prolongation of survival is rare, and factors such as quality of life, toxicity of therapy, and cost are rarely included in the therapeutic equation.

This chapter will discuss the methodologic difficulties in evaluating antitumor agents in this disease. The conflict over response criteria, the lack of reproducible bidimensionally measurable lesions, and the effects of tumor on bone, often the only site of disease at relapse, will be considered. Further, the statistical limitations of published trials which have reported a beneficial effect of treatment in spite of modest response rates will be reviewed along with possible future trial designs.

Clinical Trial Methodology

After demonstrating activity in preclinical screening systems, anticancer agents are evaluated in a series of clinical trials. The phase I evaluation seeks to define a safe and tolerated dose (MTD) in one or a variety of dose schedules. Toxicity is also evaluated. Although antitumor activity is not ignored, the number of patients with a particular tumor type is usually too small to draw any definitive conclusions. The MTD in the phase I study is used as a starting point for the phase II evaluation. While the primary objective is therapeutic benefit, such trials are designed to identify the activity of a drug or combination in a defined patient population with a particular tumor type (Simon 1985; Simon et al. 1985; Scher et al. 1986). Ideally, active agents will be evaluated further, while inactive agents will be used in the fewest number of patients.

The most crucial factor affecting the outcome of a trial is patient selection — the silent statistician (Yagoda et al. 1979). To maximize the chance of response to the study agent, entry should be restricted to patients with an ambulatory performance status (Yagoda et al. 1979; Glatstein and Makuch 1984; Simon 1985; Simon et al. 1985; Wittes et al. 1985; Scher et al. 1986), good general medical condition, adequate hematologic reserve, and adequate renal and hepatic function. Factors such as age, prior therapy—be it hormonal therapy, immunotherapy, or radiation therapy—and symptoms should also be documented to identify possible prognostic factors (Zelen 1975; Emrich et al. 1985). All sites of metastatic disease must be recorded.

Examples of prognostic factors for sensitivity to hormonal therapy and for survival include pretreatment levels of testosterone and luteinizing hormone (Harper et al. 1984), serum prolactin (Mee et al. 1984), and tissue polypeptide antigen (Lewenhaupt et al. 1985). Other examples include measured parameters in tumor specimens such as DNA ploidy (Nagel et al. 1983), androgen receptor content (Ekman et al. 1981; Trachtenberg and Walsh 1982), enzymatic profiles (Pretlow et al. 1985), dihydrotestosterone levels (Geller and Albert 1985), and nuclear roundness (Benson et al. 1984). These types of investigation are important to identify prognostic indices to be stratified in randomized clinical trials. Patients with poor prognosis can also be considered for alternative therapies.

The most serious failure of a phase II trial is rejection of a potentially useful compound. Once a drug is labeled inactive, future evaluation is unlikely. Similarly, overestimation of response rates, based on "liberal" response criteria, will permit overdevelopment of inactive agents, frequently with such agents being incorporated into multidrug regimens (Scher et al. 1986). For prostatic cancer, where disease is often limited to osseous sites, stable disease has been used as an index of therapeutic response in phase II trials (vide infra) (Slack et al. 1980, 1985). As will be discussed further, such interpretation of response is subject to too much variation for inclusion in trials designed to assess efficacy.

At the Memorial Sloan-Kettering Cancer Center (MSKCC), patients with prostatic cancer are considered for investigational therapy as first line treatment, since no significant prolongation of survival has been achieved with chemotherapy (Nesbit and Baum 1984; Silverberg 1985; Slack et al. 1986). To maximize the chance of response, only patients with minimal or no prior chemotherapy are included. While some physicians may have difficulty with this approach, giving known ineffective therapy should pose similar moral dilemmas.

Measurable Disease

Phase II trials require a clear end point of response to evaluate the effect of the study agent(s). The difficulties encountered in prostatic cancer relate to the clinical manifestations of the disease: bidimensionally measurable or unidimensional tumor masses, nondiscretely measurable disease, or disease assessable by serial chemistries. These are discussed individually.

At MSKCC, phase II trials in prostatic cancer are restricted to patients with bidimensionally measurable parameters that can be followed serially throughout the course of treatment. These include palpable lymph nodes or subcutaneous masses on physical examination; pulmonary masses or peripheral lesions on radiologic examination; hepatomegaly by physical examination, sonography, or computerized tomographic (CT) scan; and abdominal and pelvic masses by CT scan or sonography (transabdominal or transrectal). Magnetic resonance imaging (MRI) may also be of value, but data are too preliminary for serial evaluations in this disease (Buonocore et al. 1984).

Depending on the extent of the pretreatment evaluation, this may represent 5%–15% of patients considered for therapy, a highly selected group. While this approach has been criticized for selecting patients who have far advanced disease destined to do poorly regardless of therapy (Citrin et al. 1981; Logothetis et al. 1983; Torti et al. 1983) or who are not representative of the 85%–95% of patients who never develop such lesions, it is the only group in whom reliable leads can be obtained. These selection criteria are the standard policy of our group, and a similar policy has recently been adopted by the EORTC Genitourinary Group (Schroeder et al. 1984) and the University of Maryland (1985). End points such as time to progression and overall survival, including patients with nonmeasurable disease, fall outside the realm of these initial disease-oriented trials.

Evaluation of measurable disease is subject to measurement error and interobserver variation that can lead to the false interpretation of response. For lesions assessable by physical examination, investigators are advised to use lesions that are a minimum of 2.5 cm in size (Moertel and Hanley 1976; Warr et al. 1984). Tumors are not always symmetric. When using CT scans to monitor a disease site, care must be taken to align the equipment at the same starting point (Mittal et al. 1983). All radiographic material should be reviewed independently by a reference radiologist.

Unidimensional masses such as mediastinal enlargement or pleural based masses on chest X-ray should be evaluated by CT scan before inclusion as a possible measurable lesion. Examination of a local prostatic mass by rectal examination is also imprecise. In one study, estimation of prostatic size by rectal palpation prior to prostatectomy revealed a coefficient of correlation of only 0.27 (Meyhoff et al. 1981). To minimize this error, investigators of the Northern California Oncology Group (NCOG) require a 75% reduction in prostatic size by physical examination, before counting response as significant (Torti et al. 1983).

Transrectal ultrasonography may improve this situation. Investigators in the EORTC have shown a good correlation between reduction in prostatic size as measured by sonography, with reduction in acid phosphatase and survival for patients treated with androgen ablative therapy (Ekman et al. 1981). Data are limited for use of this modality in patients with hormone refractory disease treated with chemotherapy. The significance of ultrasound abnormalities (echogenic vs. echodense) in patients who have had definitive pelvic radiation, ^{125}I implantation, or radical surgery remains unclear (Dahnert et al. 1986; Rifkin et al. 1986). Serial studies using MRI are preliminary, but will be limited in part by the cost of repeated examinations (Buonocore et al. 1984). Finally, some patients have no increase in prostatic size after hormonal or definitive local therapy despite systemic progression.

The incidence of pulmonary disease at autopsy in one series was 49% (Saitoh et al. 1984), but it is often lymphangitic, where serial changes are difficult to assess (Simon 1985). Nondiscrete measurable parameters such as confluent nodules or lymphangitic spread often fall below the limit of detection by standard radiographic techniques and should not be included as the sole criteria for response assessment.

The use of bone radiographs and radionuclide bone scanning to evaluate response in bone, the most frequent site of metastatic disease, is controversial (Ihde et al. 1980; Jacobs 1983; Pabst et al. 1983; Bragg 1984). In contrast to other tumor types, prostatic cancer produces osteoblastic change in 80%, mixed osteoblastic and lytic disease in 15%, and pure lytic disease in 5% of cases (Whitmore 1973). To detect a radiographic change in a lumbar vertebra, the most frequent site of metastasis to bone, a minimum of 50% of the cancellous bone must be destroyed, an insensitive parameter (Jacobs 1983). In one chemotherapy series, only 7 of 22 (32%) responding patients showed improvement in bone radiographs (Ihde et al. 1980). Lysis or resolution of blastic bone changes, an infrequent occurrence, has been classified as response by some (Logothetis et al. 1982), and progression by others (Pollen et al. 1984a), further fueling the controversy. In most cases, osteoblastic changes do not resolve, even with response in other sites, and the status of the tumor in bone remains undetermined. In general, radiographs are of value in evaluation of progression but play little role in the evaluation of response, with the exception of the rare circumstance where a purely lytic lesion (5% of cases) recalcifies.

Radionuclide scans are more sensitive than radiographs because they reflect functional changes in bone in contrast to structural changes (Fogelman 1980). Lesions as small as 5 mm can be detected. Thus, early metastases and "new" areas of uptake can be monitored more readily (Pollen et al. 1981). While the precise mechanism of uptake is unclear, isotopes appear to concentrate in areas of increased reactive new bone formation (Condon et al. 1981; Pollen et al. 1981; Parbhoo 1983). As noted by Galasko, these agents accumulate best in early focal lesions where immature osteoid is being formed or only partially calcified. When mineralization is complete, the scan may be normal even with extensive osteoblastic change on radiograph (Galasko 1975). The lack of specificity is the result of other pathologic processes that produce similar abnormalities in bone. These include healing traumatic fractures or degenerative disease (Langhammer et al. 1978; Levenson et al. 1983). Radiographic correlation of abnormal areas is recommended. Other problems are encountered by the delay in signs of improvement in the face of clinical response and the "flare phenomenon "—paradoxical worsening in the face of clinical response and bone healing. The latter can occur in up to 15% of cases (Longhammer et al. 1978; Citrin et al. 1981; Pollen et al. 1984b). A repeat scan performed 3 months later may show improvement consistent with the clinical situation. The minimum time to improvement is considered 3 months, but in most cases it will be longer. In a study of 22 patients responding to therapy, bone scan improvement was noted in only 7 (32%) at 3 months, and ultimately in only 11 (50%) (Logothetis et al. 1982). Similarly, of 33 patients progressing on treatment, only 26 had "worsening" of the scan at the time of progression in other sites, for an overall sensitivity of 79% (Levenson et al. 1983). Some patients present with a "superscan"—symmetrically increased uptake throughout the skeleton with no renal excretion of the isotope (Constable and Cranage 1981). At first glance, the scan may be falsely interpreted as normal. Serial changes in these scans are even more difficult to evaluate. When evaluating scans, it is important to distinguish between hormone naive and hormone refractory disease. In the former, normalization of the bone scan can occur, but it is rare in the latter setting, where "responses" are often too short to allow change to be detected.

The criteria for response assessment by bone scintigraphy varies between reported trials. For example, investigators at the NCI do not consider a change in the intensity or size of a lesion as a criteria for improvement or deterioration (Levenson et al. 1983), while those at the University of California at San Diego do (Pollen et al. 1981). The National Prostatic Cancer Project (NPCP) criteria require a 50% decrease in the number of sites (Elder and Gibbons 1985), while criteria used at the University of Chicago employ a quantitation technique that requires a 50% decrease in area (Citrin et al. 1984). We have evaluated total body quantitation in a small number of patients with limited success (Scher and Yeh, unpublished data). More recently Torti et al. described a two-dimensional technique of quantitation, with evaluation of particular "regions of interest". Changes in isotope concentration were shown to correlate well with response in soft tissue and decrease in acid phosphatase for patients treated with hormonal therapy (Torti et al. 1984), and with response in soft tissue disease for patients treated with chemotherapy (Freiha et al. 1985). If these results are confirmed, more patients may be considered for trials in this disease. At present, the major limitation of these techniques is that only secondary effects of tumor on bone are assessed; tumor reduction may simply not be apparent. Further, osteoblastic healing and osteoblastic progression can look identical.

Biologic markers can be divided into two categories: those that reflect the tumor directly—such as acid phosphatase, prostate specific antigen, and the BB fraction of creatinine kinase—and those that reflect secondary effects of the tumor on the host—alkaline phosphatase, osteocalcin, and urinary excretion of hydroxyproline. Both types must be interpreted with caution.

Acid phosphatase is normally found in glandular epithelium but is also present in red blood cells, liver, spleen, kidney, and bone—primarily in osteoclasts (Pontes 1983). The activity of the enzyme in the prostate is 100-fold higher than in other tissues. Elevations in serum concentration appear when prostatic cells which produce the enzyme invade the stroma. Levels of serum acid phosphatase are dependent on a number of factors, including the method of assay (Pontes 1983; Schacht et al. 1984). Total serum levels can be measured by an enzymatic assay using a variety of substrates, of which α-naphthyl phosphate appears most reliable (Bruce and Mahan 1982). The prostatic fraction (that portion produced by the prostate) can be assayed by either an enzymatic assay, radioimmunoassay (RIA), or a counterimmunoelectrophoresis technique (Pontes 1983; Pappas and Gadsden 1984).

In general, elevations correlate with extent of disease, and 60%–70% of patients with metastatic disease have abnormal levels (Pontes 1983; Schacht et al. 1984). Absolute levels seem to correlate inversely with survival (Torti and Lum 1985), and decreases parallel improvement in disease status in patients treated with hormonal therapy (Citrin et al. 1981, 1984; Schroeder et al. 1984; Kaplan et al. 1985). Zweig and Ihde (1985) compared an enzymatic assay with two commercially available RIAs in evaluation of response by direct parameters of tumor regression: physical examination, lymphangiogram, and CT scan. In patients responding to hormonal therapy, nine out of ten decreases were meaningful for the enzymatic assay, vs. ten out of ten for each of the RIAs used.

In assessing response to chemotherapy, Paulsen et al. (1979) correlated a decrease in acid phosphatase to normal (vs a 50% decrease or no change) with an improvement in survival (98 vs 34 weeks respectively). In an NCI study, only 7 of 27 (28%) responding patients showed meaningful decreases in acid phosphatase level. In patients with progressive disease, of 48 assays performed in 16 patients, 15 on chemotherapy and 1 on hormonal therapy, 14 (27%) showed increasing levels while 15 (19%) showed decreases. No concordance was observed between the three assays (Zweig and Ihde 1985). These results confirmed an earlier study which showed that neither RIA nor enzymatic assay detected progression in a significant number of cases (Ihde et al. 1982). The authors concluded that "acid phosphatase measurements . . . cannot be relied upon as the sole basis for clinical decision making in disseminated prostatic cancer" (Paulsen et al. 1979). At MSKCC, acid phosphatase alone is not used as a criteria for entry or evaluation, and in evaluating response, only a decrease to normal is probably significant (Yagoda 1983).

Analysis using this marker is further complicated by the observation that unpredictable fluctuations have been reported in the absence of therapy (Brenckman et al. 1981). Further, elevations can occur from fecal impaction, digital rectal examination, bladder catheterization, and fever. Nissenkorn et al. (1982) noted elevations from 5 to 40 units in a 24-h period while Brenckman et al. observed fluctuations of 44%–97% around 24 h mean values when sampled on a q 3 hourly basis. No apparent circadian rhythm or correlation with activity or concurrent medication could be observed (Brenckman et al. 1981).

Elevations of the BB fraction of creatine kinase have been reported in the serum of patients with prostatic cancer (Sandhu and Conover 1980; Zweig and Ihde 1985). Sandhu et al. noted elevations in 11 of 23 (48%) patients, including five of ten (50%) who progressed on hormonal therapy (Sandhu and Conover 1980). On serial evaluation, fewer meaningful changes were observed when compared with other parameters of response. Among patients treated with hormonal therapy, all responders had decreases but only three of six progressors had increases. However, among chemotherapy-treated patients, no responders showed decreases, and of nine patients who progressed on chemotherapy, three had a greater than 50% increase while three had a greater than 50% decrease in this parameter. This suggests a limited role for monitoring the effect of therapy.

Prostate specific antigen (PSA) is a 34 000-dalton protein that is localized to prostatic epithelial cells (Kuriyama et al. 1982). It is a cell type and organ site specific molecule that is expressed independent of acid phosphatase (Pontes 1983). The reported elevation in 13 of 19 (68%) patients with benign prostatic hypertrophy in two separate series (Pontes 1983; Zweig and Ihde 1985) highlights the limited role in screening. However, in a study of 26 patients progressing from locoregional (B_2-D_1) to metastatic (D_2) disease, 24/26 (94%) showed an increase in PSA up to 12 months prior to documentation of progression by other diagnostic techniques (Killian et al. 1985). A second series evaluated five markers, including PSA, acid phosphatase, and alkaline phosphatase in relation to disease progression and survival. Seventy-nine patients with locoregional disease (group 1), of whom 40 progressed to D_2 disease, and 51 patients with newly diagnosed D_2 disease (group 2), of whom 21 progressed during the observation period, were evaluated. For group 1, only PSA and prostatic acid phosphatase (PAP) levels were prognostic for disease progression ($P=0.02$ and 0.068 respectively). For group II patients, all parameters correlated with progression: PSA ($P<0.0001$), bone alkaline phosphatase ($P=0.0007$), and PAP ($P=0.0206$). In a multivariate analysis, no parameter was significant after correction for PSA (Killian et al. 1986). Few data are available on sequential changes in response to hormonal or chemotherapy. However, Pontes et al. (1983) did observe an increase in PSA in patients treated with radiation therapy. This was felt to reflect tumor lysis.

Hydroxyproline (HP) comprises 11%–14% of the amino acid residues in collagen. It is excreted in the urine in a dialyzable fraction (5%) which consists of free amino acid or as nondialyzable HP peptides (95%) (Dequecker et al. 1983). The former is related to collagen breakdown and bone formation while the latter is related to collagen synthesis (Hopkins et al. 1983). Urinary excretion is subject to dietary variation, which can be minimized by collection of samples on a 48- to 72-h gelatin-free diet, or by collection of the second voided early morning sample (EMU) after an overnight fast (Bishop and Fellows 1977; Heller et al. 1979; Moopan et al. 1980). The latter is reported in relation to creatinine (Cr) excretion. In prostatic cancer, over 95% of patients with positive bone scans will have elevated levels (> 40 mg/24-h period) or an increase in the HP/Cr ratio (EMU HP/Cr > 4.0) (Heller et al. 1979; Moopan et al. 1980). Increased levels are not seen in patients with stage A, B, or C disease, or in benign prostatic hypertrophy (Moopan et al. 1980; Rinsho and Aoyagi 1982; Erol et al. 1983). When patients were evaluated serially in response to hormonal therapy, Mundy (1979) showed a decrease in seven of ten responders, while all four progressors showed increases. Moopan et al. (1983) reported a decrease to normal levels in six of nine responders. Hopkins et al. (1984) evaluated 14 patients who progressed after hormonal therapy, and showed an increase in 12 (86%) a minimum of 8 weeks prior to progression by bone scintigraphy. However, there is little information on the role of HP excretion in patients treated with chemotherapy. At Memorial Hospital, only 70% of patients with hormone refractory disease had elevated levels and in a preliminary evaluation HP did not correlate with "clinical" improvement (Scher 1983; Scher et al. 1985a).

Osteocalcin is a calcium binding protein synthesized post-translationally from glutamic acid residues via a vitamin K dependent CO_2 carboxylation reaction (Price et al. 1975). It appears at the time of mineral deposition (Groot and Blak 1984) and accounts for 28% of the non-collagen-binding protein in bone (Khansur et al. 1983). Serum levels are measured via radioimmunoassay. The exact role is undefined, but increased levels correlate with increased mineralization in patients with osteoporosis treated with calcium and vitamin D (Gundberg et al. 1983; Epstein et al. 1984). Increased levels have been reported in Paget's disease and metastatic cancer (Deftos et al. 1982). In patients receiving hormonal therapy, levels correlate with response. However, in a study at Memorial Hospital of patients with hormone refractory disease treated with the bone resorption inhibitor gallium nitrate, no correlation with response was observed (Lowenthal et al. 1986). Reports of a diurnal variation, where afternoon levels were 50% of fasting values, suggest a limited role (Markowitz et al. 1984). Recently, an index based on early changes (1–2 months) in osteocalcin and alkaline phosphatase levels was reported to correlate with response in bone for patients with breast cancer. These techniques have not been applied to prostatic disease (Coleman et al. 1986).

Other markers under evaluation include osteonectin [a noncollagenous protein in bone that may have a role in mineralization (Termine et al. 1981)] and α_2-HS glycoprotein [a marker of bone matrix (Quelch et al. 1984)], but these will probably show similar low efficacy in patients with hormone refractory disease. At present, indirect parameters of bone turnover seem to parallel the clinical course in patients treated with hormonal therapy, but once hormone resistant disease develops, there is no reliable indicator of response or progression. More direct assays of tumor activity will be required before reliable assessment of prostatic cancer in bone will be possible.

Response

All phase II trials require a set of criteria on which response is assessed. For prostatic cancer, the criteria are not universal, limiting comparisons of treatment results. The criteria in use at MSKCC are listed in Table 13.1. For a complete remission (CR), complete disappearance of all clinical, radiographic, and biochemical abnormalities is required. Entry is restricted to patients with bidimensionally measurable disease; restaging is performed at fixed intervals; and all sites of disease are evaluated independently.

A comparison between the response criteria employed for a partial remission (PR) is listed in Table 13.2. Significant variations are apparent with respect to evaluation of biochemical changes (acid and alkaline phosphatase), changes in bone scan and bone radiographs, hepatomegaly, use of concomitant radiation

Table 13.1. Response criteria at MSKCC

Complete remission (CR): Complete disappearance of all clinical evidence of tumor on physical examination, X-ray, and biochemical evaluation for 1 month.

Partial remission (PR): Greater than 50% decrease on physical examination or radiography of the summed products of the perpendicular diameters of all measured lesions. No simultaneous increase in size of any lesion or the appearance of any new lesions may occur.

Abdominal or pelvic masses: Greater than 75% decrease by physical examination and/or greater than 50% decrease by CTT in the sum of the products of the largest perpendicular diameters for a minimum of 1 month.

Hepatomegaly: Greater than 50% decrease in the sum of all available measurements at 5-cm intervals from the midline below the costal margin by physical examination and greater than 50% decrease in all biochemical abnormalities and filling defects on scan for 1 month.

Minor response (MR): 25%–49% decrease in the summed products of the diameters of measured lesions.

Stabilization (STAB): Less than 25% decrease or increase in tumor size or biochemical abnormalities for a minimum of 3 months.

Progression (PROG): Less than 25% decrease in tumor size for less than 3 months or greater than 25% increase in the sum of all measured lesions, appearance of new lesions, or mixed response.

Table 13.2. Criteria for partial remission

Parameter	MSKCC	NCOG	NPCP	DUKE	ECOG	SWOG	NCI	MDAH	EORTC	UMCC
Tumor mass:										
50% decrease	X	X	X	X	X	X	X	X	X	X
Acid phos:										
Normalization			X	X			X		X	Not
50% decrease	X	X		X	X		X			used
Alk. phos:										
Normalization			X	X						Not
50% decrease	X	X		X	X	NS	X		NS	used
Bone scanning	Imp.	X	X		NS		X	Imp.	X	Not
Recalcify lytic disease	NS	NS	X	NS	X	NS	NS	X	X	used
Hepatomegaly:										
50% decrease	X	X								X
30% decrease		X			X			X		
Concomitant radiation	No	No	NS	NS	No	Yes	NS	Yes	NS	NS
No new sites of disease	X	X	X			X	X		X	X
Functional status	X	X	X	X	NS	X	X	X	X	X

Abbreviations: MSKCC, Memorial Sloan-Kettering Cancer Center; NCOG, Northern California Oncology Group; NPCP, National Prostatic Cancer Project; NCI, National Cancer Institute; ECOG, Eastern Cooperative Oncology Group; SWOG, Southwest Oncology Group; MDAH, M.D. Anderson Hospital; EORTC, European Organization for the Research and Treatment of Cancer; UMCC, University of Maryland Cancer Center. NS, not stated; Imp., improved.

therapy for painful bony lesions, and functional status. For measurable disease, the summed products of *all* lesions must be considered, not only selected ones.

The response criteria for acid phosphatase, with its recognized inaccuracy (vide supra), highlight other important distinctions. For example, NCOG consider only a twice normal value as evaluable (Torti et al. 1983), and the Mayo clinic use a greater than 25% change as evaluable (Eagen et al. 1976), while the NPCP (Elder and Gibbons 1985), and NCI (Ihde et al. 1980), Duke University (Paulsen et al. 1979), and the EORTC (Schroeder et al. 1984) require normalization of an abnormal value before listing in a response category. The NPCP criteria consider a decrease to normal indicative of response, but an increase is not included in the criteria for progression (Elder and Gibbons 1985; Emrich et al. 1985). At the University of Maryland, biochemical parameters are not included in assessment of response (University of Maryland Cancer Center 1985). While the NCI and MSKCC do monitor serum parameters, no patients with only evaluable parameters such as an elevated acid phosphatase level or an abnormal bone scan are entered into phase II trials (Yagoda et al. 1979; Ihde et al. 1980; Yagoda 1983). This latter group represented 84% of patients in one recent cooperative group trial (DeWys et al. 1983).

The definitions of response also vary between trials. In the NPCP criteria, *objective regression* is used to delineate patients who obtain CR or PR status, while *objective response* includes patients with CR+PR+STAB (Schmidt et al. 1976; Emrich et al. 1985). The latter can be misleading. Response rates may also vary depending on how frequently the patient is seen. In some cases a PR of 1 or

2 months' duration is based on a single observation. If patients are seen at 3-month intervals, a response duration of 6 months may reflect only two visits (Tannock and Murphy 1983). Some investigators feel that the minimum time of response should be 3 months (Tannock 1985). To minimize these errors, a fixed schedule of visits and restaging should be part of the trial design.

The demonstration of equivalent survival patterns for patients with "objective regression" and "stabilization" of disease has been used to validate a stable response classification as a beneficial effect of therapy (Slack et al. 1980, 1985). Lesser degrees of response, such as minor response (MR) or stabilization (STAB), should not be considered clinical efficacy in phase II trials since they are subject to large measurement error and investigator bias. As an example, in the NPCP criteria, disease may be considered stable even if the indicator lesion increases up to 25% in size (Emrich et al. 1985). Such a "response" would be categorized more accurately as slowly "progressive" that cannot be accurately assessed (Tannock and Murphy 1983; Tonkin et al. 1985). Considering the growth fraction of prostatic cancer in relapse and the number of doublings required to increase the tumor burden to the point where it can be measured using currently available techniques (Issacs 1985), MR and STAB usually reflect little clinical benefit. Furthermore, tumors with a long "lead time" (interval from diagnosis to metastases and metastases to protocol) and less aggressive biologic potential have a greater chance of remaining "stable" during the treatment period, independent of therapy. As stated by Chisholm et al. (1977), "a drug that required such assistance to produce a positive result cannot be acclaimed a therapeutic success." Patients entered on clinical trials should be continued on therapy until the "time of progression," but only CR and PR should be included in the calculation of response rate.

Care must be taken to ensure that patients are adequately treated before dismissing an agent as inactive. In a phase II evaluation, some toxicity is expected, which does not always reflect an easily evaluated parameter such as myelosuppression. Further in some studies, time to response can be significant. For example, in a trial of adriamycin administered on a weekly dose schedule, the median time to regression of soft tissue disease was 4.5 weeks, the median time to maximum relief of bone pain in the 14 (67%) responding patients was 8 weeks, and the median time to the lowest acid phosphatase level was 12 weeks (Torti et al. 1983). Thus, if therapy is initiated, it should be continued for at least 4–8 weeks in order to ensure adequacy of treatment.

To ensure accuracy and minimize investigator bias, all responses should be reviewed by an independent committee. A study of leuprolide in patients with untreated metastatic prostatic cancer highlights the importance of an unbiased audit (Glode et al. 1983). Of 26 patients categorized as partial responders by the investigator, only 17 (65%) remained PR when the "response" was reviewed by an independent committee; six were reclassified as progressors.

Agents with activity in phase II evaluation are investigated for efficacy in phase III trials. These require large sample sizes and often randomization through cooperative groups. Considering the potential morbidity, the cost and difficulties in accruing patients with prostatic cancer to clinical trials, and the fact that effective combination programs depend in part on the activity of the component agents (Capizzi 1977), accurate phase II data are critical. Inflation of response rates through less stringent assessment of response will simply add to the ever growing literature of ineffective therapies.

Statistical Considerations

Modern statistical techniques incorporate decision rules to estimate efficacy in phase II trials. The most frequently used design is that of Gehan (1961). Fourteen patients are entered, and if none respond, the response rate is less than 20% with 95% confidence; for less than 10%, 25 patients are entered. If responses are observed, more patients are entered to enhance the precision. However, if patient characteristics are identified that affect response, such as prior chemotherapy, an adequate number of patients with no prior therapy must be included.

An alternative design is the multiple testing procedure of Fleming (1982). In these trials response rates are evaluated after the first ten patients are entered. If, for example, five responses are observed, the drug is considered efficacious, and additional studies designed. However, if the worst outcome of a phase II trial is to dismiss a potentially active agent, it is probably not advisable to limit entry to ten nonresponding patients. No responses in ten adequately treated patients would only allow a rejection of a response rate up to 26% with 95% confidence.

Agents with activity in phase II trials can then be evaluated further. To demonstrate an advantage for a "new" treatment, a randomized trial of the "new" vs either the "conventional" or "no treatment" control can be considered. Before starting a trial to compare two treatment programs, some estimate of the number of patients required to detect a difference based on the observed response rate for treatment A and the expected response rate for treatment B is required. This is called the power estimate and is usually determined to be between 80% and 95%. In most cases an improvement in response rate of 15%–20% would be considered a significant improvement. The beta error in clinical trials refers to the probability of not detecting a difference when in fact one exists. In general, the smaller the difference, the larger the number of patients required. For example, if one is trying to demonstrate that an experimental regimen B has a response rate greater than 20% above that of regimen A in a randomized trial, for 80% power, 91 evaluable patients per arm and for 90% power 118 patients per arm, or 236 patients, would be required (Simon 1985). In prostatic cancer, where only 10% and 20% of patients have measurable disease, 1180 and 2360 patients would be required. In this situation, other end points of response, such as time to progression or survival, may be useful.

An example of a phase II trial using survival as the end point has been outlined by Eisenberger et al. (1985). As the majority of patients present with disease sites that are difficult to evaluate, and the majority of chemotherapy trials reporting survival that include patients with nonmeasurable disease show median survival times of less than 40 weeks, those agents that produce survival distributions for all patients of greater than 50 weeks might be considered for further study. For measurable disease a CR+PR rate above 20% would also be justification for further testing. This might minimize the need for large phase III trials in the absence of clinical activity. The concept needs further evaluation but is probably best applied after efficacy is demonstrated in the selected subgroup of patients with bidimensionally measurable disease.

Statistical limitations must be considered when attempting to assess an improvement in survival. The NPCP systematically evaluated a number of compounds in hormone-resistant prostatic cancer. Although the initial reports noted an increased *mean* survival time for patients treated with chemotherapy vs. standard therapy (Scott et al. 1976; Schmidt et al. 1979; Loening et al. 1981), a more recent analysis showed no improvement in survival for the chemotherapy group. As noted by Eisenberger et al. (1985), while this may have been due to ineffective therapy, since the majority of responses were "stable," the sample size evaluated would only have allowed detection of a 70% and 80% increase in median survival time. A smaller difference may in fact be present, favoring the chemotherapy arm, which would not have been detected unless a larger number of patients were treated.

When reporting a comparison of two treatments, the results are usually considered as "significant" if the *P* value is less than or equal to 0.05. This is often accepted at face value as "clinical significance" with no consideration of morbidity, cost, or other factors that might explain the differences observed. All that can be concluded is that if there is no difference between the two treatments, then the probability of observing a difference as extreme as the data is 5%.

Another misconception reported in clinical trials is that "responders" living longer than "nonresponders" is a beneficial effect of treatment (Anderson et al. 1983; Tannock and Murphy 1983; Tonkin et al. 1985). Increasing the response rate will increase survival. However, in cases where response durations are measured in weeks, it is hard to attribute a "significant prolongation of survival" to treatment alone. In some cases, "response" selects a prognostically favorable group of patients destined to live longer independent of therapy.

When one considers how survival distributions are analyzed, the inherent bias in favor of the "responding" patients is more apparent (Anderson et al. 1983). The log rank test calculates death rates over time based on the number of patients at risk at a given time point (Peto et al. 1977). Since responders must live long enough to be classified as responders, there is an immediate survival advantage for the responding group. Patients who die early, from whatever cause, have no chance to respond and are classed in the nonresponder category. This overestimates the death rate for the nonresponder group and underestimates the death rate for the responding category (Anderson et al. 1983).

To eliminate this bias, the effect of early death can be minimized by evaluating response only after a fixed time interval and the Landmark method (Scott et al. 1976). The second technique, reported by Mantel and Byar, considers response as a time-dependent covariate. All patients start in the no response state and change categories only at the time a response is recorded (Mantel and Byar 1974). Thus, the number of patients in each category at risk for death varies over time. By comparing the survival distributions for all patients vs nonresponding patients, a beneficial effect can be demonstrated. These topics are discussed in greater detail in the review by Anderson et al. (1983).

When reporting trials, the inevaluable category should not exceed 15% of the population studied and some indication of the number of patients considered for the trial should be given. This will allow an estimate of how relevant a treatment may be for the population at large.

Chemotherapy Trials

Several recently published reviews have discussed the results of chemotherapy trials, and a detailed analysis of all trials will not be undertaken (Yagoda 1983; Eisenberger et al. 1985; Scher and Sternberg 1985; Tannock 1985; Torti and Lum 1985). Cumulative data from multiple trials, including randomized and nonrandomized evaluations of single agents in prostatic cancer, are listed in Table 13.3. Most series used the response criteria of the NPCP and did not restrict entry to patients with bidimensionally measurable disease. The most frequently evaluated parameters were bone scans and biochemical abnormalities. Recognizing the limitations of cumulative data, a 95% confidence limit was calculated. In most cases, the response rates (CR+PR) were less than 15%. For cyclophosphamide, once considered "standard" therapy, the overall response rate was 5% (7/151, 95% confidence 1%–8%).

Table 13.3. Objective response (CR+PR) (NPCP criteria = objective regression) to single agent chemotherapy in prostatic cancer [adopted from Scher and Sternberg (1985) with modifications]

Agent	# evaluable	CR+PR (%)		95% confidence limits
Adriamycin	214	31	(14%)	10%–19%
Cisplatin	209	26	(12%)	8%–17%
Cyclosphosphamide	151	7	(5%)	1%– 8%
Estramustine	561	109	(19%)	16%–23%
Methotrexate	82	6	(7%)	2%–13%
5-Fluorouracil	124	11	(9%)	4%–14%
Vinblastine	39	8	(21%)	8%–33%
Vindesine	27	5	(19%)	4%–33%
Mitomycin-C	48	10	(21%)	9%–32%
Mitoguazone	25	6	(24%)	7%–41%
Etoposide	19	2	(12%)	0%–24%
Gallium nitrate	13	1	(7%)	0%–22%

An analysis of the trials using adriamycin (ADM) as a single agent illustrate the difficulties in analyzing published reports. Of 229 cases, the overall response rate (CR+PR) was 14% (31/229, 95% confidence limits 10%–19%), yet the reported trials vary from 0% to 84% depending on the criteria used. An early report suggested a dose-response effect as 5/14 (35%) vs 0/5 patients categorized as "good risk" responded to a high vs low dose schedule (O'Bryan et al. 1977). The ECOG randomized ADM vs 5-fluorouracil (5-FU) and noted response in 23% (15/61) for ADM and 7% for 5-FU (DeWys et al. 1983). The interim analysis showed a higher response rate for the ADM group, based on ECOG criteria, and the 5-FU arm was dropped. Final analysis showed no survival difference between the two groups: 29 vs 24 weeks. In the MSKCC trial, 2/39 (5%) responded (Scher et al. 1984) while 0/12 and 0/15 patients responded in trials by the EORTC (Jones et al. 1985) and NCOG (Torti et al. 1985a) respectively. The latter results contrast with a response rate of 35% reported by the same group in 25 evaluable patients using a weekly dose schedule (Torti et al. 1983). It is of note that using NPCP response criteria for the NCOG trials, response rates of 53% and 84% were observed (Torti et al. 1983, 1985a). Also of note is that survival distributions in the two groups of patients were comparable:

median 44 and 41 weeks respectively (Torti et al. 1983, 1985a). Depending on one's bias, one would conclude that adriamycin is ineffective or highly efficacious. Considering the low response rate to ADM, it is not surprising that the addition of cisplatin (CR+PR, 12%; 95% confidence 8%–17%) or methotrexate (CR+PR, 7%; 95% confidence 2%–13%) did not enhance the response rate, response duration, or survival when compared with ADM alone (Torti et al. 1985a,b).

Agents that warrant further study include mitomycin C, reported by the EORTC to have a 21% response rate (95% confidence, 9%–32%) (Jones et al. 1985), and continuous infusion vinblastine, also reported to have a 21% response rate (95% confidence 8%–33%) (Dexeus et al. 1984). The activity of mitoguazone, with a PR rate of 24% (95% confidence 7%–41%) (Scher et al. 1985b), was not confirmed in a study by the Southeastern Cancer Study Group (Moore et al. 1987).

Table 13.4. Objective response (CR+PR) (NPCP = objective regression) for combination chemotherapy in prostatic cancer [adopted from Scher and Sternberg (1985) with additions]

Agent	# evaluable	CR+PR (%)	95% confidence limits
CTX/ADM	112	18 (16%)	9%–23%
CTX/5-FU	38	3 (8%)	0%–16%
CTX/PRED	19	7 (37%)	22%–61%
CTX/DDP/PRED	22	0	0%–14%
CTX/ADM/5-FU/	15	8 (53%)	28%–79%
+ CYTADREN	20	5 (25%)	21%–53%
CTX/ADM/5-FU	51	2 (4%)	0%– 9%
CTX/ADM/BCNU	27	7 (26%)	9%–42%
CTX/MTX/5-FU	35	1 (3%)	0%– 8%
CTX/ADM/DDP	17	7 (41%)	18%–65%
MTX/ADM	32	5 (16%)	3%–28%
ADM/MITO/5-FU[a]	62	48% response	
	80	11 (14%)	6%–21%

Abbreviations: CTX, cyclophosphamide; ADM, doxorubicin; 5-FU, 5-fluorouracil; DDP, cisplatin; CYTADREN, aminoglutethimide; MTX, methotrexate; mito, mitomycin-C
[a]M.D. Anderson criteria

The response rates and the overall survival for various combination regimens are similar to those reported with single agents (Table 13.4). The MDAH group reported on a three-drug combination of ADM, mitomycin, and fluorouracil and noted response in 48% (30/62) of patients (Logothetis et al. 1983). Although some dramatic responses were illustrated, there were three (5%) toxic deaths; the regimen should therefore be used carefully in a population "at high risk for toxicity . . ." (Logothetis et al. 1983). Two other reported trials using the same agents in a lower dose schedule have shown an overall response rate (CR+PR) of 10% (10/98) (Hsu and Babaian 1983; Saiers et al. 1985). In one trial, six patients refused additonal therapy and five toxic deaths were recorded (Hsu and Babaian 1983). More recently, this regimen was compared with cyclophosphamide in a randomized trial (Kasimis et al. 1985). Although a survival advantage was reported for the eight responders to the combination vs six responders to the single agent ($P=0.014$), overall survival was no different.

Other groups have attempted to enhance response rates through androgen stimulation. The rationale is to increase the growth fraction of the tumor and thereby enhance sensitivity to chemotherapy (Fowler and Whitmore 1982; English et al. 1986a,b). In clinical practice, the approach can be hazardous as administration of androgens can severely exacerbate pain and precipitate spinal cord compression (Fowler and Whitmore 1982). A randomized trial comparing a three drug regimen of 5-FU, ADM, and cyclophosphamide with and without fluoxymesterone (Halotestin) showed a higher response rate but equivalent survival between the two groups (Manni et al. 1986).

Many endorse the clonal selection model as the primary cause of treatment failure in prostatic cancer (Isaacs and Coffey 1982). This has provided the rationale for combined chemotherapy and hormonal therapy. Two trials comparing diethylstilbesterol (DES) vs DES + cyclophosphamide and DES vs DES + estramustine showed no benefit for the combinations (Gibbons et al. 1983; Birch et al. 1985). The approach of using chemotherapy as initial therapy was recently evaluated at the NCI (Ihde et al. 1981; Birch et al. 1985). Patients with untreated prostatic cancer were given adriamycin and cyclophosphamide. The response rate was similar to that observed in patients treated with the same agents after progression from hormonal therapy. More important, response to subsequent androgen ablative therapy was not jeopardized (Ihde et al. 1981).

Future Directions

The cumulative results of published trials make it difficult to endorse a "standard" therapy for this disease. Indeed, the true role of chemotherapy is difficult to evaluate. The limitations of hormonal therapy have been well described and while the new hormonal approaches may improve "quality of life," an important factor often neglected in clinical trials, they are unlikely to significantly change the natural history of the disease. Future progress will depend on an integration of basic biologic principles and well designed clinical trials. As more attention is given to tumor heterogeneity, metastatic potential of different subclones of a tumor, and the development of hormone resistant cells—which are either present de novo or adapt from prior therapy, be it chemotherapy or hormonal therapy—several potential trials can be considered.

First, it is apparent that several variants of the disorder exist. The first group of patients are those with untreated disease who present with bidimensionally measurable tumor masses, elevated acid phosphatase levels, and bone metastases. A second would be the select group of patients with hormone refractory disease who have bidimensionally measurable tumor masses. These patients should be considered for phase II trials with investigational agents. ·As more patients have measurable soft tissue disease in the untreated setting, more agents could be evaluated in a shorter period. This in turn would facilitate design of combination regimens. In this regard, the results reported by the NCI, showing a comparable response rate to both hormonal therapy and chemotherapy, suggest that the two groups are comparable and should provide the stimulus to further investigation (Ihde et al. 1981; Seifter et al. 1986). What remains to be determined is whether the selected patients who relapse from hormonal treatment with bidimensionally measurable tumor masses are representative of the larger population without measurable disease. The preliminary evaluation by Freiha et al. (1985) would suggest that they are. While this latter group, with nonmeasurable disease, can be considered for therapy, they should probably only be included in trials designed to test efficacy (phase III) or in extended phase II evaluations of agents that have shown promising activity in the preliminary phase II evaluation as described.

More study of basic mechanisms of bone metabolism are required and new techniques of evaluating changes in bone, both secondary to the tumor and in response to therapy, will be needed. Toward this end, an animal model of prostatic cancer which invades bone has recently been reported (Pollard and Luckert 1985).

More attention must be paid to issues of quality of life. Several new instruments have been designed for reliable assessment of symptom control (Schipper et al. 1984; Selby et al. 1984). Validation of these scales can be performed in the phase II setting and should be considered as important as accurate assessment of tumor regression. As an example, a recent study compared adriamycin/lomustine vs cyclophosphamide/5-FU (Page et al. 1985). Survival was similar to that reported with other agents; nevertheless, palliation of symptoms was recorded and a quality of life measure factored into the results. The effect of corticosteroids could also be evaluated using a similar quality of life instrument. This type of analysis can allow selection of therapy when the aim is strictly palliation.

More specific measures of tumor activity are required. We are currently attempting to confirm the in vitro and in vivo observation of increased polyamine activity in human and animal prostatic cancer (Seppanen et al. 1981; Herr et al. 1984). A clinical trial of two polyamine inhibitors, MGBG and DFMO, is ongoing (Scher 1986).

Considering the diversity of human prostatic cancer, more studies of human tumor specimens are required. Advances in biotechnologies such as monoclonal antibodies, recombinant DNA, and immune modulating growth factors may allow more specific approaches to therapy and identification of tumors with different malignant potential. The report of a prostate-derived growth factor (Bulbul et al. 1986) raises the possibility of growth regulation at the cellular level, with monoclonal antibodies to the factor(s) or their receptors. However, regardless of the treatment considered, be it hormonal therapy, chemotherapy, or a biologic response modifier, careful evaluation will be required through the phase I, II, III clinical trials mechanism.

Acknowledgment. This work was supported in part by the National Cancer Institute Contract CA-05826 and CM-57732, the Ancell Clinical Studies Fund and the David H. Cogan Fund for Prostate Cancer Research.

References

Anderson JR, Cain KC, Gelber RD (1983) Analysis of survival by tumor response. J Clin Oncol 1:710–719
Bayard S, Greenberg R, Showmutter D et al. (1974) Comparison of treatments for prostatic cancer using an exponential life table model relating survival to concomitant information. Cancer Chemother Rep 58:845–859
Benson M, McDougal D, Coffey DS (1984) The use of multiparametric flow cytometry to assess tumor cell heterogeneity and grade metastatic prostate cancer. Prostate 5:27–45

Birch A, Irwin L, Troner M et al. (1985) Diethylstilbesterol (DES) vs. cyclophosphamide (C) + DES as initial therapy for metastatic prostatic carcinoma. A Southeastern Cancer Study Group Trial. Proc Am Soc Clin Oncol 4:98

Bishop M, Fellows G (1977) Urinary hydroxyproline excretion—a marker of bone metastases in prostate carcinoma. Br J Urol 49:711–718

Bragg D (1984) Advances in tumor imaging. Hosp Pract 19:83

Brenckman W, Lastinger L, Sedor F (1981) Unpredictable fluctuations in serum acid phosphatase activity in prostatic cancer. JAMA 245:2501–2504

Breslow N, Chan CW, Thorm G et al. (1977) Latent carcinoma of the prostate at autopsy in seven areas. Int J Cancer 20:680–688

Bruce AW, Mahan DE (1982) The role of prostatic acid phosphatase in the investigation and treatment of adenocarcinoma of the prostate. Ann NY Acad Sci 390:110–113

Bulbul M, Heston WDW, Mirenda C, Fair W (1986) A prostate-derived growth factor partially purified by heparin affinity and anion exchange chromatography (abstr). Proc Am Assoc Cancer Res 27:852

Buonocore E, Hasemann C, Pavlicek W, Montie J (1984) Clinical and in vitro magnetic resonance imaging of prostatic carcinoma. AJR 143:1267–1272

Capizzi R, Keiser W, Sartorelli A (1977) Combination chemotherapy—theory and practice. Semin Oncol 4:227–253

Chisholm GD, O'Donoghue EPN, Kennedy CL (1977) The treatment of estrogen-resistant stage D carcinoma of the prostate with estramustine phosphate. Br J Urol 49:717–720

Citrin D, Cohen A, Harberg J et al. (1981) Systemic treatment of advanced prostatic cancer: development of a new system for defining response. J Urol 125:224–228

Citrin DL, Elson P, DeWys W (1984) Treatment of metastatic prostate cancer: an analysis of response criteria in patients with measurable soft tissue disease. Cancer 54:13–17

Coleman RE, Whitaker KB, Mashiter G et al. (1986) Assessment of osteoblast activity predicts radiological response in bone metastases from breast cancer (abstr). Proc Am Assoc Cancer Res 27:180

Condon BR, Buchanan R, Garvle NW et al. (1981) Assessment of progression of secondary bone lesions following cancer of the breast or prostate using serial radionuclide imaging. Br J Radiol 54:18–23

Constable AR, Cranage RW (1981) Recognition of the superscan in prostatic bone scintigraphy. Br J Radiol 54:122–125

Dahnert WF, Hamper UM, Eggleston J et al. (1986) Prostatic evaluation by transrectal sonography with histopathologic correlation: the echopenia appearance of early carcinoma. Radiology 158:97–102

Deftos LJ, Parthemore JG, Price PA (1982) Changes in plasma bone GLA protein during treatment of bone disease. Calcif Tissue Int 34:121–124

Dequecker J, Mbuyi-Muamba JM, Holvoet G (1983) Hydroxyproline and bone metastasis. In: Stoll BA, Parbhoo S (eds) Bone metastasis: monitoring and treatment. Raven Press, New York, pp 181–199

DeWys WD, Begg CB, Brodowsky H et al. (1983) A comparative clinical trial of adriamycin and 5-fluorouracil in advanced prostatic cancer: prognostic factors and response. Prostate 4:1–11

Dexeus F, Logothetis C, Hossan R et al. (1984) Phase II study of vinblastine (Vlb) in advanced hormone resistant metastatic prostate cancer (HPC). Proc Am Soc Clin Oncol 3:161

Drago JR, Santen RJ, Lipton A et al. (1985) Clinical effect of aminoglutethimide, medical adrenalectomy, in treatment of 43 patients with advanced prostatic carcinoma. Cancer 53:1447–1450

Eagen RT, Hahn RG, Myers RR (1976) Adriamycin (NSC-123127) versus 5-fluorouracil (NSC-19893) and cyclophosphamide (NSC-26271) in the treatment of metastatic prostate cancer. Cancer Treat Rep 60:115–117

Eisenberger M, Simon R, O'Dwyer P, Wittes R, Friedman M (1985) A reevaluation of nonhormonal cytotoxic chemotherapy in the treatment of prostatic carcinoma. J Clin Oncol 3:827–841

Eisenberger MA, O'Dwyer PJ, Friedman MA (1986) Gonadotropin hormone-releasing hormone analogues: a new therapeutic approach for prostatic carcinoma. J Clin Oncol 4:414–424

Ekman P, Svennerus K, Zetterberg A et al. (1981) Cytophotometric analysis and steroid receptor content in human prostatic carcinoma. Scand J Urol Nephrol [Suppl] 60:85–88

Elder JS, Gibbons RP (1985) Results of trials of the USA National Prostatic Cancer Project. Schroeder F, Richards B (eds) Therapeutic principles in metastatic prostatic cancer. Alan R. Liss, Inc., New York pp 221–242 (EORTC Genitourinary Group Monograph 2, part A)

Emrich L, Priore R, Murphy GP et al. (1985) Prognostic factors in patients with advanced stage prostate cancer. Cancer Res 45:5173–5179

English HF, Drago JR, Santen RJ (1986a) Cellular response to androgen depletion and repletion in the rat ventral prostate: autoradiography and morphometric analysis. Prostate 7:41–51

English HF, Kloszewski E, Valentine E, Santen RJ (1986b) Proliferative response of the Dunning R3327H experimental model of prostatic adenocarcinoma to conditions of androgen depletion and repletion. Cancer Res 46:839–844

Epstein S, Poser J, McClintock R, Johnston C, Bryce G, Hui S (1984) Differences in serum bone GLA protein with age and sex. Lancet I:307–310

Erol D, Adalar N, Guvencli S, Simsek F (1983) Urinary hydroxyproline levels in patients with prostatic carcinoma. Int Urol Nephrol 15:267–274

Fleming I (1982) One sample multiple testing procedures for phase II clinical trials. Biometrics 38:143–151

Fogelman I (1980) Skeletal uptake of diphosphate: a review. Eur J Nucl Med 5:473–476

Fowler JE, Whitmore EF (1982) Considerations for the use of testosterone with systemic chemotherapy in prostatic cancer. Cancer 49:1373–1377

Freiha FS, Lum BL, Spaulding J et al. (1985) Does response to chemotherapy in patients with bidimensional prostate metastases reflect tumor response in skeletal metastases? Proc Am Soc Clin Oncol 4:102

Galasko CSB (1975) The pathological basis for skeletal scintigraphy. J Bone Joint Surg 578:353–359

Gehan E (1961) The determination of the number of patients required in a follow up trial of a new chemotherapeutic agent. J Chron Dis 13:346–353

Geller J, Albert J (1985) DHT in prostate cancer tissue—a guide to management and therapy. Prostate 6:19–25

Gibbons RP, Beckley S, Brady MF et al. (1983) The addition of chemotherapy to hormonal therapy for treatment of patients with metastatic carcinoma of the prostate. J Surg Oncol 23:133–142

Glatstein E, Makuch R (1984) Illusion and reality: practical pitfalls in interpreting clinical trials. J Clin Oncol 2:488–497

Glode L, Max D et al. Leoprolide (1983) (D-Leu^6-DesGly^{10}-Pro^9-NH Et-LHRH) in the therapy of advanced prostatic carcinoma. 13th Int Cong Chemotherapy 12.1.8.A Section 242:49–52

Groot C, Blak J (1984) Electron microscopical demonstration of osteocalcin antigenicity in fetal rat bone. Am Soc Bone Mineral Res 6:12

Guinan P (1981) What is the best test to detect prostate cancer? CA 141–146

Gundberg CM, Lian JB, Gallop PM, Steinberg JJ (1983) Urinary gamma-carboxyglutamic acid and serum osteocalcin as bone markers: studies in osteoporosis and Paget's disease. J Clin Endocrinol Metab 57:1221–1225

Harper ME, Pierrepoint CG, Griffiths K (1984) Carcinoma of the prostate: relationship of pretreatment hormone levels to survival. Eur J Cancer Clin Oncol 20:477–482

Heller W, Harzmann R, Bickler R, Schmidt K (1979) Urinary hydroxyproline in healthy patients and in patients with and without bone metastases. Curr Probl Clin Biochem 9:249–258

Herr H, Kleinert E, Relyea N, Whitmore W (1984) Potentiation of methylglyoxal bis-guanylhydrazone by alpha-difluromethylornithine in rat prostate cancer. Cancer 53:1294–1298

Hopkins S, Nissenkorn I, Palmieri G et al. (1983) Serial spot hydroxyproline/creatinine ratios in metastatic prostatic cancer. J Urol 129:319–323

Hopkins S, Palmieri G, Niell H et al. (1984) Total and nondialyzable hydroxyproline excretion in stage D$_2$ prostate cancer. Cancer 53:117–121

Hsu DS, Babaian RJ (1983) 5-Fluorouracil, Adriamycin, mitomycin-C (FAM) in the treatment of hormonal-resistant stage D adenocarcinoma of the prostate (abstr). Proc Am Soc Clin Oncol 2:133

Ihde D, Bunn PA, Cohen MH et al. (1980) Effective treatment of hormonally-unresponsive metastatic carcinoma of the prostate with adriamycin and cyclophosphamide: methods of documenting tumor response and progression. Cancer 45:1300–1310

Ihde DC, Bunn PA, Cohen MH et al. (1981) Combination chemotherapy as initial treatment for stage D-2 prostatic cancer: response rate and results of subsequent hormonal therapy. Proc Am Assoc Cancer Res 22:163

Ihde DC, Belville WD, Mahan DE et al. (1982) Serum acid phosphatase in the assessment of response to systemic therapy in metastatic prostate cancer: comparison of radioimmune and enzymatic assays. Milit Med 147:949–952

Isaacs JT (1985) New principles in the management of metastatic prostatic cancer. Schroeder F, Richards B (eds) Therapeutic principles in metastatic prostatic cancer. Alan R. Liss, New York, pp 383–405 (EORTC Genitourinary Group Monograph 2, part A)

Isaacs JT, Coffey DS (1982) Adaptation vs. selection as the mechanism responsible for the relapse of prostatic cancer to androgen therapy as studied in the Dunning R-3327-H adenocarcinoma. Cancer Res 42:2353–2361

Jacobs S (1983) Spread of prostatic cancer to bone. Urology 21:337–342

Jones WG, Members of the EORTC GU Group (1985) EORTC Phase II chemotherapy studies in prostate cancer. Schroeder F, Richards B (eds) Therapeutic principles in metastatic prostatic cancer. Alan R. Liss, New York, pp 435–447 (EORTC Genitourinary Group Monograph 2, part A)

Kaplan LA, Chen IW, Sperling M, Bracken B, Stein E (1985) Clinical utility of serum prostatic acid phosphatase measurements for detection (screening), diagnosis, and therapeutic monitoring of prostatic carcinoma; assessment of monoclonal and polyclonal enzymes and radioimmunoassays. Am J Clin Pathol 84:334–339

Kasimis B, Miller B, Kaneshiro C et al. (1985) Cyclophosphamide versus 5-fluorouracil, doxorubicin, and mitomycin C (FAM') in the treatment of hormone resistant metastatic carcinoma of the prostate: a preliminary report of a randomized trial. J Clin Oncol 3:385–392

Khansur T, Yam L, Tavassoli M (1983) Serum monitors of bone metastasis. In: Stoll BA, Parbhoo S (eds) Bone metastasis: monitoring and treatment. Raven Press, New York, pp 165–181

Killian C, Yuang N, Emrich L et al. (1985) Prognostic importance of prostate-specific antigen for monitoring patients with stages B_2 to D_1 prostate cancer. Cancer Res 45:886–891

Killian C, Emrich L, Vargas, F et al. (1986) Relative reliability of five serially measured markers for prognosis of progression in prostate cancer. J Natl Cancer Inst 76:179–185

Kuriyama M, Wang MC, Lee CI et al. (1982) Multiple marker evaluation in prostate cancer using tissue specific antigens. J Natl Cancer Inst 68:99–105

Labrie F, Dupont A, Belanger A (1985) Complete androgen blockade for treatment of prostate cancer. In: DeVita VT, Hellman S, Rosenberg SA (eds) Important advances in oncology. J.P. Lippincott, Philadelphia, pp 193–217

Langhammer K, Sintermann R, Hor G, Pabst HW (1978) Serial bone scintigraphy for assessing the effectiveness of treatment of osseous metastases from prostatic cancer. Nucl Med 17:87–91

Levenson RM, Sauerbrunn BJL, Bates HR et al. (1983) Comparative value of bone scintigraphy and radiography in monitoring tumor response in systemically treated prostatic carcinoma. Radiology 146:513–518

Lewenhaupt A, Ekman P, Eneroth P (1985) Tissue polypeptide antigen (TPA) as a prognostic aid in human prostatic carcinoma. Prostate 6:285–291

Loening SA, Scott WW, Dekernion J et al. (1981) A comparison of hydroxyurea, methyl-chloroethyl-chlorohexyl-nitrosourea and cyclophosphamide in patients with advanced prostate cancer. J Urol 125:812–816

Logothetis CJ, von Eschenbach AC, Samuels ML et al. (1982) Doxorubicin, mitomycin and 5-fluorouracil (DMF) in the treatment of hormone-resistant stage D prostate cancer. A preliminary report. Cancer Treat Rep 66:57–63

Logothetis CJ, Samuels ML, von Eschenbach AC et al. (1983) Doxorubicin, mitomycin-C, and 5-fluorouracil (DMF) in the treatment of metastatic hormonal refractory adenocarcinoma of the prostate, with a note on staging of metastatic prostate cancer. J Clin Oncol 1: 368–378

Lowenthal D, Scher H, Geller N et al. (1986) Osteocalcin (OC) as a marker of bone turnover in prostatic cancer (PC) (abstr). Proc Am Assoc Cancer Res 27:160

Manni A, Santen R, Boucher A et al. (1986) Androgen priming and response to chemotherapy in advanced prostate cancer (abstr). Proc Am Soc Clin Oncol 5:96

Mantel N, Byar DP (1974) Evaluation of response-time data involving transient states: an illustration using heart-transplant data. JASA 69:81–91

Markowitz M, Gundberg C, Rosen J (1984) 24 hour fluctuations in serum osteocalcin concentration in women. Am Soc Bone Mineral Res 6:17

Mee AD, Khan O, Mashiter K (1984) High serum prolactin associated with poor prognosis in carcinoma of the prostate. Br J Urol 56:698–701

Mettlin C (1983) Epidemiology of prostate cancer in different population groups. Clin Oncol 2:187–192

Meyhoff HH, Ingemann L, Nordling J, Hald T (1981) Accuracy in preoperative estimation of prostatic size. Scand J Urol Nephrol 15:45–51

Mittal R, Korval C, Starzl T et al. (1983) Accuracy of computerized tomography (CT) in determining hepatic tumor size in patients (PTS) receiving liver transplants or resection. Proc Am Soc Clin Oncol 2:121

Moertel C, Hanley J (1976) The effect of measuring error on the results of therapeutic trials in advanced cancer. Cancer 38:388–394

Moopan M, Wax S, Kim H et al. (1980) Urinary hydroxyproline excretion as a marker of osseous metastasis in carcinoma of the prostate. J Urol 123:694–696

Mooppan U, Kim H, Wang J, Tobin M, Wax S (1983) Use of urinary hydroxyproline excretion as a tumor marker in diagnosis and follow-up of prostate cancer. Prostate 4:397–402

Moore MR, Graham SO, Birch R, Irwin L (1987) Phase II evaluation of mitoguazone in metastatic hormone resistant prostate cancer: a Southeastern Cancer Group study trial. Cancer Treat Rep 71:89–90

Mundy A (1979) Urinary hydroxyproline excretion in carcinoma of the prostate. A comparison of 4 different modes of assessment and its role as a marker. Br J Urol 51:570–579

Nagel R, Borgmann V, Al-Ahabi H et al. (1983) Premiers resultats cliniques concernant le traitement du cancer de la prostate a un stade local avance au moyen d'un puissant analogue de la LHRH: l'acetate de busereline. J Urol 89:669–676

Nesbit RM, Baum WC (1950) Endocrine control of prostatic carcinoma: clinical and statistical survey of 1818 cases. JAMA 143:1317–1320

Nissenkorn I, Mickey D, Miller D et al. (1982) Circadian and day to day variation of prostatic acid phosphatase. J Urol 128:1122–1124

O'Bryan RM, Baker LH, Gorttleib JF et al. (1977) Dose response evaluation of Adriamycin in human neoplasia. Cancer 39:1940–1948

Pabst HW, Langhammer H, Bauer R (1983) Technical problems in assessing bone scans. In: Stoll BA, Parbhoo S (eds) Bone metastasis: monitoring and treatment. Raven Press, New York, pp 85–106

Page JP, Levi JA, Woods RL et al. (1985) Randomized trial of combination chemotherapy in hormone resistant metastatic prostatic carcinoma. Cancer Treat Rep 69:105–107

Pappas A, Gadsden RH (1984) Prostatic acid phosphatase: clinical utility in detection, assessment, and monitoring carcinoma of the prostate. Ann Clin Lab Sci 14:285–291

Parbhoo S (1983) Serial scintiscans in monitoring patients with bone metastasis. In: Stoll BA, Parbhoo S (eds) Bone metastasis: monitoring and treatment. Raven Press, New York, pp 201–237

Paulsen D, Berry W, Cox E et al. (1979) Treatment of metastatic endocrine unresponsive carcinoma of the prostate gland with multi-agent chemotherapy: indicators of response to treatment. J Natl Cancer Inst 63:615–622

Peto R, Pike MC, Armitage NE et al. (1977) Design and analysis of randomized clinical trials requiring prolonged observation of each patient. Part II. Analysis and examples. Br J Cancer 35:1–39

Pollard M, Luckert PH (1985) Prostate cancer in a Sprague-Dawley rat. Prostate 6:389–393

Pollen J, Gerber K, Ashbum W et al. (1981) The value of nuclear bone imaging in advanced prostatic cancer. J Urol 125:222–223

Pollen JJ, Reznek R, Tolner LB (1984a) Lysis of osteoblastic lesions in prostatic cancer: a sign of progression. AJR 142:1175–1177

Pollen JJ, Witztum K, Ashburn WL (1984b) The flare phenomenon on radionuclide bone scan in metastatic prostatic cancer. AJR 142:773–776

Pontes JE (1983) Biological markers in prostate cancer. J Urol 130:1037–1047

Pontes JE, Chu TM, Slack N et al. (1978) Serum prostatic antigen measurement in localized prostatic cancer: correlation with clinical course. J Urol 128:1216–1218

Pretlow TG, Harris BE, Bradley EC et al. (1985) Enzyme activities in prostatic carcinoma related to Gleason grades. Cancer Res 45:442–446

Price P, Otsuka A, Poser J, Kristaponis J, Raman N (1975) Characterization of a gamma-carboxyglutamic acid-containing protein from bone. Proc Natl Acad Sci 5:1447–1451

Quelch K, Cole W, Melick R (1984) Noncollagenous proteins in normal and pathological human bone. Calcif Tissue Int 36:454–462

Richards B (1984) Clinical significance and statistical significance. In: Denis L, Murphy GP, Prout GR, Schroeder F (eds) Controlled clinical trials in urology. Raven Press, New York,.pp 17–18

Rifkin MD, Friedland GW, Shortliffe L (1986) Prostatic evaluation by transrectal endosonography: detection of carcinoma. Radiology 158:85–90

Rinsho K, Aoyagi K (1982) Urinary hydroxyproline excretion as a marker of bone metastases in prostatic cancer. Tohoku J Exp Med 137:461–467

Saiers JH, Trannum BL, Stephens R, Crawford ED (1985) Treatment of stage DII adenocarcinoma of the prostate with doxorubicin, mitomycin C and 5-fluorouracil (DMF): a Southwest Oncology Group study. Proc Am Soc Clin Oncol 4:108

Saitoh H, Hida M, Shimbo T et al. (1984) Metastatic patterns of prostatic cancer: correlation between sites and number of organs involved. Cancer 54:3078–3084

Sandhu RS, Conover RE (1980) Usually high creatine kinase BB isoenzyme and study of lactate dehydrogenase pattern in metastatic adenocarcinoma of the prostate. Clin Biochem 13:30–33

Schacht MJ, Garnett JE, Grayhack JT (1984) Biochemical markers in prostatic cancer. Urol Clin North Am 11:253–257

Scher H (1983) Memorial Hospital CIC Protocol 82–54. Ethane hydroxy 1, 1-diphosphonate in the treatment of bone metastases from prostatic cancer.

Scher H (1985) Memorial Hospital Protocol 85–25. Phase I-II trial of difluoromethylornithine (DFMO) and mitoguazone (MGBG) in hormone resistant bidimensionally measurable prostatic cancer.

Scher H, Sternberg CN (1985) Chemotherapy of urologic malignancies. Semin Urol 3:329–381

Scher H, Yagoda A, Watson R et al. (1984) Phase II evaluation of adriamycin in bidimensionally measurable prostatic adenocarcinoma. J Urol 131:1099–1102

Scher H, Tauer K, Alcock N et al. (1985a) Preliminary evaluation of gallium nitrate (GaN) on bone turnover and antitumor activity in patients (Pts) with hormone resistant prostatic cancer metastatic to bone. Proc Am Soc Clin Oncol 4:104

Scher H, Yagoda A, Ahmed T et al. (1985b) Phase II trial of mitoguazone in bidimensionally measurable hormone resistant adenocarcinoma of the prostate. J Clin Oncol 3:224–227

Scher H, Geller N, Muggia F, Rozencweig M (1986) Clinical evaluation of anticancer treatment: Phase II clinical trials. In: Muggia F, Rozencweig M (eds) Clinical evaluation of anticancer therapy. Martinus Nijhoff, Boston, pp 175–197

Schipper H, Clinch J, McMurray A et al. (1984) Measuring the quality of life of cancer patients: the functional living index—cancer: development and validation. J Clin Oncol 2: 472–483

Schmidt JD, Johnson DE, Scott WW et al. (1976) Chemotherapy of advanced prostatic cancer. Evaluation of response parameters. Urology 7:602–610

Schmidt JD, Scott WW, Gibbons RP et al. (1979) Comparison of procarbazine, imidazole-carbamide and cyclophosphamide in relapsing patients with advanced carcinoma of the prostate. J Urol 121:185–189

Schroeder FH and the European Organization on Research on Treatment of Cancer Urological Group (1984) Treatment response critieria for prostatic cancer. Prostate 5:181–191

Scott WW, Gibbons RP, Johnson DE et al. (1976) The continued evaluation of the effects of chemotherapy in patients with advanced carcinoma of the prostate. J Urol 116:211–213

Seifter E, Bunn P, Cohen M et al. (1986) Combination chemotherapy followed by hormonal therapy for previously untreated metastatic carcinoma of the prostate. Proc Am Assoc Cancer Res 27:183

Selby P, Chapman JA, Etazadi-Amoli J et al. (1984) The development of a method for assessing quality of life in cancer. Br J Cancer 50:13–22

Seppanen P, Alhonen-Hongisto L, Janne J (1981) Polyamine deprivation-induced enhanced uptake of methylglyoxal bis (guanylhydrazone) by tumor cells. Biochim Biophys Acta 674:169

Silverberg E (1985) Cancer statistics, CA 35:19–35

Simon R (1985) Design and conduct of clinical trials. In: DeVita VT, Hellman S, Rosenberg SA (eds) Principles and practice of oncology. J.P. Lippincott, Philadelphia, pp 329–350

Simon R, Wittes R, Ellenberg S (1985) Randomized phase II clinical trials. Cancer Treat Rep 69:1375–1381

Slack MH, Mittleman A, Brady MF, Murphy GP (1980) The importance of the stable category for chemotherapy treated patients with advanced and relapsing prostate cancer. Cancer 46:2393–2402

Slack N, Brady M, Murphy G et al. (1985) Stable versus partial response in advanced prostate cancer. Prostate 5:401–415

Slack N, Lane W, Prior R, Murphy GP (1986) Prostatic cancer: treated at a categorical center, 1980–1983. Urology 27:205–213

Tannock IF (1985) Is there evidence that chemotherapy is of benefit to patients with carcinoma of the prostate? J Clin Oncol 3:1013–1020

Tannock I, Murphy K (1983) Reflections in medical oncology: an appeal for better clinical trials and improved reporting of their results. J Clin Oncol 1:66

Termine JD, Kleinman HK, Whitson SW et al. (1981) Osteonectin, a bone-specific protein linking mineral to collagen. Cell 26:99–104

Tonkin K, Tritchler D, Tannock I (1985) Criteria of tumor response used in clinical trials of chemotherapy. J Clin Oncol 3:870–875

Torti F, Lum B (1985) Chemotherapy in prostate cancer. In: Garnick MB (ed) Genitourinary cancer. Churchill Livingstone, New York, pp 125–161

Torti F, Aston D, Lum BL et al. (1983) Weekly doxorubicin in endocrine refractory carcinoma of the prostate. J Clin Oncol 1:377–384

Torti FM, Martin BC, Higgins MC et al. (1984) Skeletal metastases of prostatic carcinoma can subserve the function of measurable sites in prostatic cancer trials. Proc Am Soc Clin Oncol 4:103

Torti F, Shortliffe L, Carter S (1985) A randomized study of doxorubicin versus doxorubicin plus cisplatin in endocrine-unresponsive metastatic prostatic carcinoma. Cancer 56:2580–2586

Torti FM, Flam M, Lum BL (1985) Weekly adriamycin and methotrexate in endocrine unresponsive carcinoma of the prostate. Proc Am Soc Clin Oncol 4:103

Trachtenberg J (1984) Ketoconazole therapy in advanced prostatic cancer. J Urol 132:61–63

Trachtenberg J, Walsh PC (1982) Correlation of prostatic nuclear androgen receptor content with duration of response and survival following hormonal therapy in advanced prostatic cancer. J Urol 127:466–471

University of Maryland Cancer Center Protocol #85–25 (1985) A phase II study of trimetrexate in endocrine resistant prostatic prostatic carcinoma.

Warr D, McKinney S, Tannock I (1984) Influence of measurement error on assessment of response to anticancer chemotherapy: proposal for new criteria for tumor response. J Clin Oncol 2: 1040–1046

Whitmore WF (1973) The natural history of prostatic cancer. Cancer 32:1104–1112

Wittes RE, Marsoni S, Simon R, Leyland-Jones BR (1985) The phase II trial. Cancer Treat Rep 69:1235–1239

Yagoda A (1983) Response in prostatic cancer: an enigma. Semin Urol 1:311–323

Yagoda A, Watson RC, Natale RB et al. (1979) A critical analysis of response criteria in patients with prostatic cancer treated with cis-diamminedichloride platinum II. Cancer 44:1553–1562

Zelen M (1975) Importance of prognostic factors in planning therapeutic trials. In: Staquet M (ed) Cancer therapy: prognostic factors and criteria of response. Raven Press, New York, pp 1–15

Zweig M, Ihde D (1985) Assessment of serum and enzymatic prostatic acid phosphatase and radioimmune creatine kinase BB for monitoring response to therapy in metastatic prostatic carcinoma. Cancer Research 45:3945–3952

Subject Index